D0274964

COMPLETE
Family
Nutrition

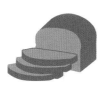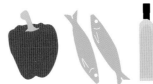

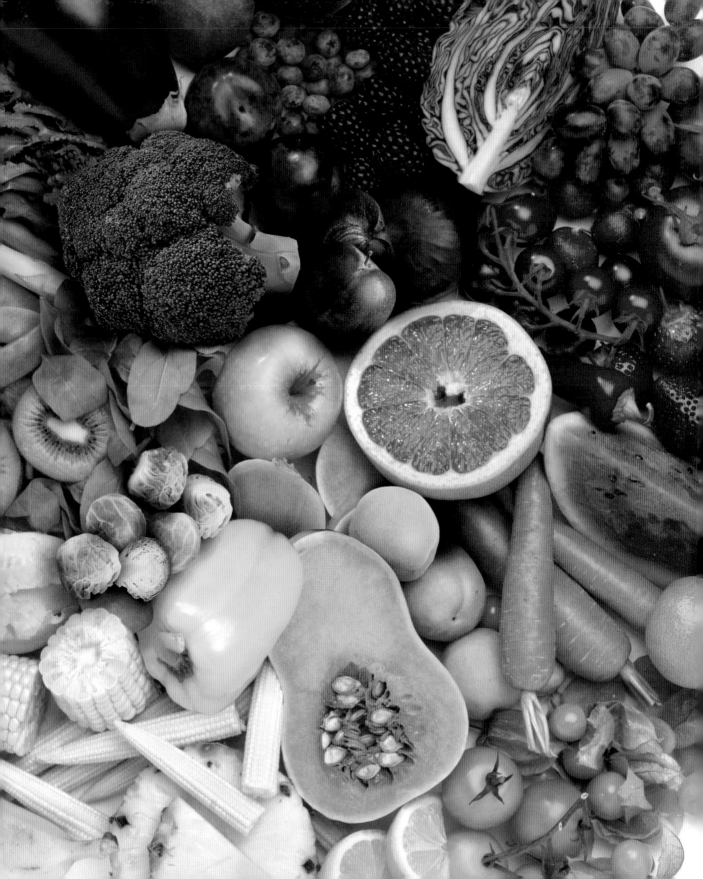

COMPLETE
Family
Nutrition

JANE CLARKE

DK

LONDON • NEW YORK
MUNICH • MELBOURNE • DELHI

Author dedication
To my beautiful Maya – for your love, your
laughs, and your patience with Mummy!

Recipe Consultant Caroline Bretherton
Senior Editor Camilla Hallinan
Project Art Editor Katherine Raj
Editors Carolyn Humphries, Diana Vowles
Designers Mandy Earey, Saskia Janssen, Simon Murrell
New photography William Reavell
Senior Jacket Creative Nicola Powling
Producer, Pre-Production Raymond Williams
Senior Producer Oliver Jeffreys
Creative Technical Support Sonia Charbonnier
Managing Editor Dawn Henderson
Managing Art Editor Christine Keilty
Art Director Peter Luff
Publishing Manager Anna Davidson
Publisher Peggy Vance

DK INDIA
Senior Art Editor Ira Sharma
Art Editor Simran Kaur
Assistant Editor Neha Samuel
Managing Editor Alicia Ingty
Managing Art Editor Navidita Thapa
Pre-Production Manager Sunil Sharma
DTP Designer Satish Chandra-Gaur

Every effort has been made to ensure that the information in this
book is accurate. However, the publisher is not responsible for
your specific health or allergy needs that may require medical
supervision, nor for any adverse reactions to the recipes
contained in this book. Neither the author nor the publisher will
be liable for any loss or damage allegedly arising from any
information or suggestion in this book.

First published in Great Britain in 2014
by Dorling Kindersley Limited
80 Strand, London WC2R 0RL
A Penguin Random House Company

Copyright © 2014 Dorling Kindersley Limited

2 4 6 8 10 9 7 5 3 1
001–192068–June/2014

All rights reserved. No part of this publication may be
reproduced, stored in a retrieval system, or transmitted in
any form or by any means, electronic, mechanical, photocopying,
recording, or otherwise without the prior written permission of
the copyright owners.

A CIP catalogue record for this book is
available from the British Library
ISBN 978 1 4093 3741 6

Colour reproduction by Scanhouse, Malaysia
Printed and bound in China by South China

Discover more at
www.dk.com

Contents

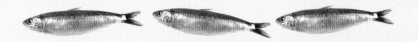

4 Different needs, *different diets*

5 Foods that *revive and heal*

6 Classic recipes *made healthy*

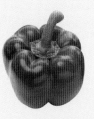

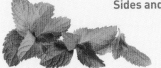

Foreword

Delicious, tempting, and nutritious food at every meal – that's something few people would say no to. Healthy food can be packed with colour, aroma, and flavour, a sensuous experience in itself, yet also full of the nutrients we need to keep our bodies healthy throughout our lives.

Eating healthily doesn't mean obsessing about the complexities of the specific nutrients in a meal, nor being faddy about food. It simply means knowing about the key foods to include in your daily diet. It's not a complicated business, and once you've grasped the principles they become second nature, so that you can just enjoy cooking to create scrumptious tastes and textures while knowing that you're doing all the right things to help your family to stay fit and healthy.

This link between food and well-being was one of the main reasons I set up my practice over 20 years ago, to inspire people of all ages to look to food to turn their health around. Many people struggle on with minor health problems, and more serious ones, not realizing that the way they eat may be lessening their enjoyment in life. Others try to eat well, but run out of ideas or get put off by conflicting advice in the media. My driving force as a nutritionist is to show how you can eat the most nourishing foods without spending hours in the kitchen and then sitting down to meals that look like some form of food penance. As I often show my 11-year-old daughter Maya while we catch up in the kitchen, there's nothing wrong with quick and simple dishes, ideally cooked from ingredients of the highest quality. A poached egg on toast can be utterly delicious, as well as full of goodness, and takes no more than five minutes to bring to the table. A big saucepan of hearty soup can be cooked in a leisurely moment, then frozen in portions to be taken out of the freezer for a quick lunch. Preparing more elaborate home-cooked dishes does take a bit longer than unpacking a ready meal, but so many processed foods are high in salt and have unnecessary sweeteners, too – and what is lost is the sense of nurturing. In preparing food to be shared around the family dining table, you are expressing love and care and creating a warmth and security that allows any problems to be shared and talked through.

Complete Family Nutrition is designed to be a guide to the nutritional needs of all the family, from babyhood all the way to old age. Modern life is increasingly pressured, and today it's often the case that both parents of a young family have to cope with the stresses of work as well as running a home – but putting nourishing and delicious meals on the table need not be an added burden. In this book you'll find the basic principles of good nutrition clearly laid out, along with plenty of tips on how to tailor the food and drink you prepare so that it meets your own individual needs and those of all the members of your family. There are times in life, such as puberty, pregnancy, the menopause, and old age, when our nutrition needs a bit of adjustment to provide added minerals or vitamins. You'll find them all covered here, along with simple food choices we can make to minimize the impact of common food allergies and reduce the risk of key health issues – and while serious illnesses such as cancer and heart disease need medical intervention, you can do your bit at home, too, by providing a diet designed to boost the immune system, restore stamina, and alleviate as many side effects as possible.

Ending with 50 classic recipes given healthy twists that everyone will love, this book lays down a nutritional pathway for life – a pathway of food to be celebrated in all its deliciousness, variety, and rewards.

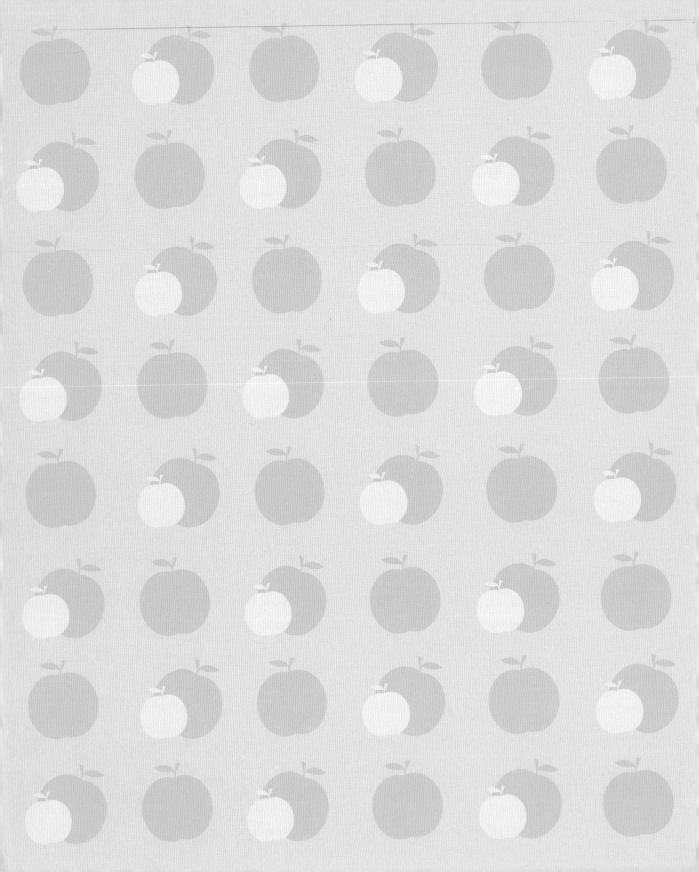

1

What your *body needs*

Food for *life*

We all need to eat a certain amount of food to survive, of course, but this is only half the story. Savouring the array of colours, aromas, textures, and flavours of good food goes hand in hand with ensuring we get all the nutrients we need to enjoy life to the full.

When you eat a nourishing, carefully balanced diet, your body obtains the fuel (or energy) and the nutrients it needs to accomplish every bodily task – the ones that you ask of it and the ones that go on behind the scenes. The food-energy balance is crucial. In a nutshell, to stay at the same weight, the energy you take in from food (measured in calories) needs to be the same as the amount of energy you use through the day. If you eat more calories than you burn, the energy is stored as body fat; if you eat fewer calories than you need for fuel, your body burns fat to use as energy. Exercise is essential, not just to keep the heart pumping and the circulation and digestion working but also to burn up any extra calories, while a good diet is vital to meet the demands that energetic exercise makes on your body. But life shouldn't be about counting calories – this book shows you how to get into great eating habits with delicious combinations of food that will tempt you on to a path you can stick to.

Beginning with the basic building blocks on the following pages, you'll see your body requires a full range of nutrients to maintain good health. At a glance, they are **carbohydrates** for energy; **proteins** for growth and repair; **fats** for warmth, energy, and healthy body functioning; **vitamins, minerals, and phytonutrients** for general health and well-being; and **fibre** for a healthy gut. The final, vital element is **water** – without it, your body can't survive.

Different foods offer different combinations of these nutrients, which can make ticking all the right boxes seem a little daunting at first. A good place to start is the UK government's **"eatwell plate"**, which shows the percentages of the major food groups that should make up our daily diet. They are: potatoes, bread, rice, pasta (wholegrain where possible), and other starchy carbohydrates, 33 per cent; fruit and vegetables, 33 per cent; milk and dairy, 15 per cent; meat, fish, eggs, beans, and other non-dairy sources of protein, 12 per cent; foods and drinks high in fat and/or sugar, no more than 7 per cent. Throughout this chapter you'll find more details about these food groups and the nutrients they provide, which foods are the best sources for those nutrients, how much you need, and lots of scrumptious tips to try.

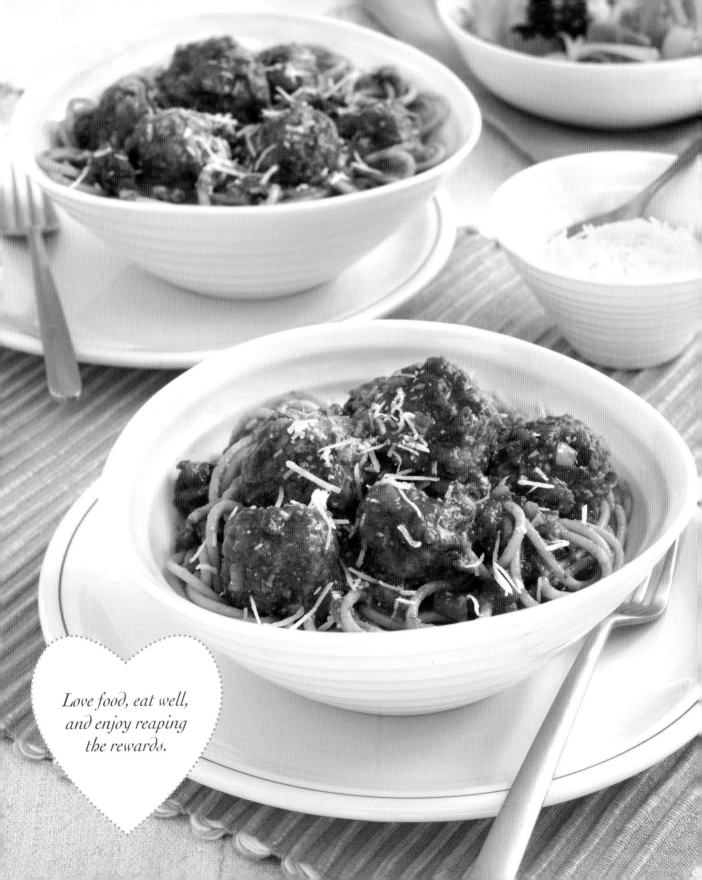

*Love food, eat well,
and enjoy reaping
the rewards.*

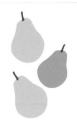

Getting to grips
with the food groups

Different countries have differing ideas about how much of each type of food we should eat. Even so, no matter where we live, we need a varied, balanced diet containing all the different food groups. Making sure they're present in everyday meals soon becomes second nature.

Carbohydrates

The body needs starchy (also known as complex) carbs to convert into glucose energy. They include potatoes, yams, cereals and grains such as wheat, oats, rye, and rice, plus foods made from them, such as bread, pasta, and couscous. Wholegrains are best as they contain all the goodness, including fibre. We should eat at least five portions a day, or a third of the food we eat. Sugars (glucose and fructose in fruit, vegetables, and honey; lactose in milk; and sucrose, which is table sugar) are simple carbohydrates. They provide fast but not sustained energy. Avoid adding table sugar, which has no useful nutrients. See pp14–15.

Fruit and vegetables

We have our first tastes of fruit and vegetables as purées when we are weaned. We're used to grabbing a banana as a quick and nutritious snack to keep us going during exercise or just because we're peckish. With so many glorious, colourful varieties and differing flavours, textures, and nutrients, these fabulous plant foods play a huge role in a healthy lifestyle. They provide masses of vitamins, minerals, and phytonutrients (see pp28–33), as well as carbohydrates and fibre. We should all eat at least five portions a day, so that fruit and vegetables make up a third of our daily food. See pp16–17.

Fibre

There are two types of fibre. The insoluble type of fibre is from the husks of cereals and other grains (the bran), in pulses and seeds, and in the skin of vegetables and fruit. It isn't digested but moves through our systems and keeps the digestion working in peak condition, preventing constipation among other things. The other type, soluble fibre, is found in fruit, vegetables, pulses, nuts, and grains. It absorbs water in the gut and then works to lower cholesterol in the blood, helping to prevent heart disease, and to keep our energy levels constant. That's why we need, depending on our age, about 24g (³⁄₄ oz) of fibre a day. See pp22–23.

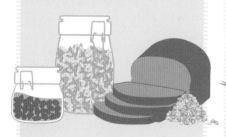

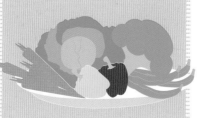

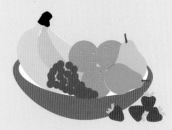

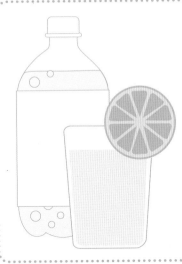

Drinking water

Our bodies rely on water to keep everything functioning properly. We can't survive without it. Most people don't drink enough: an average man should consume around 10 glasses of water a day, a woman 8 glasses, and children 6–8 small glasses (see pp38–39). Non-alcoholic drinks also count, but avoid sugary ones as they contribute to obesity and tooth decay. Cut back on caffeine, as one of its drawbacks is that it's a diuretic (see pp98–99).

Occasional treats

There are moments in life when a slice of cake or a comforting pudding is just what you want. If you make them yourself, with nourishing ingredients such as wholemeal flour, oats, fruits, seeds, and nuts, they'll actually be good for you, too. See the yummy recipes on pp232–247.

Proteins

Proteins are made up of building blocks called amino acids. Not only do proteins make every cell, but they also help to repair any damage and maintain every part of the body in good working order. Our bodies make some amino acids but others we need to eat. Some foods, such as meat, fish, eggs, poultry, soya products, and dairy produce (see right) provide complete proteins, containing all of the eight amino acids we need. Most plant proteins, such as pulses, nuts, and seeds, are not complete so we must eat a mixture to ensure we get all of the essential amino acids, in two to three portions a day. See pp18–19.

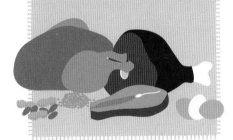

Milk and other dairy

Milk provides nearly all the essential nutrient groups, since it contains proteins, carbohydrates, vitamins, minerals, fats, and water. The most important element of milk – and cheese and yogurt – is calcium, which is vital for healthy teeth and bones. If you can't eat dairy produce, you can get calcium from other milks, such as almond, hemp, oat, or soya, and other soya products, such as tofu. Some of these are fortified with calcium, as they don't have as much as cow's milk. Dairy produce is high in saturated animal fats, so from the age of two, low-fat versions are sensible for our two to three portions a day. See pp26–27.

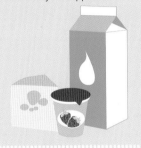

Fats

Fats should always be eaten in moderation as they are all very high in calories and, if we have too much, can make us put on weight. Yet they are vital to keep us functioning well, to provide energy, and to protect our organs. Some fats are better than others. Saturated fats, found mainly in animal produce, can clog our arteries, causing heart disease. We should eat less of these "bad fats". Polyunsaturated and monounsaturated fats – found in oily fish, nuts, seeds, vegetable oils, and some fruit, such as olives and avocados – have the opposite effect, so it's best to go for these "good fats". See pp24–25.

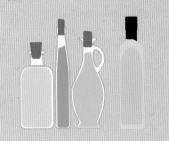

Energy-delivering *carbohydrates*

Carbs are broken down by our bodies into glucose for energy and are the basis of a healthy diet. Generally, they are classified as complex or simple, depending on their structure. They all come from plant foods and from dairy produce, such as milk, but some are better for you than others. So eat a good variety of carbs to put a spring in your step.

All carbohydrates are made up of chains of sugar molecules. Simple carbs are made up of one or two molecules – monosaccharides and disaccharides. Complex carbs have more molecules in their chains, known as polysaccharides.

Complex carbohydrates

Complex carbs contain starch, which gives them their floury, hearty texture, glycogen, which the body stores as energy, and fibre. They tend to give you a more consistent (slow-release) energy supply, making you less likely to become tired and grumpy (which can happen if you eat a lot of simple carb-rich foods). They are found in most plant foods – particularly grains, pulses, and starchy vegetables, such as

potatoes. When grains are processed to make white flour, polished rice and so on, a lot of the goodness is removed along with the bran, which is an important insoluble fibre (see p22). Although a bowl of white pasta with a delicious sauce can hit the spot of an evening, and will still give you energy, try not to make these more refined starchy foods the only carbs in your diet. It's better if you lean more towards wholegrains for maximum goodness and health benefits. So, where possible, choose wholemeal breads and pasta, wholegrain cereals, and brown rice. But white is not all bad, as refined white flour is often fortified with calcium, iron, and B vitamins to put back some of

the goodness. The elderly and the under-fours shouldn't eat too many wholegrains as the bulk can fill them up before they've eaten enough nutrients – fortified white bread can be better.

Simple carbohydrates

Simple carbs are basically sugars, which take several forms: glucose and fructose, found in honey, fruit, and vegetables; lactose (a mixture of glucose and galactose), found in milk; and sucrose – table sugar. They give a quick burst of energy but it doesn't last. Table sugar is high in calories (the measurement of how much energy a food can produce) but it has no useful nutrients, so these are "empty calories". Better to sweeten with fruit or a tiny drizzle of honey.

Know your grains

WHEAT

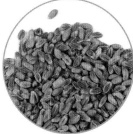

Choose wholemeal **wheat** flours (milled whole grains) for breads and baking. Use wholegrains like rice; cracked/bulgur for sides and salads; and flakes for muesli and baking.

OATS

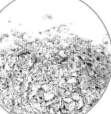

Add whole **oats** to stews; use rolled for porridge, muesli, in flapjacks, breads, and crumbles; and oatmeal (fine, medium, coarse, and pinhead) for baking, coatings, and porridge.

MAIZE

Maize is mostly coarse-ground as golden cornmeal (polenta). Cook as a hot porridge or let it cool, cut in slabs, and grill or fry. Also use for cornbread and tortillas.

BROWN RICE

Brown rice is wholegrain and nutty, with bran left on. Most types are available: short-grain, long-grain, risotto, basmati, and Thai jasmine. All take longer to cook than white.

RYE

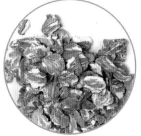

A very high-fibre grain, **rye** is sold rolled (good for porridge or muesli), whole (boil and use like rice) or milled as dark, wholegrain flour or light, refined flour, for baking.

MILLET

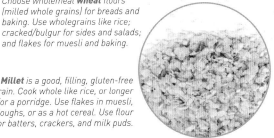

Millet is a good, filling, gluten-free grain. Cook whole like rice, or longer for a porridge. Use flakes in muesli, doughs, or as a hot cereal. Use flour for batters, crackers, and milk puds.

QUINOA

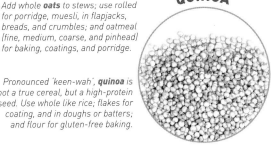

Pronounced 'keen-wah', **quinoa** is not a true cereal, but a high-protein seed. Use whole like rice; flakes for coating, and in doughs or batters; and flour for gluten-free baking.

BARLEY

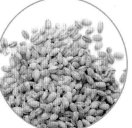

Pearl **barley** (bran on or polished), and pot barley (husk removed), are good for orzotto, and in soups and stews. Infuse, strain, and flavour for barley water. Use flour for baking.

WILD RICE

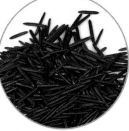

Wild rice is not really rice but the seeds of an aquatic grass, cured and dried. Use as rice (boil until they split slightly and are pleasingly chewy). Also available mixed with long-grain.

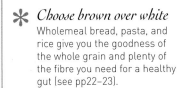

Top tips for carbs

✱ *Choose brown over white*
Wholemeal bread, pasta, and rice give you the goodness of the whole grain and plenty of the fibre you need for a healthy gut (see pp22–23).

✱ *Eat wholegrain cereals*
Go for porridge, muesli, or wholewheat breakfast cereals. Avoid those high in salt and added sugar: read the labels.

✱ *Eat plenty of fruit and veg*
Our five-a-day are packed with carbs (see pp16–17). Leave the skin on, if edible, for maximum fibre (see pp22–23).

✱ *Avoid tooth decay*
All carbs can cause cavities. Worst are refined sugars, dried fruits, and pure juices. Best avoid added sugar; brush and floss twice daily.

REALITY **CHECK**

✓ *Daily calories*
The energy you need depends on your age and lifestyle (see p41). For an average adult male, it's 2,500 kcals; female, 2,000 kcals; children aged 5–10, 1,800 kcals.

✓ *From five to adult*
About 50 per cent of daily calories should come from carbs; 39 per cent from starchy, complex ones. The GDA is 300g for men; 230g for women; 220g for 5–10-year-olds.

✓ *Children under five*
When growing so rapidly, children's calorie or fat intake should not be restricted, but still avoid added sugar. Offer a wide variety of foods.

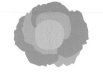

Fruit *and vegetables*

Fruit and vegetables are almost like tapestry yarns, all colourful and enticing, which should be woven through our meals to create a glowing and nourishing backdrop to our body's performance. They should make up about a third of the food we eat each and every day.

In the UK we recommend five portions a day, but other countries believe it should be more. France, for example, recommends 10 portions a day, as do the Canadians (between five and 10 portions); Denmark says six is the right amount; and Japan advises that we should consume a massive 13 portions of vegetables and four portions of fruit every day! Such is the strength of passion scientists share that fruit and vegetables provide such a plethora of essential life-giving and life-maintaining nutrients.

They don't have to be served on their own or as a side dish. Try combining in delicious soups and smoothies, in salads, as crudités with dips, and in stir-fries, stews, and casseroles. You don't have to go for fresh every day either, as canned, frozen, dried, and

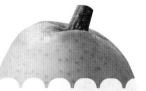

Raw
Fruit and vegetables, especially if high in vitamin C, which is sensitive to heat, are delicious raw. Try rainbow-coloured pepper strips, and sticks of cucumber, carrot, and celery with some hummus; or a crisp, colourful mixed salad, including some avocado for a touch of protein, drizzled with a little olive oil and lemon juice, with a grinding of black pepper. A platter of fruits with a pot of yogurt to dip into is a glorious, healthy pleasure, too.

Canned
Canned fruit and vegetables, in natural juice or water (avoid those with added salt or in sugar syrup), are a convenient and healthy alternative to fresh. Although some nutrients are reduced in the process (such as vitamin C), most remain intact. Some products, such as tomatoes, carrots, and corn, have higher antioxidant properties after canning. Many people find their softer texture comforting and easy to eat.

Frozen
Fruit and vegetables home-frozen soon after picking and commercial ones, which have to be frozen within a couple of hours of harvesting, are as nutritious as fresh. They're tasty and convenient. Frozen berries are especially good for making smoothies, or for cooking into a compôte with other fruits, such as plums and rhubarb, which can be stored in enticing, clear jars in the fridge for a sweetie moment.

Enjoy seasonal fruit and vegetables when you can. Eat as many different ones as possible – as part of a meal and as perfect, healthy snacks when you're peckish.

precooked vegetables, say in a soup, can be just as nourishing and nutritious.

Your five-a-day

Fruit and vegetables provide carbohydrates (see pp14–15), vitamins, minerals, and phytonutrients (pp28–33), and fibre (pp22–23). Some fruit and vegetables – particularly avocados, dried fruits, sweetcorn, and legumes (peas and beans) –

also provide a good amount of protein (pp18–21). When added together, your daily portions should weigh at least 400g (14oz), but don't become too obsessed with measuring them out. For instance, if you have a glass of freshly squeezed juice and a banana with breakfast, a snack of fruit later in the morning, a salad with your lunch, and vegetables with your supper, you'll easily hit the five-portion target. Bear in

mind, though, that a glass of juice counts as only one-a-day, however much you drink, as you need to eat whole fruit for the fibre content.

Mix and match

Eat a variety of fruit and vegetables, as they each have their own gorgeous, individual tastes and textures and their unique nutritional properties (pp34–35). For instance, lightly wilted, green, earthy spinach is rich in vitamin K, iron, and folate, whereas a scrummy bowl of tomato and orange soup is packed with vitamin C and other antioxidants (p32).

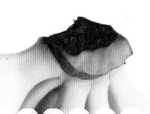

Dried

Dried fruits have concentrated flavour and nutrients as the water content has been driven off. Some paler ones, such as apples, apricots, peaches, pears, and sultanas, have a sulphur-based preservative added to help keep their colour. If you suffer from allergies, buy unsulphured ones. They are all a great source of energy. Add to breakfast cereals, use in compôtes and baking, or nibble for a healthy snack.

Cooked

Cooking some fruit and vegetables makes it easier for us to absorb their nutrients as it helps to break down the plant cell walls. When cooked, they can be served cold, if you like – for instance, poached peaches in apple juice, with a dollop of thick yogurt; chargrilled asparagus spears with a splash of balsamic vinegar; or roasted butternut squash and courgettes, with a few slices of torn buffalo mozzarella, drizzled with olive oil.

Sneaking them in

Whether you have fussy eaters or just want to include more fruit and veg, try any of these. Purée mixed stewed fruits, such as raspberries and apple or pear and banana, and fold through thick yogurt. Add grated carrot to tomato sauce for pizza topping or with pasta. Throw finely chopped spinach into any casserole – it melts into the juices. Boil root veg or leeks with potatoes, then make fluffy mash.

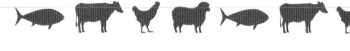

Proteins for *growth*

Making up a large part of all body cells, proteins ensure everything works properly – inside and out – and help growth, maintenance, and repair of tissues. We need to eat two or three small portions every day, whether it be a juicy steak, a piece of cheese, or a dollop of hummus.

Proteins are divided into two groups: complete proteins, explained in detail below, and plant proteins, (see pp20–21). All of them are made up of amino acids, which are linked together in a different order or chain, so each protein has its own sequence. There are eight essential amino acids we must eat, as the body can't make them, and around 12 non-essential ones that are also in food but which the body can make for itself – it only takes them from food when it needs to. However, children have a problem making enough of some of these non-essential amino acids to meet their needs, so a good range of proteins in their diet is very important. When we digest proteins, they are broken down into the separate amino acids and used for different functions in the body. Complete proteins, found mainly in animal produce, have all eight essential amino acids.

Protein v saturated fat

Unless we're vegetarian or vegan (see pp118–121), we tend to get most of our proteins from animal sources. The plus is that these proteins have every amino acid we need to eat and they're delicious. The downside is that some also contain high amounts of saturated fat, which is known to cause heart disease and strokes. You don't need to – and shouldn't – eat red meat every day: instead, go for fish, skinless poultry, or a mixture of vegetable proteins (see pp20–21). Also try supplementing meat with vegetable proteins. For instance, if you make a chilli con carne, double the amount of red kidney beans and halve the amount of meat – just as tasty but half as much saturated fat (and

Food (100g /3½oz)	Protein	Total Fat	Saturated Fat
Turkey breast (no skin), roast	29.8g	1.4g	0.4g
Rump steak (no fat), grilled	28.6g	6.0g	2.5g
Chicken breast (no skin), roast	26.5g	4.0g	1.2g
Trout (no skin), steamed	23.5g	4.5g	1.0g
Prawns (cooked, peeled)	22.6g	1.8g	0.4g
Cod (no skin), steamed	17.4g	0.7g	0.1g
Eggs (1 medium), boiled	6.4g	4.6g	1.3g

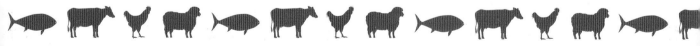

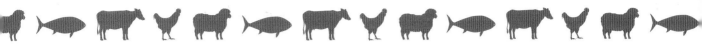

cheaper, too). You need only three small portions of protein a day (see pp40–43). If you eat more, it can be used for energy, but any that is not needed is stored as body fat.

Meat

Beef, pork (including bacon and ham), lamb, goat, veal, venison, and offal are all packed with protein, B vitamins, zinc, and iron. These days, animals are often bred to contain less fat than used to be the case, which is a plus for our health, if not for the quality and flavour of the meat. Always choose lean cuts, and remove excess fat before cooking. Spoon off any fat from the surface of stews or casseroles, and don't eat the crackling (if you can bear not to). Goat and venison are lowest in saturated fat. Cook goat like lamb, and venison like beef.

Poultry

All birds are a great source of protein, as well as B vitamins, zinc, potassium, and phosphorus. Duck and goose are good sources of iron, too. The dark meat has the higher concentration of minerals but it does contain more saturated fat than the white (although most of the fat is in the skin, so remove before eating). Birds are tender, so particularly good for quick-cooking, such as in low-fat stir-fries with plenty of vegetables and noodles or rice.

Fish

Fish and shellfish from sustainable sources have huge health benefits. Oily fish, such as mackerel and trout, are high in omega 3 fatty acids (see pp24–25). Although they contain low levels of pollutants, we should eat at least one portion – and up to four – a week, unless pregnant, trying for a baby, or a nursing mum (see pp50–51).White fish and shellfish are lower in fat but still high in protein, and more easily digested. Eat as much as you like except for sea bass, bream, turbot, halibut, and brown crab meat (for the same pollutant reasons). Do still enjoy them, but not every day. Fish are best steamed, baked, or grilled, and make the most of canned ones (in oil or water, not in brine, as we need to cut down on salt).

Eggs

A super, easy-to-eat source of protein, packed with other vital nutrients, eggs are ideal for quick, delicious meals. The yolks contain cholesterol (see p174) but this is not thought to affect levels in the blood so, unless advised by a doctor, there is no need to limit your intake. Raw or runny eggs can cause food poisoning, so they should be avoided by babies under 12 months, the sick and the elderly, and pregnant women.

A note about dairy

Milk, cheese, and yogurt also contain complete protein but are classed as dairy, a separate food group (see pp26–27). They're great for quick meals, such as a jacket potato with some grated cheese and a side salad; or a breakfast smoothie of a banana, some berries, yogurt, milk, and a spoonful of oats.

REALITY **CHECK**

 GDAs for adults
- Men and women aged 19–50, 55g per day.
- Men and women aged 50+, 53g.
- Most of us eat more protein than we need. It should be only 2–3 servings a day (see pp40–43).

 GDAs for children
- 1–3 years, 15g
- 4–6 years, 20g
- 7–10 years, 28g
- 11–14 years, 42g
- 15–18 years, 55g

GDA: Guideline Daily Amount

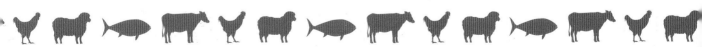

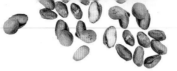

Protein from *plants*

Key sources

Pulses

Dried peas, beans, and lentils (including soya) are a great base for main meals, being rich in protein, complex carbohydrates, B vitamins, minerals, and soluble fibre. If you mix them with some nuts, seeds, grain, or a little meat, cheese, or yogurt, you know you will have good-quality protein meals. Chickpeas are good as a snack, too, roasted and then seasoned with spices.

Soya

Soya beans provide nearly as many essential amino acids as animal proteins do. They are rich in A and B vitamins, calcium, phosphorus, potassium, and iron. They also have large amounts of phytonutrients (see pp32–33) that benefit health. They are available as fresh (edamame) and dried beans and are also made into many products (see Soya sources, below right).

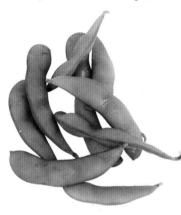

Mix and match

Vegetarians need to combine vegetable proteins each day to get all the essential amino acids. As wholegrains also contain protein, combos are easy, such as hummus with pittas or pesto with pasta.

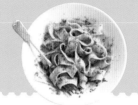

Nuts and Seeds

Both nuts and seeds have 10–25 per cent protein, depending on the variety, and are rich in E and some B vitamins, minerals, and healthy, unsaturated fats. Nuts can help protect against heart disease and diabetes. Both are great for snacks but can also be turned into many delicious dishes. Grind nuts for nut butters or with oil, herbs, and spices for pestos; add chopped nuts to tomato sauce for pasta or mix with pulses for burgers; throw both into salads, stir-fries, rice and noodle dishes.

Speciality grains

All wholegrains contain some protein but quinoa, amaranth, and buckwheat provide complete proteins, ideal for vegetarian meals.

More seeds, please

* **Pumpkin**
  Large, green seeds with a nutty flavour and high in protein, iron, zinc, and phosphorus. Good raw or toasted in sweet and savoury dishes. Use the oil in dressings.

* **Sesame**
  Good for protein, calcium, iron, and niacin. Also ground for tahini, as a dip, and to enrich hummus, soups, and stews. A dash of sesame oil adds flavour.

* **Sunflower**
  Small seeds, rich in potassium and phosphorus, but also valuable for protein, iron, and calcium. Sprinkle over salads, add to cereals and in baking.

* **Linseeds**
  Also called flax, the richest plant source of omega 3 fats and high in fibre, protein, and minerals. Best soaked first. Add to cereals, yogurt, or smoothies.

SOYA SOURCES

Miso
Tempeh
Tofu
Soya beans (fresh / dried)
Soya mince
Soya milk

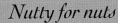

Nutty for nuts

* **Almonds** High in monounsaturated fat, with protein, fibre, vitamin E and some B vitamins, calcium, and most other minerals. Available whole, flaked, ground, and as almond milk.

* **Brazil nuts** The highest source of selenium; one nut exceeds your daily RDA. Also high in monounsaturated fats, other minerals, protein, and B and E vitamins.

* **Cashews** Lower in fat than most other nuts, and also contain protein, carbohydrates, fibre, B vitamins, iron, and zinc. Eat raw or roasted but unsalted.

* **Hazelnuts** Good source of protein, fibre, calcium, magnesium and other minerals, and vitamin E. Buy whole raw, ready-toasted, and chopped.

* **Peanuts** These groundnuts are legumes, not true nuts. They're high in monounsaturated fat, protein, B and E vitamins, and antioxidant phytonutrients. Avoid salted ones.

* **Pecans** High in poly- and monounsaturated fats, they are also a good source of protein, vitamin A, some B group, and most minerals. Available whole and ready-shelled.

* **Pine nuts** Creamy little seeds of pine trees, rather than true nuts, rich in protein, calcium, and magnesium. Good toasted lightly to enhance their nutty flavour.

* **Pistachios** Rich in potassium and, also, a good source of iron, magnesium, calcium, protein, fibre, vitamin A, and folate. Avoid salted ones.

* **Walnuts** Good source of omega 3 fatty acids and rich in folate, magnesium, potassium, iron, and zinc. Buy whole, or shelled (walnut pieces are often cheaper than halves).

Plant proteins are delicious, healthy options but you must eat a wide variety to get all your amino acids. Non-vegetarians can mix pulses, nuts, or soya with just a little meat or fish, for the best of both worlds.

Pulse (100g / 3½oz)	Protein	Calories
Soya beans	14.0g	141 kcal
Green/brown lentils	8.8g	105 kcal
Chickpeas	8.4g	121 kcal
Red kidney beans	8.4g	103 kcal
Split peas	8.0g	118 kcal
Red lentils	7.6g	100 kcal
Butter beans	7.1g	103 kcal
Haricot beans	6.6g	95 kcal

The body's **trillions of cells** are mostly made of proteins. Although the body makes some proteins itself, we must eat others so that it can **grow**, **heal**, and **function well**.

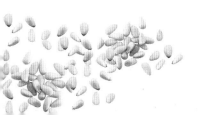
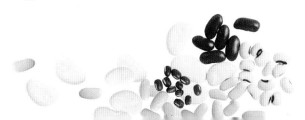

Full of *fibre*

A well-known health buzzword, fibre is needed for efficient digestion, and to keep the heart and gut healthy. It helps regulate the amount of glucose in our blood, keeping our energy levels up and aiding concentration and the ability to learn. It also reduces the chances of developing diabetes and certain cancers.

Two forms of fibre

The two types of fibre are insoluble and soluble, and we need both. Insoluble fibre (also known as roughage) is found in the husks of wholegrains, in seeds and pulses, and in the skin of fruit and vegetables. It doesn't dissolve, but passes through the digestive system (see p37), keeping the gut healthy and preventing constipation. Soluble fibre is found mainly in fruit, vegetables, pulses, and grains, such as oats. It dissolves in water and is fermented in the colon to a gel. It helps lower cholesterol (see pp174–175) and slows glucose absorption, which helps keep our energy levels constant (see pp91, 172–173).

Feeling full

Foods high in dietary fibre often take longer to chew and swallow. The fibre slows down the rate at which they pass through the gut and therefore they take more time to digest. As they stay in our tummies longer, we're left feeling satiated and hunger pangs don't return so quickly.

5 ways to eat more fibre

1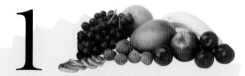

Eat more fruit

Enjoy the best of every season in all their glorious colours, tastes, and textures. Keep the skin on, if edible, or cook them. Try baked apples, stuffed with dried fruits, so that you get that lovely, almost caramel-like, baked skin with the soft apple purée inside to provide a great dose of fibre.

2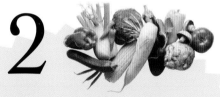

Eat more vegetables

Again, make the most of the seasons for the tastiest vegtables. Eat them raw, steamed, roasted or lightly boiled in just a little water. Brassicas, such as broccoli, are tops for fibre. Potatoes are classed as starchy carbs – not one of your five-a-day but, with skins on, a great source of fibre.

{ Most adults eat only just over half the **fibre** they should. The key is more **vegetables**, more **fruit**, and more **wholegrains**. }

3

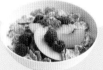

Choose high-fibre breakfast cereals

Many commercial breakfast cereals are made with refined grains and packed with added salt and sugar. Muesli can be really healthy but is often sweetened with sugar, so read the labels. Go for wholegrain cereals, preferably with little or no added salt and sugar. Or make your own scrummy granola – see p188.

4

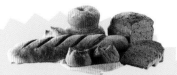

Go for wholegrain bread

For most adults, brown, nutty loaves made from wheat, spelt, rye, and/or barley (sometimes with added nuts, seeds, or dried fruit) are the best breads to choose as they're packed with fibre. But it's OK to eat fortified white bread sometimes, and young children under four shouldn't eat wholemeal all the time (see right).

5

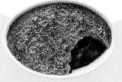

Home bake

Cook your own puddings and pies, such as an apple and blackberry crumble with a wholemeal flour and oat topping, instead of the classic white flour. For pastry, try half white and half wholemeal for a lighter option. Get the kids to help, too – baking wholemeal muffins, bread, or their own pizzas.

Great for weight control

Because fibre helps you feel full-up longer, it can be a brilliant help with weight control. Before you resort to a starvation regime, try a diet rich in fibre, then you won't feel so hungry. Just think, all those verdant veg, sweet, juicy fruits, and heavenly baked products – from a multi-seeded loaf (but don't slap on too much butter) to a warm, wholemeal muffin, bursting with dried fruits – give you lovely doses of fibre and are a good route to a slimmer, healthier you.

Fighting disease

If you eat plenty of fibre, your gut will be healthy and teeming with "good" bacteria (see p36), which decreases the risk of colorectal cancer and helps prevent diverticulitis and diabetes. When the soluble fibre forms a gel with water in the intestines, it also binds cholesterol to the stool for excretion, leaving less cholesterol in the blood and reducing the risk of heart disease.

REALITY **CHECK**

 Adults and children
Government guidelines per day are adults and over-14s, 24g ; children aged 4–6 years, 12g; 7–10, 16g; 11–14, 20g. If you plan to change to a higher fibre diet, increase fibre intake gradually, to let the body adjust, and drink plenty of water to balance that absorbed by the fibre.

 Under-fours and the elderly
Children under four and the elderly shouldn't have all wholegrains. The high fibre can fill them up before they have eaten enough nutrients. It can also upset a sensitive younger or older gut. So eating fortified white bread and white pasta and rice is OK, too.

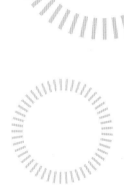

Fats, *the whole story*

We all need fats in our diet – especially children and older people.
It's about finding the good fats, eating the right amount of them,
and seeing them for their essential roles but, as with all
nutrients, not overloading the body with too much.

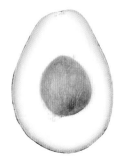

It's important to know which are the better fats for us to eat, and incorporate them in sensible amounts in our diets, rather than think we always have to put low-fat foods in our shopping basket. There are three types: saturated (found in animal and dairy produce, and, also, in coconut and palm oil), polyunsaturated (in fish and vegetable oils), and monounsaturated (in avocados, plant oils, nuts, and seeds). Saturated fats raise the "bad" sort of cholesterol in our blood (see p174), so it's better to go for unsaturated ones.

What are fats for?

Fats, which are found mainly in fish, meat, dairy, and plants, are essential for brain function, particularly for helping children to learn and concentrate, and for maximizing the function of an ageing brain. They form a large part of all cell membranes and also provide insulation, to help regulate our body temperature and keep us warm.

Fats are an important source of energy and are also necessary for the absorption of fat-soluble vitamins A, D, E, and K. We need to modify the amount we eat, though, as any excess is stored as body fat.

Good fats and bad fats

We should reduce the amount of saturated fat in our diet, as it can clog our arteries with cholesterol, so opt for lean meat, don't eat the skin of chicken, and go easy on the cheese. But don't forget that dairy produce also contains calcium and other minerals and vitamins, so do include 2–3 portions a day. Eat more polyunsaturated fats for omegas 3 and 6 (see right), and monounsaturated fats, which reduce the level of bad cholesterol in the blood. Avoid the trans fats (hydrogenated fats) found in some processed foods, as they, like saturated fats, increase bad cholesterol and decrease good cholesterol.

Do low-fat options help?

For adults, because we need to watch our saturated fat intake, we are recommended to have semi-skimmed or skimmed milk, and reduced-fat yogurts, cream, and cheeses. The problem with some low-fat options is that they can have added sugar and fillers to emulate the taste and texture of the missing fat, so they can end up being as high – or even higher – in calories. Always read the labels. There is also the

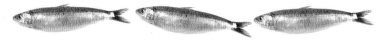

notion that you can eat more of something because it is low in fat. For some people it may be better to have a smaller amount of a high-fat food and savour every mouthful than to have a larger amount of an adulterated low-fat product. But, if you prefer them, are watching your weight, or have a big appetite, low-fat options probably are better.

Is butter ok?

Butter is a good source of calcium as well as other minerals and vitamins. It is also the best-tasting fat to use in baking, sauces, and some sautéing. However, it is high in saturated fat, so use it in moderation and only put a scraping on bread or crackers. Olive oil spread is a good alternative, or make your own nut butter (see p185) for a delicious non-dairy version. You can also try making "butters" simply from cooked and puréed dried beans or fresh peas for tasty, wholesome bread spreads.

Omegas – the super fats

Omega 3 fatty acids help maintain healthy brains, spinal cord, and eyes, regulate blood pressure and clotting, and may also help prevent heart disease. They're found in all oily fish, such as salmon, trout, mackerel, herrings, pilchards, and sardines, and in fresh or frozen (not canned) tuna. They also occur in linseeds (flaxseeds), pumpkin seeds, soya, and walnut and rapeseed oils, but aren't so readily processed in the body. Omega 6 fatty acids, found in eggs, nuts, seeds, avocados, and vegetable oils, are essential for growth, cell structure, and boosting the immune system.

Which oils to use?

All oils contain a mixture of monounsaturated, polyunsaturated, and saturated fats. The graph below shows you the proportions. Coconut oil is very high in saturated fat so use in moderation. For frying, choose one with a high smoking point, like rapeseed, sunflower, or extra light olive oil (but don't reheat, as it will deteriorate, producing carcinogens and unhealthy trans fats). Olive and sunflower are best for dressings. Remember, they are all 100 per cent fat, and 99 calories per tablespoon, so don't overdo it.

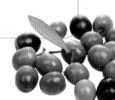

The fat content of vegetable oils

Percentages of specific fats

	0% 10% 20% 30% 40% 50% 60% 70% 80% 90% 100%
OLIVE	
RAPESEED	
CORN	
SUNFLOWER	
COCONUT	

Vegetable oils

Monounsaturated fat
Polyunsaturated fat
Saturated fat

REALITY **CHECK**

 Daily fat limit for adults
• Men should have no more than 95g fat, of which only 30g should be saturated fat.
• Women should have no more than 70g fat per day, of which only 20g should be saturated fat.

 Fat intake for children
Fat is vital for growth and development, so do not restrict fat for children under 2 years. As a guide, children aged 1–3 should eat a variety of foods, with about a third of calories coming from fat. Children aged 4–18 should get between a quarter and a third of their energy from fats.

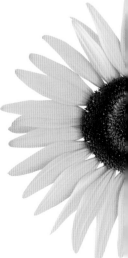

Dairy *foods*

Milk, yogurt, fromage frais, quark, and other soft and hard cheeses provide us with easily absorbed calcium, protein, vitamins A, B$_2$ and B$_{12}$, as well as other vitamins and minerals – all of which are essential for growth, development, and healthy teeth and bones.

Everyone should be encouraged to consume three portions of dairy produce every day (see pp40–43). They play a vital role in a healthy diet. Butter and cream are classed as fats, not dairy, so they aren't included here. It's worth noting that cheeses can be high in salt, and flavoured yogurts and fromage frais are often packed with sugar, so check the labels and choose wisely for your family.

If you have allergy problems (see pp126–127), you will need to select alternatives – you may be able to tolerate other dairy sources or go for non-dairy choices. The other wonderful thing about dairy foods is that they can be very comforting if the body is a little out of sorts. A small bowl of yogurt, drizzled with honey, can be just what the body craves when your appetite's gone or your tummy's playing up.

Fat content

We're encouraged to eat low-fat options. Whether you do depends on how much you like them. Bear in mind that most of the fat in dairy food is saturated fat (see pp24–25), which, if eaten to excess, can lead to furring of the arteries – in children as well as in adults. There is no difference, fat-wise, between a smaller amount of a full-fat food and a larger amount of a low-fat one. It takes more willpower not to overindulge in the richer, high-fat food but as it is more stomach-satisfying, you may be able to eat less of it.

Cow's milk

Children should have whole milk and milk products up to the age of two, but then they can change to semi-skimmed until they're five, at which point you can switch them to skimmed if you prefer – especially if they drink a lot and you want to reduce their fat intake. Adults should opt for low-fat milk, too, as it's an easy way to reduce saturated fat consumption. UHT milks are just as nutritious and can be a handy and cheaper standby to ensure you never run out. Alternatively, you can freeze fresh milk.

Other dairy milks

Some people prefer milk and yogurts made from other dairy milks such as goat's, sheep's, or lactose-free cow's milk. Sheep's milk is slightly higher in calories than goat's and cow's milk, whereas the fats in goat's milk are slightly different, and some children and adults find it easier to digest. Then again, the levels of calcium, iron, magnesium, phosphorus, sodium, and zinc are higher in sheep's milk. So which milk you choose can depend on taste preference, cost, and which one best suits your digestion.

Dairy facts

DID YOU KNOW?

Only **20%** of primary schoolchildren and **30%** of teenage children in the UK have their three servings of dairy a day.

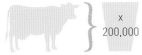

} x 200,000

1 cow can give 200,000 glasses of milk in her lifetime

ABSORBING CALCIUM

Caffeine inhibits calcium absorption, so don't drink tea, coffee, or cola with meals. If you don't get enough calcium, your body will take it from your bones, which can cause rickets in children or osteoporosis in later life.

REALITY **CHECK**

 Calcium for children

As children grow and develop they need more calcium. 1–3 year olds, 350mg; 4–6 year olds, 450mg; 7–10 year olds, 550mg; 11–18 year old girls, 800mg; 11–18 year old boys, 1,000mg. As a guide, a 200ml glass of milk has around 230mg; a 30g stick of Cheddar, 126mg; a small pot of yogurt, 225mg; a scoop of vanilla ice cream, 65mg; and a little fromage frais, 43mg.

Calcium for adults

The UK Department of Health recommends 700mg per day. We should be able to get all we need from a balanced diet (see pp40–43) but elderly people, in particular, may be advised to take a calcium supplement along with vitamin D to help its absorption.

Cheese

Cheeses are a brilliant alternative to meat, fish, eggs, or pulses for protein. They all vary in fat content but it's better to choose cheese that you love and then just make sure you don't eat too much of it if it's a high-fat one. That said, Edam is lower in fat than most hard cheeses, which makes it a good choice. It also helps to cut the rind off soft cheese, such as Brie, as this significantly reduces the fat content. Use a strong-flavoured cheese for cooking so that you'll need less to get the desired taste.

Yogurt

Don't always assume that low or reduced-fat is the only way to go. Low-fat, flavoured yogurts and fromage frais can be very high in added sugar and thickeners. For children, especially, it may be better to go for the plain, full-fat ones and add your own, natural sweetness if you need to – ideally using fresh or puréed fruit, or (from the age of one) a small drizzle of honey. In cooking, full-fat yogurt works best as it can be cooked without curdling. But low-fat is fine for dressings, dips, and cold desserts.

Non-dairy choices

Almond milk, rice milk, and coconut milk are popular as dairy alternatives. Choose unsweetened, plain varieties, as sweetened and flavoured options contain significant amounts of sugar. Soya products are also common alternatives; however, some research suggests we should limit soya intake due to its oestrogen-like properties (see p74). Some non-dairy milks are fortified with calcium but it isn't so easily absorbed, so get more calcium from fortified bread, broccoli, nuts, and fresh or canned fish.

Vital *vitamins*

Vitamins, along with minerals (see pp30–31), are essential for health. They're only needed in tiny amounts, so most people should get all they need from food (see individual entries for exceptions). However, as our bodies can't make most of them, it's important to eat a varied diet to make sure you get enough.

Water-soluble vitamin

Fat-soluble vitamin

Two types

Vitamins are classified by whether they are soluble in fat or water. Fat-soluble ones (A, D, E, and K) are stored in the body. If there's an excessive build-up, it can be harmful, but that's unlikely if you eat a balanced diet. Water-soluble ones (C, all the B vitamins, and folic acid) cannot be stored in the body (except B_{12}) so they need to be consumed daily.

VITAMIN A

ROLE: There are two types – retinol and beta-carotene – vital for growth, healthy skin, teeth, and vision. Vitamin A strengthens the immune system and is a powerful antioxidant (see p32) against heart disease and cancer.

SOURCES: Retinol from liver, oily fish, egg yolk, dairy, fortified low-fat spreads; beta-carotene from red, yellow, orange and green fruit and veg.

RDA: (mcg/day) Men, 700; women, 600; children aged 1–3 years, 400; 4–10 years, 500; 11–14 years, 600.

VITAMIN B_1

ROLE: Also known as thiamin, vitamin B_1 is needed for energy production, heart function, and healthy digestive and nervous systems. Also aids general growth and development and helps children concentrate.

SOURCES: Wholegrains, legumes (such as peas and fresh soya beans), brown rice, nuts, seeds, pork, and offal.

RDA: (mg/day) Men, 1.0 (over 65, 0.9 and 15–18, 1.1); women, 0.8; children aged 1–3 years, 0.5; 4–10 years, 0.7; 11–14 years, 0.9.

VITAMIN B_2

ROLE: Also known as riboflavin, this vitamin is needed in order to release energy from food, digest fats and proteins, protect the nervous system, and maintain mucous membranes.

SOURCES: Dairy, fish, meat, offal, eggs, yeast extract, and fortified cereals.

RDA: (mg/day) Men, 1.3; women, 1.1; children aged 1–3 years, 0.6; 4–6 years, 0.8; 7–10 years, 1.0; 11–14 years (boys), 1.2, (girls), 1.1.

VITAMIN B_3

ROLE: Niacin – or nicotinic acid – plays a major role in helping convert food into energy, develops and maintains the nervous and digestive systems, and helps in the manufacture of DNA.

SOURCES: Meat, fish, pulses, eggs, nuts, wheat, maize, and fortified breakfast cereals.

RDA: (mg/day) Men, 17; women, 13; children aged 1–3 years, 8.0; 4–6 years, 11; 7–10 years, 12; 11–14 years (boys), 15, (girls), 12; 15–18 years (boys), 18, (girls), 14.

VITAMIN B_5

ROLE: Pantothenic acid is needed for the conversion of proteins, fats, and carbohydrates into energy and for making vitamin B_{12}, cell membranes, and haemoglobin in red blood cells.

SOURCES: Pantothenic means 'from every side' and is found in most plant and animal foods. It's particularly high in wholegrains, nuts, meat, oily fish, yogurt, mangetout, mushrooms, avocados, cauliflower, Brussels sprouts, and fortified breakfast cereals.

RDA: Eat a wide variety of foods daily.

RDA: Recommended Dietary Allowance

VITAMIN B₆

ROLE: Also known as pyridoxine, this vitamin is needed for strong nervous and immune systems, to digest proteins, and to fight infection.

SOURCES: Poultry, offal, eggs, oily fish, potatoes, sweet potatoes, bananas, nuts, and wholegrains.

RDA: (mg/day) Men,1.4; women, 1.2; children aged 1–3 years, 0.7; 4–6 years, 0.9; 7–10 years, 1.0; 11–14 years (boys), 1.2, (girls), 1.0.

VITAMIN B₁₂

ROLE: Needed for growth and development, releasing energy from food, and to maintain a strong nervous system. It's important in the production of energy, and, with folic acid, for healthy blood cells.

SOURCES: Red meat, such as beef, lamb, and pork, offal, seafood, eggs, and dairy produce. The only vegetable source is yeast extract.

RDA: (mg/day) Adults, 1.5; children aged 1–3 years, 0.5; 4–6 years, 0.8; 7–10 years, 1.0; 11–14 years, 1.2.

FOLIC ACID

ROLE: A B vitamin, also called folate. It helps make healthy red blood cells and reduces the risk of defects in the central nervous system of unborn babies. For women, a 400mcg supplement is recommended if trying for a baby (as is vitamin D) and up to 12 weeks pregnant.

SOURCES: Leafy greens, asparagus, broccoli, Brussels sprouts, liver, pulses, wholegrains, and fortified bread and breakfast cereals.

RDA: (mcg/day) Adults, 200; children aged 1–3 years, 70; 4–6, 100; 7–10, 150.

VITAMIN C

ROLE: Also called ascorbic acid, this is a powerful antioxidant (see p32), protects against infection, and helps wounds heal. It is easily destroyed during food preparation and by heat.

SOURCES: Best in kiwi fruits, berries, fresh currants, pomegranates, citrus fruits, potatoes, winter squashes, sweet and chilli peppers, cruciferous vegetables, and brassicas.

RDA: (mg/day) Adults, 40; children aged 1–10 years, 30; 11–14 years, 35.

VITAMIN D

ROLE: It is important for the absorption of calcium and phosphorus, and for building and maintaining healthy bones and teeth. It also boosts the immune system and helps muscle function.

SOURCES: Largely manufactured in our skin when it's exposed to sunlight, but also in oily fish, eggs, and fortified low-fat spreads and cereals.

RDA: Enough from some sun and a balanced diet. Take a supplement if under 5, pregnant, breastfeeding, over 65, or lacking in exposure to sunlight.

Maxing your vitamins

❋ *Freshly prepare*
Fruit and vegetables start to lose nutrients as soon as they are cut, so it's best to prepare just before use when possible.

❋ *Don't overcook*
Many vitamins are damaged by heat so boil veg briefly in just a little water; microwave; steam; or stir-fry with a splash of oil.

❋ *Store sensibly*
Keep fresh food in a cool, dark place or in the fridge, unless it is ripening, as many vitamins are light-sensitive.

❋ *Supplement advice*
It's better to glean vitamins and minerals from your food, unless you require an amount that can't be reached through food and your doctor or health professional recommends certain supplements.

VITAMIN E

ROLE: An antioxidant (see p32), vitamin E is needed for healthy skin and heart and for a strong immune system. This vitamin is also used in topical creams to reduce scarring.

SOURCES: Vegetable, nut and seed oils, avocados, almonds, dairy produce, seeds, eggs, soya and wholegrains, and fortified low-fat spreads.

RDA: (mg/day) Men, 4.0; women, 3.0; there is no RDA for children.

VITAMIN K

ROLE: Mainly needed for blood clotting and healthy bones. Babies are given an injection of vitamin K at birth, as their body supply doesn't kick in immediately. Watch intake if on blood-thinners.

SOURCES: Most is produced in the gut but also in vegetable oils, cereals, green leafy vegetables, particularly broccoli, grapes, and plums.

RDA: (mcg/day) 1 per 1kg body weight, so if you weigh 65kg, you need 65mcg; infants, 10 per kg body weight so, if weight is 20kg, they need 200mcg.

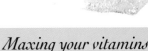

Mighty *minerals*

Minerals are essential for health. They're the same ones found in rocks and metal ores. We glean minerals by eating plants that have taken them from the soil and animals that have eaten the plants, and, to a lesser extent, by drinking water. Some key minerals are listed here but we also need copper, iodine, chromium, fluoride, sulphur, and other trace elements.

How much?

Some minerals are needed in larger quantities than others but each one is just as important. A balanced diet supplies enough for most people but requirements vary according to age, health, gender, and particular conditions, such as pregnancy. So the RDAs given here are a guide only.

Water has a unique mineral content, depending on its area of origin.

CALCIUM

ROLE: Calcium is essential for bones and teeth and to help our muscles contract, including the heart. Lactose, the sugar found in milk (a rich source), aids its absorption. Although spinach is also a good source of calcium, it contains oxalic acid, which makes it harder to process, so you shouldn't rely on spinach for your daily dose. If you eat three portions a day of dairy, you should get enough calcium, but a wide variety from the list below is better.

SOURCES: Dairy produce, whitebait, sardines and canned fish (if you eat the bones), green leafy vegetables, okra, soya products, almond milk, nuts, seeds, tahini, dried fruits such as apricots, and fortified bread.

RDA: (mg/day) Adults, 700; children aged 1–3 years, 350; 4–6, 450; 7–10, 550; 11–18 (boys), 1,000, (girls), 800.

IRON

ROLE: Iron is important for growth and development and crucial in the formation of healthy blood cells, which carry oxygen around the body and, therefore, helps us to feel healthy and energetic. Iron from animal products is easier to absorb than that from plants but if you have plenty of foods rich in vitamin C (like orange juice with your breakfast cereal), it helps enormously.

SOURCES: Liver, lean red meat, shellfish and canned fish, egg yolks, fortified breakfast cereals, dried fruit such as prunes, apricots, and figs, nuts, seeds, dark leafy greens and seaweed, baked beans and other pulses, and oat and wheat bran.

RDA: (mg/day) Men, 8.7; women, 14.8 (over 50, 8.7); children aged 1–3 years, 6.9; 4–6, 6.1; 7–10, 8.7; 11–14 (boys), 11.3, (girls), 14.8.

MAGNESIUM

ROLE: Magnesium helps the body process fats and proteins and build strong healthy bones and teeth. Along with calcium, sodium, and potassium, it also facilitates muscle contraction and the transmission of nerve signals, and helps to control the level of calcium in the blood. It can also be a useful aid to relaxation and sleep.

SOURCES: Cabbage (best raw), okra, globe artichokes, sweet potato, wholegrains, meat, game birds and poultry, haggis, dried fruits, especially figs, sunflower and sesame seeds, and nuts, such as Brazils, cashews, almonds, and peanuts.

RDA: (mg/day) Men, 300; women, 270; children aged 1–3 years, 85; 4–6, 120; 7–10, 200; 11–14, 280; 15–18 (boys), 280, (girls), 300.

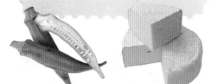
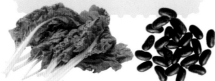

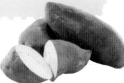
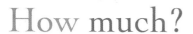

Calcium helps **weight loss**. Increased calcium in **your diet** makes your body break down more fat and store less of it. Result: **less body fat**.

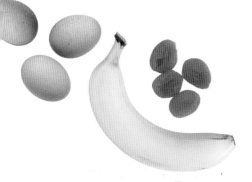

PHOSPHORUS

ROLE: Vital for healthy bones and teeth, phosphorus also helps store energy needed by body cells. It is essential for the manufacture of DNA, too. As it's found in all animal and plant proteins, provided you have your daily two or three portions, and include plenty of calcium-rich foods, you'll get enough. The body needs vitamin D (see p.29) to process phosphorus.

SOURCES: Wholegrains, dairy produce, red meat, poultry, seafood, pulses, soya products, Quorn, nuts, and seeds.

RDA: (mg/day) Adults, 550; children aged 1–3 years, 270; 4–6, 350; 7–10, 450; 11–18 (boys), 775, (girls), 625.

SELENIUM

ROLE: Selenium works alongside other antioxidants (see p32), such as vitamin E (see p29) and is essential for normal function of the immune system and thyroid gland. It is thought to help protect against cancer, enhance male fertility, and regulate asthma.

SOURCES: Brazil nuts, liver, shellfish, caviar, fish (especially canned tuna), mushrooms, garlic, egg yolk, sesame and sunflower seeds, wheat germ, and wheat, oat, and rice bran.

RDA: (mcg/day) Men, 75; women, 60; children aged 1–3 years, 15; 4–6, 20; 7–10, 30; 11–14, 45; 15–18 (boys), 70, (girls), 60.

POTASSIUM

ROLE: Potassium works in conjunction with sodium and chloride to regulate the amount of water and acid/alkali balance in the body. It also helps the nerves and muscles to function properly, lowers and controls high blood pressure, keeps the heart healthy, and eases fatigue, irritability, and confusion. Elderly people are more at risk of too much potassium in their body, as their kidneys are less able to excrete excess.

SOURCES: Many fruit and vegetables but especially bananas, oranges, tomatoes, chard, spinach, mushrooms, fennel (best raw), beetroot, and potatoes, as well as pulses, soya products, bran and bran breakfast cereals, meat, poultry, game, and fish.

RDA: (mg/day) Adults, 3,500; children aged 1–3 years, 800; 4–6, 1,100; 7–10, 2,200; 11–14, 3,100.

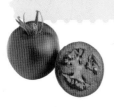

ZINC

ROLE: Although needed in miniscule amounts, zinc is still essential in normal cell division, growth, and repair, for the immune system, too, and for the development of the reproductive organs and hormones – oysters are a great source of zinc, hence their reputation for being an aphrodisiac. Zinc also helps regulate moods and appetite, including the sense of taste and smell, and assists in the breakdown of carbs, proteins, and fats.

SOURCES: Fish and shellfish, lean red meat, poultry, wholegrains, wheat germ, nuts (especially Brazils), seeds, haricot and soya beans, eggs, and dairy produce.

RDA: (mg/day) Men, 9.5; women, 7.0; children aged 1–3 years, 5.0; 4–6, 6.5; 7–10, 7.0; 11–14, 9.0.

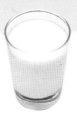 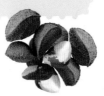

SODIUM CHLORIDE

ROLE: Sodium chloride is salt, and is naturally present in most foods. Both elements (sodium and chloride) are crucial in controlling the amount of water in the body and its acid/alkali balance. Salt also helps muscular contraction. Most people eat too much, which can cause higher blood pressure, heart disease, and strokes. Processed food often has a lot of salt, although manufacturers are now reducing their levels. Check labels: if you see sodium levels in grams, multiply this by 2.5 to get the salt content. The RDA for salt below is the most you should eat.

SOURCES: All foods, particularly high in shellfish and processed foods, and table salt.

RDA: (g/day) Adults and children over 11, 6; children 1–3, 2; 4–6, 3; 7–10, 5.

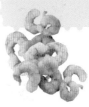 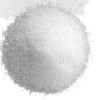

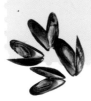

Phytonutrients

All plant foods (fruit, vegetables, wholegrains, nuts, seeds, and pulses) contain thousands of natural chemicals, which help to protect them. Known as phytochemicals, or phytonutrients, they may keep us functioning properly, too, and help to prevent many serious diseases.

There are thousands of phytonutrients in the plant foods we eat – *phyto* comes from the Greek word for plant. They are divided into many groups, one of which is the polyphenols, which are the most abundant type of antioxidants in fruit and vegetables. We need antioxidants, which also include vitamins A, C and E, selenium, zinc, copper, and manganese, to combat free radicals – unstable molecules made by oxygen in our bodies and also by unhealthy lifestyles. The free radicals attack the DNA, then attach themselves to healthy cells, damaging them, which can lead to heart disease and some cancers.

There may be as many as 100 phytonutrients in one serving of fruit or vegetables, providing specific protective roles for both minor and major health problems. They are another reason to eat plant-based foods, but it's not just there that you'll benefit from these amazing chemicals – they're also in teas (black, green, rooibos, and white), and red wine.

FLAVONOIDS

ROLE: These water-soluble compounds are powerful antioxidants with antivirus, anticancer, anti-allergy, and anti-inflammatory properties. Anthocyanins, prominent flavonoids, also add the purple, red, and blue hues to plants.

SOURCES: They are found in all fruit and vegetables but some plants' flavonoids have particular health benefits. Tea and red grapes may help to reduce cholesterol; cranberries and blueberries fight urinary infections.

CAROTENOIDS

ROLE: They give the yellow, orange, and red pigment to fruit and vegetables. Powerful antioxidants, carotenoids (such as lycopene – see above right – and capsanthin, in chillies and sweet peppers) may also help to prevent heart disease and some cancers and boost the immune system. Lutein has a role in protecting eyes. Orange-yellow beta-carotene is changed by the body into vitamin A (see p28).

SOURCES: All red, orange, yellow, and dark green vegetables and fruit.

PHYTOESTROGENS

ROLE: Found most notably in soya, phytoestrogens resemble mammalian oestrogen. Soya is widely consumed in the Far East, where rates of breast cancer, osteoporosis, and other serious health conditions are lower than in the West, so it is thought phytoestrogens may have a beneficial role. Research suggests that large amounts of soya may not be good for us, so it's best to limit soya intake, as part of a balanced diet.

SOURCES: Soya beans and products such as tofu and soya milk, yogurt, and chickpeas.

ELLAGIC ACID

ROLE: This polyphenol protects plants against infection and pests, and has now been shown to help fight breast and skin cancer and cancer of the colon, prostate, pancreas, and oesophagus. It also has anti-inflammatory and antioxidant properties, and plays a role in eliminating toxins from the body. Cooking doesn't destroy it, so it's even present in fruit jam.

SOURCES: Pomegranate, berries, grapes, currants, and some nuts, including walnuts and pecans.

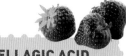

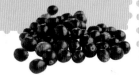

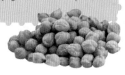

We love tomatoes!

Tomatoes are one of the healthiest foods around. Lycopene, a carotenoid in tomatoes, is thought to help in the prevention of heart disease and cancers of the cervix, stomach, breast, lung, colon, and prostate. Lycopene is most effective if the tomatoes are cooked and/or processed – sun-dried tomatoes are the tops but roasted, or in soup, sauce, purée, and ketchup are all good. But don't let this stop you tucking into them fresh, as you'll still get great benefits.

Choose ripe fruit
Generally, the redder and riper the skin, the more lycopene the fruit will contain. They're full of vitamins and minerals, too.

Eat with healthy fats
Lycopene is fat-soluble, so eat tomatoes with a drizzle of olive oil, or with sliced avocado, for instance, for fast absorption.

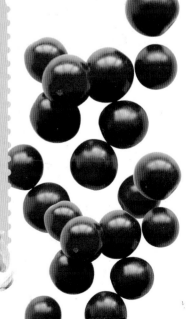

GLUCOSINOLATES

ROLE: Derived from glucose and containing sulphur, glucosinolates are in nearly all brassica plants. They are thought to protect against several cancers and also have antiviral, antibacterial, and anti-inflammatory properties. To preserve them in your food, steam, stir-fry, or microwave brassicas rather than boiling.

SOURCES: Cabbages, turnips, swede, pak choi, cauliflower, watercress, Brussels sprouts, radishes, and horseradish.

PHYTOSTEROLS

ROLE: Also called saponins, phytosterols (plant stanols and sterols) are known to reduce both blood cholesterol levels and hardening of the arteries. They also have antioxidant properties. Phytosterol supplements, however, are not recommended while pregnant or breastfeeding, or for children under five, as the developing brain needs cholesterol.

SOURCES: Nuts, seeds, and their oils, olive and corn oils, whole grains, broccoli, red onions, carrots, Brussels sprouts, and berries.

SULPHIDES

ROLE: These sulphur-containing phytonutrients are present in all members of the allium family and are thought to boost cancer-destroying enzymes in the body. Mincing, slicing, or chopping onions, for example, and then letting them stand for 5–10 minutes before fast cooking such as sautéing enhances their health-giving properties as this activates the phytonutrients.

SOURCES: Onions, shallots, leeks, spring onions, garlic, wild garlic, and chives.

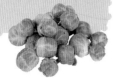

Eat a *rainbow*

Packed with phytonutrients (see pp32–33), fruit and vegetables are appealing on the plate and crucial to health. Eat a wide range of colours and types each day and treat your plate like an artist's palette. Each colour gives different nutrients – so the greater the mix, the more goodness you'll get.

PURPLES

Fruit and vegetables such as blackberries, plums, beetroot, and aubergines contain anthocyanins, a flavonoid that is good for the heart and eyes and may help reduce the risk of gum disease and mouth cancers.

BLUEBERRIES are rich in antioxidants and help prevent urinary tract infections.

Beetroot's phytonutrients are particularly beneficial for detoxifying the liver.

GREENS

From kiwi fruit to okra, broccoli to cabbage, there is a vast range of green foods. They contain carotenoids, which help maintain healthy eyesight and can also reduce the risk of heart disease and some cancers.

PEAS ARE PACKED with vitamin B1, beta-carotene, niacin, folate, vitamin C, and protein.

Broccoli is a superfood, rich in folate, beta-carotene, vitamin C, fibre, and cancer-fighting phytonutrients.

PHYTONUTRIENTS · MINERALS · VITAMINS · ANTIOXIDANTS · WATER

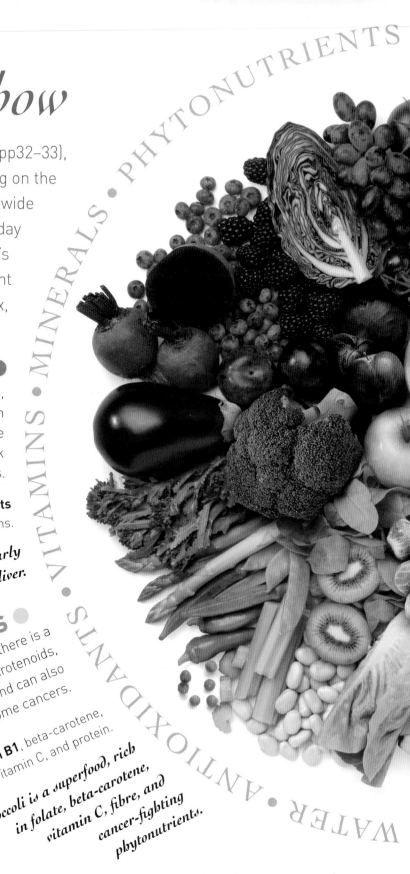

TASTY • SATISFYING • MOSTLY VERY LOW FAT • HIGH IN FIBRE

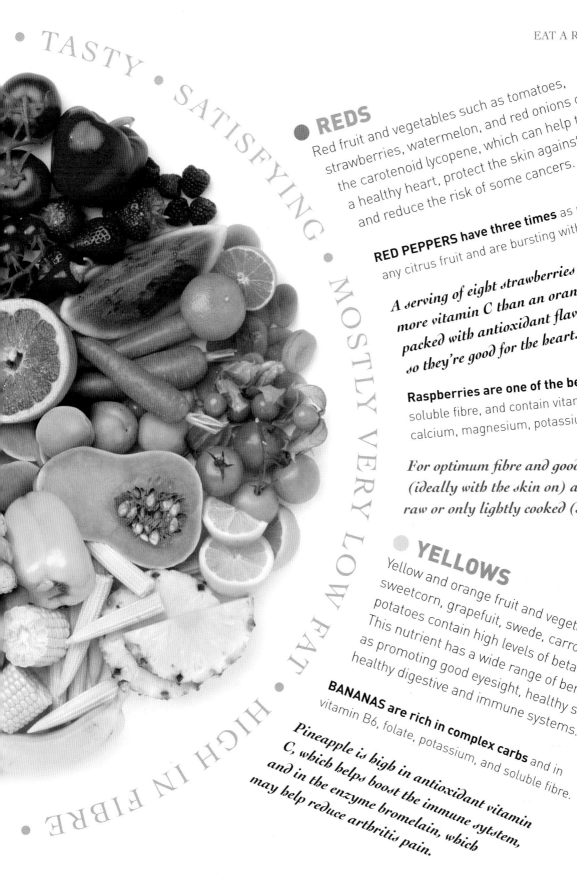

REDS

Red fruit and vegetables such as tomatoes, strawberries, watermelon, and red onions contain the carotenoid lycopene, which can help to promote a healthy heart, protect the skin against UV rays, and reduce the risk of some cancers.

RED PEPPERS have three times as much vitamin C as any citrus fruit and are bursting with beta-carotene.

A serving of eight strawberries provides more vitamin C than an orange. They're packed with antioxidant flavonoids, too, so they're good for the heart.

Raspberries are one of the best fruits for soluble fibre, and contain vitamins C and E, calcium, magnesium, potassium, and iron.

For optimum fibre and goodness, eat fruit (ideally with the skin on) and vegetables raw or only lightly cooked (see pp16–17).

YELLOWS

Yellow and orange fruit and vegetables such as sweetcorn, grapefuit, swede, carrots, and sweet potatoes contain high levels of beta-carotene. This nutrient has a wide range of benefits such as promoting good eyesight, healthy skin, and healthy digestive and immune systems.

BANANAS are rich in complex carbs and in vitamin B6, folate, potassium, and soluble fibre.

Pineapple is high in antioxidant vitamin C, which helps boost the immune sytstem, and in the enzyme bromelain, which may help reduce arthritis pain.

Probiotics and *prebiotics*

Our guts teem with bacteria, or gut flora – some good, some bad. If the bad take over, we may get an upset tummy, diarrhoea, or worse. This is where probiotics and prebiotics come in. They work in different ways to keep our gut and digestion functioning in tip-top form.

Probiotics are the good or "**friendly**" **bacteria** that we can build up by eating certain foods. The most common is *Lactobacillus*, which is found in probiotic drinks, bio yogurts, and other cultured milks, such as buttermilk, and in fermented products, such as sauerkraut, kimchi, tempeh, and miso. Purposely increasing the levels of bacteria in our body may seem strange, but we need the friendly kind as they can keep the bad bacteria under control. With more good bacteria in there, **our gut behaves much better**, with symptoms such as bloating and diarrhoea far less likely. Everyday life conspires against us maintaining a healthy balance of gut flora. Stress tends to disturb the balance, as does drinking too much alcohol, eating badly, or taking antibiotics to clear up infections – so we need to choose our food with an eye to counteracting the effects of these common events.

Probiotic bacteria change the acidity in our stomach and many help to prevent the growth of germs. No one knows how many of them survive the digestive process before they reach the colon, where they really get to work (see opposite). That said, they are definitely worth having as they **aid digestion** by breaking down tough fibres, enzymes, and other proteins in food, boost the immune system, and ease upset tummies and the symptoms of lactose intolerance and irritable bowel syndrome (IBS).

Prebiotics, on the other hand, don't contain any of the good (or bad) bacteria, yet bring real benefits. A type of carbohydrate, they are not easily digested, so they move through the gut into the colon, where they **encourage good bacteria to grow**. The best sources include tomatoes, bananas, Jerusalem artichokes, chicory, soya beans, asparagus, and alliums such as leeks and onions. **Eat them as fresh as possible**, as levels of prebiotics decline with time.

When you introduce more prebiotics and probiotics as part of your diet, your gut may initially be a little more windy and unsettled, but this should sort itself out within a few days.

The inside story

Digestion is the incredible process of changing food into a form that our body can absorb and use as energy or for repairing and building cells. When you eat, your teeth grind food into small pieces to start breaking it down. As it is moved through the digestive system by the muscles, the food is processed by different enzymes. The nutrients are all absorbed and the waste is excreted.

1. See and smell

The look or smell of what you are about to eat triggers signals to your brain that food and drink are on the way. Your brain sends back impulses that make your mouth water (with saliva), your stomach contract (hunger pangs), and your intestinal glands produce digestive enzymes ready to start work – all before you take your first bite.

2. Taste and chew

When food enters your mouth, the taste steps up the digestive process. Your teeth and tongue grind and mix the food with saliva, which starts to break down any starchy carbs into sugar (glucose). When you swallow, muscle contractions send the small pieces of food, mixed with more saliva, down your oesophagus (gullet) and into your stomach.

3. Digest

In your stomach, muscle contractions break the food into ever smaller pieces. Glands release a blend of enzymes, hydrochloric acid, and mucus, which begin the digestion of proteins and fats into amino acids and fatty acids. The food, now a thick, soupy mass called chyme, is pushed along to the small intestine for absorption.

Stomach

4. Absorb nutrients

In the small intestine, digestive juices finish breaking down carbs into sugar, dissolve fats into water, and complete the separation of proteins into amino acids. As muscles push the chyme along, special cells in the intestine walls absorb glucose, amino acids, fatty acids, vitamins, minerals, and phytonutrients, and the blood carries them around the body.

Small intestine

5. End of the line

Muscle contractions move undigested food and other waste material to the colon (or large intestine). Like a giant sponge, it absorbs water from this material and squeezes it into compact faeces, after resident colonies of friendly bacteria (see opposite) have digested the last few amino acids. The rectum then pushes the faeces out of the body.

Colon

Drinking *water*

Research and everyday experience show that if we drink enough water we feel much healthier. It is also thought that if we sip water regularly during the day it helps to keep the brain more alert. Children should be encouraged to drink plenty of water, too.

Why do we need water?

Every cell in our body needs water to function. In fact, the body is made up of around 60 per cent water. It controls body temperature and prevents dehydration when we sweat. Water also helps to move nutrients around the body, aiding their absorption, and assists in ridding the body of toxins and other waste products. If you drink plenty of water, you are less likely to suffer from constipation, urinary infections, colon cancer, and kidney stones.

Do you and your family get enough?

The amount of fluid we drink differs enormously, and it can be hard to always hit the water target. Try for a glass an hour as a good guide. For the first few days the kidney and bladder will react such that you need the loo more often, but this usually settles down. To check that you or your children are getting enough water, look at the colour of the urine. If it's very pale, it's fine – the darker it is, the more fluid needs to be drunk.

When children say they are hungry, they may in fact be thirsty, so give them a glass of water – particularly if it is nearly mealtime, or they'll end up eating a snack and not their meal. When you feel thirsty, you are already dehydrated, so make sure you drink plenty then. If you don't, you are likely to suffer from a headache and dry mouth and eyes, feel tired, and find you cannot concentrate for long.

Does it have to be water?

All drinks count, but water is the healthiest. Sweetened soft drinks and pure fruit juice contain large amounts of sugar, which can cause tooth decay and obesity (see pp92–93). Children who consume large quantities of sweet drinks eat less at mealtimes, so they may not get all the essential nutrients they need. If you give children water from the start, they won't crave the sweet drinks.

Tea and coffee also count towards your fluid intake but it's best to cut down on caffeine, as it is a stimulant, acts as a diuretic, and suppresses the absorption of calcium. Choose caffeine-free instead.

An easy way to increase your intake

Keep a small bottle of water with you to sip at all times. With mineral water, read the label to ensure it has less than 20mg sodium per litre, to keep salt levels in check, especially for children. Sparkling is refreshing but still water suits a sensitive stomach.

Ways to jazz up water

Cinnamon can have a natural anti-inflammatory effect on the body and help to reduce pain. Snap a couple of sticks and infuse in boiling water. Sweeten with a little honey, if you like.

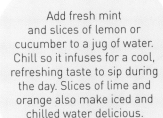

Add fresh mint and slices of lemon or cucumber to a jug of water. Chill so it infuses for a cool, refreshing taste to sip during the day. Slices of lime and orange also make iced and chilled water delicious.

Make a fresh mint tisane, ideally with peppermint. Crush some leaves in a cup, pour on boiling water, and leave to infuse for 5 minutes. You can also freeze whole stems of fresh mint, and place straight into boiling water.

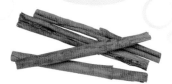

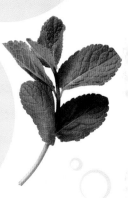

Freeze fresh berries in water in ice cubes. Float in sparkling water and add a straw, for a pretty, fruity treat. You can do the same with the leaves of fresh mint or other herbs, too.

If you have a surplus of lemons or other citrus fruits, juice them, pour the juice into ice cube trays, and freeze. Adding the cubes to a glass of water gives you a lovely, fresh, lemon-tasting infusion.

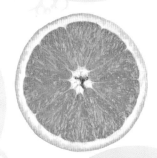

Buy a root of fresh ginger, grate it, and freeze it packed in ice cube trays. Just take one cube out and pop it straight into a cup of boiling water. Ginger is good for the digestion and for alleviating nausea.

REALITY **CHECK**

✓ *How much for adults?*
Generally it's about 8–10 glasses a day. Women should drink about 1.6 litres (2¾ pints) a day, and men more like 2 litres (3½ pints). You need extra if it's hot or humid, or if you are pregnant or breastfeeding. If doing hard exercise, you need roughly 1 litre (1¾ pints) per hour.

✓ *How much for children?*
School-age children should aim to drink about 6–8 small glasses of water or other non-sugary liquids during the day. Under-fives need roughly half to three-quarters of this amount – depending on how active they are.

Herbal and caffeine-free teas such as rooibos don't have a diuretic effect, which means you can drink them more often as part of your daily water intake. See pp98–99 for some more examples of caffeine-free drinks.

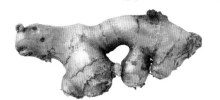

How *much to eat*

There's no such thing as fixed quantities of food that will suit everyone, and even in your own life there will be times when you seem to need more food than usual. Here are some ideas to help you work out how much you need to eat of all the food groups in order to stay at a healthy body weight and maintain energy throughout the day.

You are what you eat

The energy you need is a bit like that of a car. If you drive at an even, average speed, you don't use as much fuel as when you roar down the motorway in the fast lane. Likewise, someone with a sedentary job has lower energy needs than growing teenagers or very active adults – which doesn't just mean those who go to the gym, but also those with physically energetic jobs or parents rushing around after small children.

When you look in the mirror your body shape and size will probably tell you whether you're eating too little or too much (unless your doctor has diagnosed an underlying medical problem). If you're looking very slim and are also constantly tired, it may be that you need to eat a little more. Alternatively, you may well feel better just by tweaking the balance of the different types of foods, such as eating more starchy carbs (see pp14–15) for slow-release energy, or more fruit and vegetables (see pp16–17) for extra vitamins and minerals.

The daily portion chart opposite should be treated as a motivational and informative tool only. Don't worry about hitting the desirable balance every day – for most of us, daily meals can't always follow an exact routine, especially where caring for young children is involved. Instead, try to get the balance roughly right over the course of the week.

What is a portion?

A portion is the average serving of any food. It's the sensible amount to eat, so children will eat smaller portions, and very active people larger ones. If you really love a particular food, whether it be chocolate cake or a thick chunk of cheese, it's all too easy to tuck into far more than you need. So don't keep eating until you're feeling full to bursting. Aim to get up from the table thinking you could have eaten a bit more – that last potato or piece of apple pie. Your body doesn't need it, and instead of it making you feel good, you'll just have a horribly full and sluggish sensation.

Your at-a-glance guide

The chart opposite gives you an easy guide to government recommendations for a healthy diet. It isn't necessary to start weighing out your food – nor would that be a good way to lead your life – but if you can get used to recognizing what the sensible amount is, you can manage your meals much more effectively. This

Food group	Daily portions	What is one portion?
Starchy carbohydrates	5–14 (depending on your lifestyle)	Slice of wholemeal bread • 1 medium potato • 3 tbsp wholegrain breakfast cereal • 2 tbsp cooked rice • 3 tbsp cooked pasta (75g/2½oz raw)
Vegetables	2–3 (as part of the minimum 5 a day)	80g (2¾oz) or 3 heaped tbsp raw, cooked, frozen, or canned veg (preferably in water with no added salt or sugar) • 1 dessert bowl of mixed salad
Fruit	2–3 (as part of the minimum 5 a day	2 small plums • 1 medium apple • slice of large melon • ½ avocado or banana • handful of grapes or berries • 1 heaped tbsp dried fruit • 1 glass pure juice
Dairy	2–3	200ml (7fl oz) milk: whole, semi-skimmed, 1%, or skimmed milk • 150g (5½oz) yogurt • 125g (4½oz) cottage cheese • 40g (1½oz) hard cheese
Protein	2–3	85–100g (3–3½oz) poultry or lean meat • 140g (5oz) fish • 2–3 tbsp pulses • 2 medium eggs • 2 tbsp peanut or other nut butter • 3 tbsp nuts or seeds
Fats	Eat sparingly (as part of your overall diet)	A thin scraping of butter-type spreads on bread • 1–2 tsp olive, seed, or nut oil drizzled on a salad • a light brushing of oil on food for grilling or frying

is particularly useful when you're eating out, as restaurants and fast food outlets increasingly offer extra-large portions. They may look like good value for money, but clearing your plate without realizing just how much is on it could be to the detriment of your long-term health.

Managing your plate

If you know you eat too much, put your food on a smaller plate so that you can't get so much on it. Also, make sure you dish up with a proper tablespoon, not the largest spoon you have. You should also cut down on the fatty and sugary foods. As a general rule, eat more vegetables, ideally raw or steamed, without high-calorie sauces or dressings. While an extra portion of fruit is also helpful, overdoing it can pose a problem with too much sugar.

Calories per day

Besides giving you all the nutrients you need, food is used by your body as fuel for energy. This is measured in calories (kcals); each food has a calorific value per gram. By adding them all up in a day, you can work out how many calories you've eaten. If you consume more than you use in energy, they are stored in the body as fat. If you consume fewer than you use, your body burns its fat for fuel and you lose weight. The calories children need varies, too, depending on whether they're very active, going through a growth spurt, or getting over an illness or injury (in which case you should roughly double their intake to help them recover their strength). See the British Nutrition Foundation's guide to the estimated average requirements (EARs) of different age-groups for a healthy weight: http://www.nutrition.org.uk. If you have any concerns about calories and weight, ask your GP what is appropriate for you and your children. Babies should be weighed by health professionals once a month up to the age of six months, then once every two months up to one year old.

Count to 5

As well as the mantra of eating five portions of fruit and vegetables a day, think about the five food groups at each meal and remember that everyone should eat five times a day: three main meals, and a mid-morning and mid-afternoon snack.

Every member of your family – from a just-weaned baby or young schoolchild to a rapidly developing teenager and their parents – needs to eat regular, healthy meals. This will give them the mental and physical energy to maintain concentration, grow, recover quickly from illness, and generally enjoy life to the full.

Eating foods from the five main groups (see pp12–13) five times a day will bring all these benefits. Here are some delicious suggestions for the three main meals, plus some healthy snacks in between, to keep your energy levels topped up. The food groups aren't entirely separate, as most foods contain lots of different nutrients. Keep fats to a minimum, as many foods (such as dairy) already include what you need. If you prefer to have your main meal in the middle of the day, just swap the lunchtime and evening ideas around. Remember to drink lots of fluid with, and between, meals, too (see p13).

For breakfast

1. A portion of dairy for calcium, such as a glass of milk, or milk on cereal, or a bowl of plain yogurt or fromage frais with a little honey.

2. Two portions of different-coloured fresh fruit (one could be a glass of fruit juice) and/or dried fruit, in a smoothie or compôte, on cereal, or with yogurt.

3. A wholegrain ingredient, for fibre and starchy carbs, such as wholemeal toast, porridge or other wholegrain cereal, or a handful of nuts and seeds on your yogurt.

4. For a protein-rich start to your day (you don't need it if eating dairy), an omelette or a boiled or scrambled egg.

5. A little fat, which could come from your portion of dairy or, if you're having toast, just a scraping of butter.

At lunchtime

1. A protein-rich food, such as roast chicken (without skin), or canned tuna or sardines, or thinly sliced lean ham or roast beef, or hummus, baked beans, or cottage cheese.

2. A wholegrain fibre and starchy carb hit, such as some wholegrain bread or crackers, brown rice cakes, or a wholemeal bagel or pitta bread.

3. Two different-coloured vegetables and/or fruit – such as cherry tomatoes and carrot sticks, or a bowl of vegetable soup plus a pear, or a bowl of mixed salad and two satsumas, or coleslaw in a sandwich and a small bowl of fruit salad.

4. A small portion of dairy, if you haven't had cheese, such as a plain yogurt.

5. A little fat (from dairy, fish, or meat), or a scraping of butter or drizzle of olive oil.

In the evening

1. A protein-rich element, which need not be meat, chicken, or fish – it could be a lentil curry, chickpea stew, falafel, beanburgers, or marinated tofu.

2. One (or more) vegeables – raw, or steamed, stir-fried, roasted, or casseroled.

3. Starchy carbs – for instance, some brown rice, pasta, or couscous, or a jacket potato.

4. Some dairy, such as yogurt raita with your curry, or grated cheese on pasta or a jacket potato, or a fromage frais for dessert.

5. A small amount of fat from chicken, fish, or dairy, or just a splash of oil for cooking.

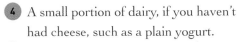

Healthy snack suggestions

✳ **Homemade crisps.** Slice root veg, apples, or pears wafer thin, dry in a very low oven, and store in an airtight container.

✳ **Breadsticks,** with or without a little hummus (see p185) or nut butter (see p224) to dip.

✳ Homemade, unflavoured **popcorn**. Children love to help make it. Store in a sealed container.

✳ Little hard-boiled **eggs**, such as quail's or bantam. Shell, store in the fridge, nibble with black pepper.

✳ A handful of **toasted pumpkin seeds** and dried cranberries or blueberries.

Variety is the spice of life and makes for delicious, healthy eating.

2

What you and *your family need*

Nutrients *now*

While we need the full spectrum of nutrients throughout our lives, the amounts change according to age. A good, balanced diet helps to optimize everyone's health, but we need to know which nutrients require special attention at each period of life. Get started with this overview, then see the stage-specific detail throughout this chapter.

Babies

THE FIRST 12 MONTHS

Your baby needs only breast milk (or formula) up until 6 months. However, every baby is different and yours may be ready to start trying some solids earlier. See pp48–55 for advice on breast and formula feeding and baby's first foods.

KEY NUTRIENT NEEDS

Breast or formula milk provides all the nutrients your baby needs up until 6 months: fat, protein, lactose (milk sugar), vitamins, and minerals. Cow's milk isn't suitable as a drink for your baby until he or she is a year old.

Vitamins A, C, and D are vital for your baby's growth. From 6 months to 5 years, give vitamin drops to be on the safe side. Your health visitor will advise.

Milk is still first from 6 months. Breast or formula milk should be the main source of nourishment up to a year old, to ensure your baby gets enough vital nutrients. As you build up a range of solids in the five food groups (see pp12–13), your baby still needs 3–5 milk feeds a day (500–600ml/16–20fl oz).

Toddlers

FROM 1 TO 3 YEARS

As a parent, you'll know that children this age are bursting with energy. They need plenty of fuel from starchy carbs and fats. They also need proteins, dairy produce, fruit, and vegetables to build a healthy body with strong bones, teeth, and muscles. See pp56–59.

KEY NUTRIENT NEEDS

Vitamins A, C, and D are vital for growth and healthy teeth, bones, muscles, and immune system. Vitamins C and D help in the absorption of iron, and the latter of calcium, too. They're in meat, liver, oily fish, eggs, fruit, and vegetables.

Calcium is essential for strong bones and teeth. The best source is dairy produce, but you'll also find it in green leafy veg, soya, nuts, and seeds.

Iron and zinc are vital minerals. Iron is needed to carry oxygen round the body in the blood, and for various bodily processes. Zinc is vital for hormones, growth, repair, and the immune system. These minerals are in lean meat, fish, pulses, dairy, leafy greens, nuts (not whole for under-5s), and wholegrains.

Schoolchildren

FROM 4 TO 11 YEARS

At this stage, children need three good meals a day and a couple of snacks in between to give them the energy to get through a strenuous school day and to continue to grow and develop. Some nutrients boost their concentration, too. See pp60–63.

KEY NUTRIENT NEEDS

B vitamins play a huge role in releasing energy from the food we eat, boosting concentration, and building healthy cells and strong nervous and immune systems. These vitamins are found in meat, poultry, fish, pulses, nuts, wholegrains, and green veg.

Calcium is just as important now as earlier on in life – your child is still growing and developing all the time. See Toddlers (left) for food sources.

Zinc and vitamins A, C, and E boost a child's immune system in the early school years and help heal after bruises and scrapes. These nutrients are found in lean meat, poultry, fish, eggs, red, yellow, and green fruit and veg, pulses, nuts, seeds, and wholegrains.

Teenagers

FROM 12 TO 18 YEARS

Adolescence is a time of massive change, with hormones running amok and growth spurts. Issues of body image (see pp106–109), mood swings, relationships, and exam stress may all come into play. A healthy, balanced diet helps get them through. See pp64–67.

KEY NUTRIENT NEEDS

Iron is crucial for healthy blood. A lack of it can cause fatigue and anaemia. Girls lose iron during their periods but boys, too, need iron in their diet. Beef, liver, wholegrains, leafy greens, nuts, eggs, and pulses are all rich in iron.

Calcium is needed for rapidly growing bones; a deficiency now could lead to osteoporosis later. Vitamin D (see pp29, 30 for sources) helps process it.

Protein is needed more than ever now for muscle growth and maintenance. Key sources are meat, fish, eggs, and dairy, but it's also in pulses, nuts, seeds, and soya products. If your teenager is vegetarian, offer a whole mixture of vegetable proteins for essential amino acids (pp118–121).

Adults

FROM 19 TO 70 YEARS

Adulthood can bring pregnancy, children, careers, menopause, and the risk of age-related diseases. We need to focus on a healthy, balanced diet and staying active to try to reduce that risk. Both men and women need to boost certain nutrients in their 50s. See pp68–77.

KEY NUTRIENT NEEDS

Omega 3 fatty acids, particularly in oily fish, such as salmon and sardines, and also in seeds, soya, walnuts, and their oils, may help to alleviate symptoms of the menopause (see p25) and lower the risk of heart disease.

Phytonutrients in purple, orange, and red fruit and vegetables may protect the skin (see pp162–165). Those in garlic and leafy greens may boost sex drive.

Magnesium and calcium strengthen bones and so help prevent osteoporosis, which affects 1 in 3 women and 1 in 5 men. The best sources of calcium are dairy foods and also leafy greens, soya products, nuts, and seeds. Brazil nuts, cashews, and dried fruits are the top magnesium-rich foods.

Later years

OVER SEVENTIES

Our diet still needs to contain proteins, carbohydrates, vegetables, fruit, some dairy, and some fat, but we particularly need plenty of fibre and fluids for a well-functioning digestive system. Some vitamins and minerals are more important than ever. See pp78–79.

KEY NUTRIENT NEEDS

Vitamins B_5 and B_{12} and folic acid are all important to increase energy and alertness, and avoid anaemia. Try to have a mixed diet including red meat, dairy, eggs, seafood, leafy greens, bananas, nuts, and fortified cereals.

Vitamins C and D are both important. Vitamin C heals and repairs, so try to eat plenty of fruit and vegetables. A vitamin D supplement will help absorb calcium.

Iron, zinc, and calcium are key minerals. Lack of iron can lead to lethargy and anaemia, so try to eat red meat, green vegetables, and dried fruit. Zinc helps regulate appetite. Meat, shellfish, wholemeal bread, and pulses are good sources. Bones need plenty of calcium: a supplement may be advised.

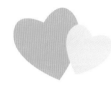

Breastfeeding *your new baby*

By the time they give birth, many mums will have reached a decision about whether they want to – or feel they will be able to – breastfeed their baby. There are, of course, instances when breastfeeding isn't possible or appropriate, but if you can breastfeed, even for a few days, there are lots of health benefits for you and your baby.

What's in your milk?

Breast milk provides everything your baby needs to thrive for the first six months. You produce three types of this perfect food. **Colostrum** is the initial milk, made during late pregnancy and for the first few days of the baby's life. It's high in protein, antibodies, some vitamins and minerals, and hormones. These nutrients encourage "good" bacteria in the gut (see also p37) and help the baby pass his or her first stools. The colostrum is then followed by **transitional milk** – higher in fat and lactose (milk sugar) but lower in protein and minerals. From day 15, the milk becomes **mature milk**, the composition of which changes as each feed progresses. Babies take most of their milk in the first 5–10 minutes but only 50 per cent of the calories per feed. The milk produced later in the feed – the hind milk – is the richest, so let your baby feed until satisfied.

Baby benefits

Breast milk is a living fluid containing active cells that mop up bacteria and viruses, as well as antibodies tailored to fight the infections your baby comes into contact with. These valuable components are missing from substitutes such as formula. Breastfeeding thus provides babies with some **protection** while their own immune system is developing. So even if you don't want to breastfeed for long, this is one reason why it's such a good idea to give it a go for at least a week or two if you can. There is clear evidence that babies who are breast-fed may be less susceptible to immune system disorders, diabetes, allergies, and sudden infant death syndrome (SIDS). They also have fewer ear infections and fewer bouts of gastroenteritis, and are less likely to develop colitis (inflammation of the colon) and diseases such as bacterial meningitis.

Good for mum too

There are many reasons why breastfeeding your baby is a bonus for you as well as for him, if you are able to do it. Whether you manage it for months, for just a few days or even for one day, it can be a great opportunity for you to **connect and bond** with your baby. Breastfeeding also helps your womb to contract towards its normal size, and since milk draws on the fat deposits you've laid down during pregnancy, your body is far more likely to return to its pre-pregnancy shape and size. Breastfeeding is also **less work** than bottlefeeding. Instead of having to sterilize and prepare bottles, your breast milk is always available fresh, usually in the right amounts (apart from when you're having problems producing enough) and at the right temperature, ready to be used whenever your baby is hungry, wherever you are.

Getting started

You should start suckling your baby within the first two hours of giving birth to give him the colostrum (see "What's in your milk?" far left). His sucking will also encourage milk production (see below). Find the hold that works best for you. Sit or lie down comfortably, with your back supported. Cradle him in your arm, supported by a cushion if that helps. Try to relax as much as possible as this will help the milk flow and keep your baby calm, too.

Milk production

Prolactin, the milk-making hormone, becomes active as soon as the placenta is delivered. Two to five days after the birth, your transitional milk will come in, replacing the colostrum. If you don't breastfeed, production slows down and then stops altogether. Your body will only keep on making milk if it's removed from your breasts, since that's the signal that your baby needs more.

Looking after yourself

Your midwife or breastfeeding counsellor will give you advice on how to latch your baby on to the breast in order to reduce the chance of your nipples becoming very sore or damaged, which can lead to infection. Your nipples might be a little sore at first while both you and your baby adjust to the process of breastfeeding, but if he latches on properly you shouldn't find it painful. Make sure you eat well (see pp50–51) and get as much rest as possible so that you make plenty of milk.

Feeding on demand

At first, you'll find your baby asks for feeds a lot and may not sleep for long. He may have as many as 10–15 breastfeeds over 24 hours and it's unlikely that you'll establish any sort of routine before he's at least six weeks old. However, as time goes on, feeds are likely to become more predictable, though there may be occasional days when he enjoys a "feed in" where all he wants to do is breastfeed.

How much?

Start on one side, then when he's had enough (usually 10–20 minutes), stop and gently burp him. Now offer the other side. He may or may not take it all, but this isn't anything to worry about. Always offer the second side first at the next feed as it encourages even milk production.

REALITY CHECK

 Is it going well?
If your baby is happy and contented after a good feed, and doesn't fight when latching on or when being taken off the breast, all is well.

 Is he getting enough milk?
You can't see how much milk he is having, but if he is gaining weight, it's fine. Don't give him bottles, too.

✓ **Is he gaining enough weight?**
Getting some rest usually helps to boost your milk production. But if you are worried your baby isn't thriving, talk to your health visitor.

Can I store breast milk?

For bottlefeeding, expressed breast milk can be kept in sterilized containers in the fridge for up to five days, or in sterile freezer bags in the freezer for up to six months, then fully defrosted (but not in a microwave) before use.

Switching to a bottle

Some mums wean straight to a feeder cup but if you change to bottles, do it gradually over two weeks, one feed at a time. Your milk supply needs time to decrease, and your baby has to get used to the feel of a teat and the taste of formula. If you have a partner, suggest that he gives the bottle, so that your baby doesn't smell your milk and want only his familiar feed instead. See also pp52–55.

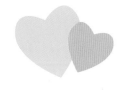

Eating for you
and your new baby

Your body will take everything it needs to make the perfect milk for
your new baby, but by eating well, you yourself will fare so much better.
You are more likely to feel less drained emotionally and physically, and
more able to cope with the demands of a small baby.

What should I be eating?

After you've given birth, the
backdrop of your diet should be
as for any other woman –
nutritious and varied – but you
also need to make sure you take
in enough of all the major food
groups to nourish both you and
your baby. Even if it's hard to find
time to eat, never skip meals and
eat regular, healthy snacks in
between. Even grabbing a cereal
bar and a banana on the run is
better than not having anything.

How much extra?

1st month	+450 kcals a day
2nd month	+530 kcals per day
3rd month	+570 kcals per day

Note: If that's too much, just try
300–400 extra calories per day

Do I need more food?

You don't need to eat much more,
but when you're breastfeeding,
your body prioritizes your baby's
milk in its use of nutrients. Unless
you eat enough, you'll be the one
lacking in nourishment. You need
some extra calories (see below left)
but how many depends on how
much weight you put on during
pregnancy and your metabolism.

Can I diet?

You shouldn't diet while you're
breastfeeding, as this can leave
you and your baby depleted
and exhausted. Your body will
naturally return to its normal
weight, within a few months to
a year. If progress is slow, keep
a food diary and see whether
you can make some healthier
tweaks to your diet.

How much water?

You need plenty of water and
other fluids. As when you were
pregnant, you should drink 2 litres
(3½ pints) a day – that's at least 8
glasses. Keep a cold drink beside
you, such as still or sparkling
water, or milk, to sip while you are
breastfeeding. It's not a good idea
to have a hot drink with your
baby so close. See pp38–39 for
other fluid ideas, and go easy on
sugary drinks – even no-added-
sugar fruit juices are high in sugar.

If you are thirsty or your urine
is dark, you are not taking in
enough fluid, so drink something
right away. Lack of fluids can
make you feel more tired, ratty,
and headachey than you would
otherwise be. It can also play
havoc with your digestion and
lead to constipation.

Eating sensibly and well is vital to both your health and that of your baby. Try to make time to relax and enjoy a meal, but even eating on the go is better than not eating at all.

Are tea and coffee ok?

A cuppa can get your sanity back, but if you are breastfeeding, too much caffeine may keep your baby awake. Sensitive mums may also feel more stressed and jittery, and may be kept awake at the wrong moments. Best advice is to limit caffeine drinks to occasional treats rather than every day. Go for caffeine-free or decaf tea and coffee most of the time (see p99).

What about alcohol?

If you drink alcohol, even in small amounts, some will pass to your baby if you are breastfeeding. Ideally don't drink it at all. 1 or 2 units, once or twice a week, are unlikely to harm him, but might affect how easily he feeds. If you want to drink more on a special occasion, express your milk first.

Any foods to avoid?

If your baby has colic, bloating, or wind, it may be a reaction to something you've eaten. Other symptoms could be diarrhoea, vomiting, bronchitis, runny nose, skin rashes, or wheezing. Foods that may cause problems are cow's milk or other dairy, eggs, wheat, citrus, caffeine, chocolate, garlic, brassicas, or cucumber. Only drop them from your diet if they cause problems, not "just in case".

Which fish?

Fish is rich in protein and omega 3 fats but you need to watch the type and quantity you eat. Oily fish – such as salmon, fresh tuna, sardines, pilchards, herring, trout, and mackerel – contain pollutants, some of which will pass from the fish you eat into your breast milk. Do eat them, as the benefits outweigh the risks, but stick to two 140g (5oz) portions a week. You can eat as much canned tuna and white fish as you like (except rock salmon, sea bass, bream, turbot, halibut, and brown crab meat, which have the same pollutant problems as oily fish).

Are peanuts OK?

There's no evidence that eating peanuts while breastfeeding may cause your baby to develop an allergy. Eat them as part of your normal, balanced diet. However, if there is a history of peanut allergy in your immediate family or that of the baby's father, check with your GP or health visitor first. (See also p134.)

Do I need supplements?

You should be able to glean nearly all the vitamins and minerals you and your baby need from your diet. Vitamin D is the exception. It's difficult for your body to make enough at this time. Take a 10mcg supplement each day. If you're not getting enough nourishment, you may also need to consider a tailored breastfeeding vitamin and mineral supplement – but check with your GP or health visitor before taking any supplements.

Keep a cold drink, such as still or sparkling water, milk, or pure unsweetened fruit juice beside you to sip regularly when you are breastfeeding.

Formula *feeding*

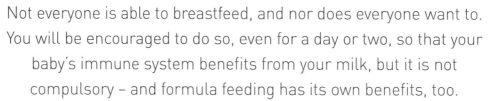

Not everyone is able to breastfeed, and nor does everyone want to.
You will be encouraged to do so, even for a day or two, so that your
baby's immune system benefits from your milk, but it is not
compulsory – and formula feeding has its own benefits, too.

What is formula milk?

Formula milks are usually dried, and you reconstitute them with cooled boiled water – although "ready-to-feed" formula is also available in cartons and sachets, which can be useful when you are out and about. These milks are normally derived from **cow's milk** and are created to be as close to breast milk as possible.

Some things in breast milk cannot be replicated, such as the antibodies your baby gets from you, and the enzyme lipase, which breaks down fat globules in the milk to make it more digestible (so formula milk is harder for your baby to digest than breast milk). Otherwise formula milks contain **everything your baby needs** for optimum nutrition: carbohydrates, proteins, unsaturated fats, and all the essential vitamins and minerals. Some also have added omega fatty acids (see pp24–25) to boost your baby's brain and nervous system development. Others have pro- and prebiotics to encourage a healthy gut (see pp36–37). The different types of formula milk are listed opposite.

Moving to formula

At what point you make the transition from breast milk to formula is a personal and often difficult decision, but talking with your breastfeeding care team or your health visitor will help.

Once you switch, you can rest assured that your baby is still getting all the key nutrients she needs to grow and develop. As formula milk has a controlled amount of vitamins and minerals, you should not need to give her a multivitamin supplement, but see opposite for more about vitamin D. Make up the formula exactly to the instructions, and then your baby should gain weight steadily.

There isn't one standard formula to fit all. If your baby has special dietary needs, there will be one to suit her (see opposite). If she doesn't thrive on the first one you try, seek advice from your health visitor.

The benefits of formula

Holding the baby close, skin to skin, at feeding time is a bonding experience for baby and parent, and with a bottle-fed baby this becomes something that dad can share. You will also be able to leave the baby with someone else without having to express your milk first, and Dad can take turns at doing the night-time feeds, too, allowing you to rest. You won't have to cope with leaking and possibly sore nipples, and what you eat and drink won't directly affect the baby. While you will have to spend time sterilizing bottles and measuring amounts, formula takes longer to digest than breast milk, so feeds may be less frequent. You'll be able to see exactly how much milk your baby is taking at any feed – her weight gain is the biggest reassurance of all, and that is true of both breastfed and bottle-fed babies.

How much?

- Average daily milk intake is 150–200ml (5–7fl oz) per 1 kg (2¼lb) body weight.

- Newborn and early on, your baby will only take 30–60ml (1–2fl oz) at each little feed.

- As she grows, she will work up to 120–180ml (4–6fl oz) a feed.

- From around 6 months until she is fully weaned, she may take 180–240ml (6–8fl oz) at a feed.

Choosing your formula

Always choose a recognized infant formula. The main types for babies under six months old are:

Whey-rich formula, based on cow's milk and the closest to breast milk in nutritional content, is the most common, and recommended for most babies from birth.

Casein-rich formula, suitable for babies from birth, though it is usually marketed as being for hungrier babies as the casein is less easily digested, and so will keep your baby feeling fuller for longer. Use only on medical advice.

Soya-based formula, for babies who can't tolerate cow's milk formula, usually because of lactose intolerance (see pp126–127). Give it only on medical advice.

Special formulas are for babies with various problems. They include higher-calorie formulas for premature babies, predigested ones for babies who can't digest breast milk or usual formulas, and hypoallergenic ones for babies allergic to cow's or soya milk.

Follow-ons Instead of weaning onto cow's milk at a year old (see pp54–55), you can buy protein- and iron-rich formulas. There is no need to if your baby eats well.

Weaning

When you introduce solid foods (see pp54–55), your baby's daily intake of formula milk will gradually decrease to about 720ml (24fl oz). Once she is established on solids, she should be having about 600ml (20fl oz) of formula milk per day alongside a varied diet until she is a year old. She can then change to whole cow's milk, or follow-on milk, if you prefer it.

Extra water

Offer your baby a little boiled, cooled water in between feeds, as this can prevent her becoming dehydrated and will get her used to the taste of plain water.

Vitamin D

Since infant formulas include all the necessary nutrients your baby needs during the first six months, you don't need to give her anything extra. When she is on solids, and drinking less than 600ml (20fl oz) formula or changing to cow's milk, she should have vitamin D drops. Check with your health visitor or GP first.

Other milks

Neither goat's milk formula nor goat's follow-on formula are nutritionally complete enough to be a substitute for infant formula. The same goes for coconut, oat, rice, and nut milks, which should not be given before 6 months old.

REALITY **CHECK**

 Follow instructions
Make up the formula precisely to instructions. Too little milk powder gives your baby too few calories; too much will upset her tummy.

 Water
Use freshly boiled, cooled tap water, not filtered or pre-softened. Bottled water has too many minerals unless the label states it's suitable for babies.

 Test the temperature
Stand the bottle in hot (not boiling) water to warm. Shake a little milk on the back of your hand to check it's at body temperature.

 Use fresh
Make up feeds just before they are needed, not in advance. If you are going out, take boiled water and formula in separate containers.

 Don't freeze
Never freeze made-up formula milk. Throw away any left over after a feed.

Weaning your *baby*

The first steps towards getting your baby to eat real food can feel daunting. There will be good days when he'll be excited about trying new tastes and others when he'll show no interest at all. This is nothing to worry about – he'll soon get the hang of this new idea.

When to begin weaning will depend on the individual baby. Guidelines say by 6 months, and never before 17 weeks, as he may struggle to digest the nutrients. Your baby may want to progress to solid foods more quickly than suggested below, so follow his signals and your instincts. If you start earlier than 6 months, don't give foods containing wheat, gluten, nuts, peanuts or peanut products, seeds, liver, eggs, fish, shellfish, cow's milk, and soft or unpasteurized cheese, as they could cause food allergies (see pp124–135). Stick to baby rice cereal, and/or first tastes of fruit and veg, until he is 6 months old. After that, so long as you avoid a few foods (see far right), and never add salt (to avoid damaging his kidneys) or sugar (to avoid tooth decay), you can wean him in the way that works best for you both. Breast milk or formula are still his main source of nourishment until he is eating enough to drop feeds. Your GP or health visitor will do regular weight and health checks.

Food hygiene

There's no need to be obsessive about cleaning, as exposure to everyday germs is a vital part of the development of your child's immune system. But when it comes to food preparation and spoilage, be sure to keep utensils, cutlery, and crockery scrupulously clean and store food properly to keep it safe and fresh.

The very first foods

By around 6 months, you need to introduce your baby to solid food. Baby rice is a good, bland starter, mixed with either breast milk or formula so it's very runny. You can give the rice on its own, or mix it with a little vegetable or fruit purée, thinned with cooled, boiled water. Begin with just one "solid" a day, offering 1–2 teaspoonfuls at the start of your baby's usual feed, or halfway through. If you leave it until the end, he'll be full and not interested. As your baby gets used to the feeling of a little texture in his mouth, you can make the purées thicker. It's fine to start him on something fruity, such as banana or stewed apple, but try a savoury hit such as potato first, so he doesn't get used to just sweet foods. Offer new tastes one at a time, once every three days, so that you can spot if something disagrees with him.

From 7 to 9 months

When your baby is roughly 7 months old, he can move on to more complicated textures and tastes. By the time he is 9 months old he should be strong enough to sit in his own chair, he may have a few teeth, and he'll be happy to chomp through some finger foods, such as pieces of raw, soft fruit or cooked pasta shapes. It's a good idea to start reducing the amount of milk feed he has, so that he's hungry when you offer him solid food, but you should still expect to give him 500–600ml (16–20fl oz), or 3–4 feeds, of breast milk or formula each day until he's a year old. The nutrients in the milk provide a cushion while you're getting him to eat normal food. You can add milk to his food, but if you give it to him by breast or bottle you can also make it a time to cuddle.

It's important to offer sips of water in a feeder cup as he now has less fluid in the form of milk. If you choose to give fruit juice, do not give more than 175ml (6fl oz) a day that has been diluted 1 part juice to 10 parts of water. Do not make it stronger, as the sugar it contains can damage his emerging teeth.

Once your baby is happy eating solids, start to include protein foods such as eggs (well cooked), cheese (not blue), minced chicken, fish, and meat, or lentils and other pulses, slowly introducing lumpier textures. Offer a range of foods from all five food groups. They contain different amounts of nutrients, so the more variety the better.

From 9 to 12 months

Meals should be pretty much chopped or mashed up adult food now, but don't cook with added salt or sugar. Your baby will probably be eating three meals a day and a couple of snacks, such as fruit or rice cakes. You still need to include 500–600ml (16–20fl oz), or 3–4 feeds, of breast milk or formula each day. He will love finger foods, to hold himself, but give him a spoon so he starts learning to feed himself. Never leave him unattended, as he could choke. It will be a messy time, but fun to watch as his taste buds develop and he shows his enthusiasm for new food.

{ Share a voyage of discovery as your baby **learns all about food**. }

Foods to avoid

* **Certain milks**
Do not give your baby under one any cow's, sheep's, goat's or soya milk to drink – only your breast milk or formula.

* **Popcorn and crisps**
These are choking hazards and tend to be high in salt.

* **Nuts**
While eating nuts when you're breastfeeding won't cause a problem, don't feed products containing nuts to a baby under the age of six months, in case it leads to an allergic reaction. Pieces of nuts and whole nuts should be avoided until your child is five years old because of the risk of choking.

* **Whole grapes**
Whole grapes and cherry tomatoes, too, can slip down the throat and cause choking. So cut them in half, and keep an eye on your baby while he is eating. Do this for toddlers, too.

* **Honey**
Avoid all honey until your baby is a year old because of the slight risk of infant botulism. It's better to sweeten sharp fruits with apple juice, mashed banana, breast milk, or formula.

* **Hard fruit and veg**
Small pieces of raw, hard fruit and veg can cause choking. Give them soft, lightly cooked, or canned in natural juice.

* **Raw and runny eggs**
Well-cooked eggs are fine from 6 months, but don't give soft-cooked eggs, or dishes made with raw eggs (such as mayonnaise, ice cream, or mousses) until a year old as there's a risk of food poisoning.

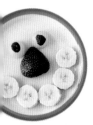

What do *toddlers need?*

Increasingly active, your child is busy exploring and learning about her world. Food plays an important part in her life as she discovers new tastes and textures, and learns to feed herself. With simple routines in place, eating should be fun, not a battle.

First birthday onwards

Your toddler is now sharing in your healthy (and salt-free) family meals, and coping with a wide range of textures. Most children love feeding themselves, but don't give her whole grapes or small citrus segments just yet. Cut everything up small at first or slice into short, thin sticks so there is no risk of her choking, and never leave her alone while she is eating.

Switching milks

You can now switch from breast milk and formula to cow's milk for drinking – whole, not semi-skimmed, as your child needs the extra fat for energy and growth. When she's two, you can go over to semi-skimmed, but don't offer skimmed milk until she's five (and then only if you wish). You can also start to use goat's, sheep's, rice or soya milk (see pp26–27), but their fat content and other nutrients are different from whole cow's milk, so you need to ensure that you give your toddler a good varied diet (see pp12–13).

Good eating habits

Try to get into a routine of three meals a day and a couple of nutritious, tasty snacks, all at regular times. There's a huge difference between a toddler who is in the habit of sitting down and having, say, a rice cake and a banana or a little bowl of halved grapes as a snack, and one who toddles around with a packet of something permanently in her hand. Your child needs to know that food comes at certain times of the day, that she sits and eats it, and then it's over. Try not to fall into the trap of giving her a random snack to pacify her. She probably isn't hungry – it's more likely she is thirsty, so offer water first. If that doesn't work, give her a cuddle, then something different to play with to distract her.

If you have your main meal in the evenings, cook for the whole family at once if you can and eat together so that your toddler sees the enjoyment of food as part of her family life. If this isn't possible, always make sure you sit down with her when she eats – even if you're only having a cup of tea. Don't leave her eating in front of the TV on her own.

Hands on – it's fun

A toddler who is always fed from a jar will almost inevitably think that's where all food comes from. But if she sees you, for instance, peeling a banana and mashing it before you give it to her on a spoon, she'll understand that food is much more interesting than that. Involve her as much as you can in its preparation. If you encourage her to select and put

How much?

- **At least 4 servings a day of starchy carbohydrates** A serving is ¼–½ slice bread or 2–3 tbsp cooked rice or pasta.

- **2 servings a day of protein** A serving is about 30g (1oz) cooked meat, chicken, fish, or pulses, or 1 tbsp smooth nut butter.

- **2–3 servings a day of vegetables** A serving is 2 tbsp peas, carrots, or beans, 3 cherry tomatoes, or 2 cauliflower or broccoli florets.

- **2–3 servings of fruit** A serving is ½ apple, pear or banana, a satsuma (cut in pieces, not whole segments), or a handful of grapes.

- **2 servings a day of dairy foods or at least 350ml (12fl oz) whole milk** A serving is a small pot of yogurt or 40g (1½oz) cheese.

pieces of prepared fruit in a little bowl, wash a new potato before it's cooked, or cut a cooked carrot (with a plastic or toddler knife), she'll engage with the food and enjoy it much more. Let her help with baking, too, away from the oven – rolling out pastry, putting topping on pizza dough or cutting out cookie shapes.

New textures

Some children are picky about new textures at first and refuse to eat. If need be, keep puréeing, mashing, or mincing for a while, then try again. Finger foods such as bite-sized sandwiches may help as your child can pop them in her mouth herself.

Some children refuse to eat all but one or two things. This isn't anything to worry about: toddlers will eat when they're hungry and nearly always grow out of food fads. Don't be alarmed if yours is too busy to eat very much some days, finding everything else more exciting – it's normal. However, if she seems unwell or you are worried, seek medical advice.

Balanced nutrition

Apart from whole nuts, nothing's off the menu – you just need to watch out for fruit stones and too much salt or sugar. Every meal, even a snack lunch or supper, should contain foods from all the food groups (see pp12–13 and serving sizes above). Main meals can be the same as yours (but take out her portion before adding salt to the rest). Just chop or mash as necessary.

Starting the day right

Breakfast is important – the last meal was a long time ago and energy levels need restoring. Porridge is ideal. Sweeten with a little honey or, preferably, sliced banana, chopped dried fruits, or compôte. Toast and other bread options are great, too. Spread with a little butter (or butter-type, full-fat spread) and a pure fruit spread, or a smooth nut butter on its own or with banana on top. Or, now that your child is more than a year old, give her a runny boiled egg with soldiers to dip into it. Give salty foods such as sausages or smoked fish only occasionally, and avoid sugary cereals.

End of the day

Allow an hour or two after your child's evening meal so she can digest it before bedtime. Avoid sugary foods, which can make children too active. They love a wind-down bedtime ritual: bath, pyjamas, story, and a cup of warm milk before being tucked in.

REALITY **CHECK**

 Sometimes unhealthy is OK There are times when we all have to resort to not-so-healthy options. If you're generally giving your toddler a balanced diet, she'll be fine.

 Don't offer alternatives If your toddler won't eat what you give, don't rush around getting something else. She'll probably enjoy her next meal.

 Don't get stressed If you look and appear anxious, it will rub off. Try to keep mealtimes calm. Eating together can help, as everyone is interacting.

Tips for tasty *first foods*

Good nutrition is vital for rapidly growing babies and toddlers, but you also need to offer them a range of new foods in a form that appeals to the eye, mind, and tastebuds. Few will reject sugary treats, but getting them to appreciate the right stuff instead takes a bit more thought.

First foods for babies

To make a change from baby rice, use a blender to grind plain porridge oats down to a very fine powder that you can then mix with vegetable or fruit purées.

Puréed apple is a popular first weaning food, but other soft, ripe fruit, such as banana, papaya, or avocado, are also good, and can be mashed with some breast or formula milk.

Make vegetable purées (such as carrots, swede, parsnips, sweet potato, courgette, or butternut squash) for the whole family, remembering not to add any salt. Mash up the vegetables on their own or with olive oil or butter, and freeze them in separate portions for the baby – an ice-cube tray is ideal here.

As your baby gets older, make purées thicker, and leave in some little pieces of vegetable or fruit, so that he can enjoy the textures and start to chew.

Even if your baby doesn't have any teeth yet, it's good for his mouth and tongue muscles to tackle something more than soft baby rice. As well as purées, you can also give him cooked vegetables, such as pieces of carrot, to chew.

Try mashing stronger-tasting vegetables, such as broccoli, green beans, and peas, into some potato, sweet potato, baby rice, or oats.

Frozen vegetables and fruits often contain more vitamins and minerals than fresh (unless you grow your own) and save time, too. Just steam or microwave a few frozen vegetables and blend them to the sort of consistency your baby likes.

From 6 months, give your baby berries such as strawberries and raspberries. They can upset some babies' tummies, so it's best to start with just small amounts and see how your baby copes.

Dried fruits are fine from 6 months, but offer just a little at a time, as they can have a laxative effect. Don't give him dried fruit on its own, as it'll be too sweet – try soft prunes (such as Agen prunes) with a little pear, or pieces of soft dried fig with puréed apple.

Soups can be a very successful way of getting your baby to eat a good variety of foods, all in one bowl. Either blend the soups, or leave them with bits in, so he can enjoy the texture and start to chew.

Dairy products such as fromage frais, yogurt, and a variety of cheeses (but not blue) are great for your baby, but remember you need to stick to the full-fat versions.

Once your baby is 6 months old, you can give well-cooked white rice instead of baby rice. Mash the grains well so they're not too big. A basic risotto (salt-free) can also be frozen in small individual portions, clearly labelled.

First foods for toddlers

Once your child reaches his first birthday, he can eat the same range of nutritious food as you. Start the day with a breakfast that includes carbohydrate, protein, fat, and some fruity vitamin C. As protein and fat take longer to digest than carbohydrates, he'll feel satisfied for longer.

Avoid cereals marketed at children, which often contain too much sugar and salt. Instead, go for porridge, unsweetened muesli, or cornflakes and other cereals, checking the labels for salt and sugar quantities.

Porridge is a wonderful food – you can make it with milk or water, as well as soya, oat, or rice milk. You can also use toasted oat flakes and add yummy ingredients. If you need some sort of sweetness, add a little honey, fruit spread, date syrup, brown sugar, or fructose powder, which has a lower GI value (see p91) than cane – or fresh, puréed, poached, or dried fruits.

Fruit smoothies are fun, especially if you can involve your toddler in choosing which fruits go in the blender. Use fresh fruits and add some frozen berries (available year round and easy). Dilute the smoothie roughly 50:50 with water to protect his tummy and teeth from the fruit's natural sugar and acids, and serve with a straw.

As far as fresh fruit goes, toddlers usually like most varieties because they enjoy their sweet taste. Try giving your child everything from clementines, mangoes, figs, and kiwis to bananas, apples, and pears. Blend pure fruit purées and freeze them to make ice lollies or ice creams.

Even if the lunchtime meal is a light one, make sure it still contains some protein as well as carbohydrate. Chicken, meat, fish, eggs, beans, and lentils are all high-protein foods – baked beans or scrambled eggs on toast are quick and nourishing options.

To provide variety and make them more appealing, serve vegetables in different guises – roast, stuffed, puréed, and so on. Because they'll be a little different in taste and texture, your toddler will be less likely to decide never to eat a particular vegetable at all.

If a new vegetable doesn't go down well, try it 10 or 12 times, with a few days in between. If your child still doesn't like it, blend or purée foods to disguise them in soups or pasta sauces, or mash small amounts into potatoes.

Eating with fingers is fine. Your toddler will most likely make a beeline for brightly coloured peas and sweetcorn or chunks of soft carrot in his food, so make sure they are visible and don't worry if he picks them up in his fingers.

Good snacks to take along when you're out and about include breadsticks, rice cakes, oatcakes, unsulphured dried fruits, and fresh fruits, sliced up and put in a little bag for convenience. Remember to take a small bottle of water, too.

Slices of Parmesan cheeese go well with your snacks of rice cakes and fresh or dried fruit while you're out and about. Parmesan can also be a good thing for your toddler to nibble while you get his food ready. The salty taste is not really salt, but the proteins that have broken down in the milk as it matures.

For snacks at home, try a small bowl of soup; a small portion of hummus with raw vegetable sticks; a couple of slices of cheese with fig, apple, or pear; rice cakes with unsweetened pure fruit spread, nut butter, or a little fish pâté; a small slice of cake made with wholemeal flour; a plain muffin or bagel (white or wholemeal) with a little honey and sliced banana; or a small portion of baked fruit, such as apple, pear, or apricot.

What your toddler eats and drinks before he goes to bed can affect how he sleeps. The wrong foods and drinks may make him restless or give him tummy-ache, but if you feed him relaxing, filling foods his body will wind down. Avoid high-GI foods (see p91) and opt for pasta, rice, couscous, or other starchy food, along with milk to drink.

What do schoolchildren need?

Children often have their own strong opinions on food, and eating routines may fall by the wayside as their social lives develop. Even so, it is still possible to keep a healthy diet on the go – and it's never too late to establish good foundations for good eating habits.

Regular meals

For some parents, mealtimes are not an issue and their children happily chomp through whatever is put in front of them. For others, though, it can be stressful. If you haven't done so already, now is the time to establish proper mealtimes. Your child needs to eat regularly to help keep her energy levels constant so that she functions to her optimum. She is growing and developing all the time and needs not only energy but all the right nutrients to give her the best of everything. She will be eating much more than a toddler now. Needs vary as children grow, but see right for average portions and sizes. The meal pattern should be much the same – three good meals a day and two nutritious snacks in between. Aim to have meals together, so your family can chat about how the day has gone. You will soon pick up whether there is a problem at school or with friends, and hear about the good things that have happened. Try to avoid leaving your child eating alone in front of the TV with a tray on her lap, since sharing mealtimes helps children to develop their social skills, including good table manners.

Breakfast is vital

It is a long time since your child's last meal, so it is absolutely vital that she eats properly before going to school. Research has shown that children who do not eat breakfast are lower achievers, with poorer behaviour and brain function. Avoid breakfast cereals that are high in sugar and salt and give your child wholegrain ones, adding fresh or dried fruit and/or yogurt. Eggs and toast are often popular, especially eggy bread – try topping it with sliced fruit or fruit purée, or go savoury, adding a little ham, cooked tomatoes, or mushrooms. If on some mornings she won't eat at all, make a fruit smoothie with yogurt or milk, and add a tablespoon or two of instant oat cereal for grain.

Food fads

Your child won't like all foods, but don't accept her refusing a certain ingredient or dish at first taste as final. Persevere with it on other occasions. After 8 or 10 refusals, accept that she means it and try offering it in a slightly different guise – you need it to

How much?

• **5–11 servings a day of starchy carbohydrates** A serving is 1 slice bread or 2–3 tbsp cooked rice, couscous, or pasta.

• **2–3 servings a day of protein** A serving is 85–100g (3–3½oz) lean meat or chicken,140g (5oz) fish, or 3 heaped tbsp pulses (cooked).

• **2–3 servings a day of vegetables** A serving is 3 tbsp cooked vegetables, or a dessert bowl of mixed salad.

• **2–3 servings of fruit** A serving is 1 apple, pear or banana, half a grapefruit, 2 satsumas, a handful of berries, or a wedge of melon.

• **2–3 servings a day of dairy foods** A serving is a small pot of yogurt, 40g (1½oz) cheese, or 200ml (7fl oz) skimmed milk.

work for all the family. Variety is important at this age, as the more foods she becomes used to now, when her willpower perhaps hasn't kicked in quite as much as it will do later, the more likely she is to continue eating them, getting plenty of nutrients from a broad range of foods. Often family celebrations or having one of her friends for tea can be a way of showing your child that eating meals can be a real pleasure. Be devious, if necessary. Sneak in the vegetables she thinks she doesn't like, perhaps by blending them into a favourite soup. Bite-sized pasties with a filling of finely chopped veg and mince are enjoyable, or finger food such as chicken legs or fish goujons. Anything that is really easy to eat goes down better – try one-pot meals that need only a spoon or fork, such as pasta or rice dishes, shepherd's pie with lots of vegetables in it, or tasty stews.

Snacking

Healthy snacks are important to keep your child's energy levels up. Discourage fatty, salty crisps, sweets, and other sugary foods and instead offer her any of the tasty snacks mentioned on p43 and p63, or a couple of wholegrain crackers with nut butter or a few thin slices of cheese or lean ham. Alternatively, make her a home-baked treat (see pp240–247).

Unhealthy snacks, eaten too often, can be a problem when your child is with her friends. If you notice that her weight is out of kilter with her height, see pp102–105 on helping your child to lose or gain weight sensibly.

A tired child

If you notice your child lacks vitality and is not very happy, it could be at a time of a growth spurt, when her energy levels are sapped. Keep a diary of what she's eating and drinking, and what her symptoms are. You may notice that she doesn't respond well to a lot of pasta, for instance. This isn't necessarily an allergy, but her body reacting to the intake of too much of the same food, especially if it is rich. Fibre is important but check she isn't having too much, preventing her from absorbing enough nutrients from food (see pp22–23).

All-important water

If your child is listless or not performing well at school, it could be due to lack of fluids. Keep a drink diary to check – she should be having 6–8 small glasses a day. See pp38–39 for more drink ideas, and encourage her to take a bottle of water to school to sip throughout the school day.

Encourage exercise

Energetic activity will keep your child's body and mind fit and healthy. It stimulates endorphins in the brain, which give us the feel-good factor, too. Encourage her to walk a lot and play outdoor games and sports. Exercise will also help to tire her physically, so by the end of the day she should fall into a better sleep pattern (see pp142–143) and wake refreshed the following morning.

Packed *lunches*

Whatever the reason your child takes lunch to school, it is really important that the food provided is tasty, easy to eat, nutritious, and balanced. Not everything has to be home-made, but in most cases it makes things cheaper and healthier.

Parents sometimes make the choice to send their children to school with a packed lunch because they suspect their children aren't choosing healthy options from the menu offered, or because they don't think the school menu is all that healthy, or perhaps because their children have certain special requirements as a result of food allergies or intolerances, or strong dislikes of a wide range of foods. Parents of vegetarians or vegans may also feel happier knowing there is something nutritious and tasty in their child's school bag.

Why nourishment counts

The school day is long, especially if before- and after-school clubs and childcare are tagged on. The demands on children's energy are great, physically and mentally, as their brains too need a plentiful supply of nutrients from their three meals a day plus snacks. If children don't eat enough of the right foods, their mood can dip, lethargy kicks in, the ability to concentrate takes a nose-dive, and they just don't flourish.

It is also true that if children put something into their stomach that doesn't feel comfortable – too salty, fatty, or sugary – the gut can start complaining and tummy aches can appear. If the food is too heavy, all the body wants to do is sleep, so the trick is to put food in your child's packed lunch that is nourishing and sustaining enough to get him through the day until he reaches home but, at the same time, easy to eat and easy to digest.

Check that your child is happy to eat a packed lunch – no matter how delicious you make it, some children prefer to have something similar to, or even exactly the same as, everyone else's lunch.

Quick snacks to pack

* **Banana, apple, or pear** are easy to eat and full of vitamins and gentle fibre

* **Dried fruits** such as raisins, apricots, and apples (ideally without sulphur dioxide preservative)

* **Berries, citrus, or stone fruits**, cut up or segmented

* **Yogurt or fromage frais**, ideally natural

* **Dried muesli bar**, without any added sugar, ideally home-made (see p245)

* **Unsalted raw or roasted nuts** or nuts and raisins – if no allergy and if the school allows (but not for under-fives, as they might choke)

* **Rice cakes** (the plain and seeded varieties), oatcakes, or wholemeal pitta breads

* **Small pot of hummus** and raw vegetables such as carrot sticks for dipping

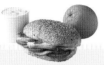

Sandwiches

There are many bread choices, from traditional white and wholemeal to sourdough and all sorts of grains, such as spelt, rye, and multigrain. Try also soft or crusty rolls, flat breads, pitta pockets, and dark rye-type pumpernickels. There are some good gluten-free breads on the market, too, or make your own (see two recipes on pp240–241). Choose fillings that aren't too messy: lean, cooked meat; fish; a hard-boiled egg moistened with a little yogurt or mayonnaise; grated or soft cheese; or hummus or other bean paste. Add salad, too, or good-quality, home-made coleslaw (see p231).

Crackers and dips

Children like the crunchiness of crispbreads, crackers, and breadsticks. There are lots of types to choose from: plain, wholemeal, oat, rye, seeded, or the Scandinavian crisp rolls. Some of them can be salty, so check the labels. Apart from having with chicken, cheese, or ham, children also enjoy dipping them into a small portion of hummus (bought or home-made – see p224), guacamole, ricotta mixed with some yogurt and herbs, or nut butter, if the school allows (see p185). Wrap them in foil to keep them crisp. Pack some veggie sticks or cherry tomatoes, too.

Soups and stews

Hot lunches can work very well if you buy one of the large-rimmed vacuum flasks – look for ones for individual servings, which are more compact. Pasta, soups, stews, and casseroles, with plenty of vegetables in them, can be made the night before, then heated until piping hot in the morning and popped in the flask to fill a hungry stomach at lunchtime. Soups can be one of the easiest hot treats (see pp210, 214) and make a sandwich lunch far more satisfying. You can, of course, buy good-quality fresh and canned soups, too – many are delicious, but check the label for salt and sugar levels.

Salads

Don't think cold just means bread or crackers, as cold lunches can be a sealed plastic bowl of salad based on pasta, rice, couscous, quinoa, chickpea, potato, or even sweet potato. Add tempting things such as egg, lean roast meats, ham or chicken; cooked chickpeas or red kidney beans; baked beans, or canned tuna or salmon; diced or crumbled cheese; cooked mushrooms; prawns or smoked fish; and plenty of chopped raw salad, or cooked vegetables. Moisten the whole with just a little mayo (made lighter by blending with plain yogurt) or with a touch of vinaigrette-style salad dressing.

Batch and freeze

Another good idea is to get ahead at the weekend by batch-cooking extra quantities and then freezing in small, one-portion bags. They need only a defrost and thorough heat-through in the morning (a microwave is a real asset here) before you transfer them to a warmed flask for the school bag. Chapter 6 provides lots of delicious and nourishing recipes specially chosen to appeal to all the family – including chunky home-made soups (pp210, 214), soothing risottos (p218), mild curries and scrumptious casseroles (pp203, 220), or the simplest of pastas in a tasty tomato sauce (p215).

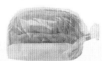

Slice and freeze

Divide up packs of rolls, and wrap separately. Sliced loaves can be frozen in their plastic bag and slices removed as you need them. This ensures you always have fresh bread for your sandwiches and can make lunch more exciting than two slices of bread daily all week until the loaf is used up or stale. You can also freeze sandwiches already filled if you wrap them well – take a frozen pack out in the morning (or, if the weather is really cold, the night before and put in the fridge). By lunchtime it will be thawed. Fillings to freeze are plain meat, cheese, or fish. Pack salad separately, fresh.

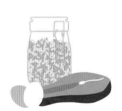

What do teenagers need?

Teenagers can't wait to explore and achieve, but their self-confidence can take a knocking as their bodies change and they work out how to change with them. Moods may dip as hormones kick in. By treading carefully and feeding them well, you'll help to get them through.

A sensitive time

Teenagers are touchy creatures at times. Their bodies are changing rapidly and they may feel they are plagued by spots, lanky hair, or an ungainly frame. Mood swings are almost inevitable (see pp66–67). Encourage your teenager to eat a healthy diet, reassuring him that if he eats plenty of fresh fruit and vegetables, the vitamins and minerals will do wonders for his complexion, hair, and general sense of wellbeing.

Tweak the quantities

While body shapes can change dramatically during the teenage years, most typically hips and breasts develop in girls, while boys fill out with more muscle, become broader in general, and shoot up fast. The balance of what they should eat from the five food groups (see pp12–13) doesn't need to change significantly, but quantities do. Teenagers are in a time of rapid growth and they need the higher end of the servings (see panel). Boys don't need to start eating whole chickens to reach their protein requirement, nor will it lead to the desired six pack – that only comes from doing plenty of exercise (see pp114–115). However, the average 15–18-year-old boy or girl does need more calories than at any other time in their life (unless they go on to be a professional athlete).

Upping the iron

Girls in particular need a diet rich enough in iron to make up for the monthly iron losses during their periods. Lean red meat, such as steak, is one good source (see p30 for others), but it shouldn't be a major part of the diet. Red meat can be high in saturated fat. It's best to eat meat with plenty of vegetables or salad instead of the classic chips. Period time for girls can be tough, with stomach cramps, bloating, and fluid retention, so make some cooked vegetables for your teenager to dip into and persuade her to eat foods rich in omega 3 (see pp24–25). For more food tips for period pains see pp154–155.

If your teenager has decided to become vegetarian or vegan, she (or he) may also need an iron supplement if they're having difficulty with their diet. See pp120–121 for advice on meat, fish, and dairy-free diets.

How much?

• **5–11 servings a day of starchy carbohydrates** A serving is 1 slice of wholemeal bread or 2–3 tbsp cooked brown rice or pasta.

• **2–3 servings a day of protein** A serving is 85–100g (3–3½oz) lean meat or chicken,140g (5oz) fish, or 3 heaped tbsp pulses (cooked).

• **2–3 servings a day of vegetables** A serving is 3 tbsp cooked vegetables, or a dessert bowl of mixed salad.

• **2–3 servings of fruit** A serving is 1 apple, pear or banana, ½ grapefruit, 2 satsumas, a handful of berries, or a wedge of melon.

• **2–3 servings a day of dairy foods** A serving is a small pot of yogurt, 40g (1½oz) cheese, or 200ml (7fl oz) skimmed milk.

Body image

Girls need to be careful that in their desire to be slim they don't restrict their fat and protein intake too much, as this can stall the start of their menstrual cycle, which can affect fertility and bone health later in life. Boys, too, are becoming increasingly body-conscious. A throwaway comment from a parent or a schoolmate can sometimes set a teenager on the path to an eating disorder. That said, it doesn't help, either, to avoid discussing body image issues with your teenager for fear of getting it wrong – silence is worse than anything and being unable to talk through fears with a parent can only make the teenage years feel lonelier. Try to keep your advice constructive, but take care to discourage crash dieting – it might lead to short-term weight loss but can damage health. If you are worried they're starting to carry too much weight or too little, see pp106–109.

Get them cooking

Teaching your teenager a few simple meals, such as an omelette or a quick stir-fry with egg noodles, will stand him in good stead in the future and give him a bit of independence if he isn't eating at the same time as you. A microwave oven can be a boon, as a meal can be quickly heated up at odd times of the day or night without input from a parent.

It's easy to cook extra portions of the meals you make, such as a bolognese sauce, meatballs, falafel burgers, or a spinach and ricotta filo bake. Your teenager can heat them up when she's hungry, and perhaps cook some pasta or rice or grab a chunk of wholegrain bread to go with them.

Skin perfection

Spots can really knock teenage self esteem. Omega 3 helps here – girls can have a couple of portions of oily fish a week, and boys up to four a week. Eating fresh fruits for vitamin C is a good idea, too. Zinc can help heal a spotty skin – good sources include chicken, nuts, almond milk, and eggs – and good hydration also has benefits. For more tips on a healthy skin, see pp162–163.

Sleep issues

Going to sleep far too late, then spending all morning in bed doesn't help energy levels or moods. Encourage a good night-time routine: a soporific starchy carb supper, such as pasta and sauce, the computer and mobile turned off at an agreed hour, and a warm, milky drink. See also pp142–143.

REALITY **CHECK**

 Keep well stocked up
Store nourishing foods such as eggs, home-made soup, cooked chicken, cheeses, and salad stuffs in the fridge, along with wholegrain bread and bagels in the bread bin or freezer. In the cupboard, have packets of wholegrain cereals, dried fruit, and nuts, cans of baked beans, quick-cooking egg or rice noodles, and ingredients for easy sauces, such as passata and herbs. Make sure there are plenty of bananas and other fruit to have on the side. That way you'll ensure your son especially can healthily satisfy his often voracious appetite.

Food for mood swings

One minute teenagers are happy and everything is fine, then it can all change in an instant, and as a parent you can often be in the firing line. What's needed is a sympathetic ear and good, wholesome food to help them cope. Amino acids from proteins can help to ensure that the levels of endorphins – the mood hormones – are boosted.

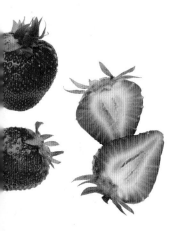

A banana and a few Brazil nuts a day are a great blend of mood-lifting nutrients.

Watch the high-GI foods

Teenage low moods can be exacerbated by a diet heavy with refined sugar and high-GI snacks, such as cakes, biscuits, and fizzy drinks (see p91). Encourage your child to **reduce his or her sugar intake** (see pp92–93), including the so-called **energy drinks**. Alcohol can aggravate mood swings. If your child is starting to have a drink or two, make them aware of the impact and try to persuade them not to.

Go for fruit instead

Point your teenager towards dried fruits and nuts and make sure **the fruit bowl is always full** of attractive-looking fresh fruit. Stock up on fruit compôtes (see p186) and on frozen berries, too, which they can either nibble while still frozen or make into a smoothie with some yogurt or almond milk (p97).

Ensure meals aren't being skipped

Moods are not helped by an empty stomach. If your child has got into the habit of grazing instead of sitting down for a proper meal, you might need to insist **they join you to eat**. It's vital they have some protein-rich foods, such as an omelette (see the recipe on p190), roast chicken and roots (p209), a bowl of mixed bean soup (p214), or chicken noodle soup (p210).

Breakfast is vital

Try not to let your child skip breakfast. Even if they get up late, **they need fuel**. Eggs and oily fish such as salmon provide amino acids for helping to start the day off on a good-mood note, so some scrambled egg and smoked salmon could work a treat. See also the delicious breakfast recipes on pp186–191.

How to deal with a broken heart

Going off food can often be a sign of teenage heartbreak. The pain your child is going through can even make them feel nauseous. Try to get them to eat **something simple**, such as poached egg on toast, or a smoked salmon and cream cheese sandwich, or pasta with a fresh tomato sauce (p215), or a bowl of fresh fruit salad with some Greek yogurt.

Chocolate comfort

Chocolate can help to ease the anguish, so you could try making some irresistible chocolate brownies (see p236). Or for another real treat, how about a **bowl of strawberries** (or other fresh fruit available) with a couple of squares of melted 70 per cent-cocoa **chocolate** to dip them in?

{ Your teenager is still growing and still needs you. Be ready to give plenty of TLC, and good food to get them through. }

Easing the anxiety

If your teenager is having an anxious time, check they're **not overdoing the caffeine**, as it will lower their mood. Encourage them to drink more water (see p39 for refreshing options), and to eat small meals that are rich in protein and vegetables. Think about oats, too – they're good for stabilizing moods, and can be soothing on the stomach. A bowl of porridge or a glass of oat milk could work wonders.

Exam nerves

If your child feels too sick before an exam to eat, try oat biscuits with nut butter (see p185), or a smoothie with added yogurt and some ground almonds or oats (p191), or add those to some stewed apple (which can be made the night before).

What do *I need?*

Be mindful of what you're putting in your body and ask yourself if that mouthful is going to nourish you. If the answer is no, think twice and question whether you really want it. It's amazing how just a brief pause for thought can get you on track to eating more healthily.

Men and women have different nutritional needs. Men tend to have larger bodies, with more water, muscle, bone, and organ tissue than women, and a higher metabolic rate. They therefore need more calories for energy, more protein to build and repair the muscles and tissues, and more fat. Their needs for carbohydrates and fibre are the same, as part of a balanced diet and sensible portion sizes (see pp40–41).

If you are concerned about how your diet makes you feel, try writing everything down in a food and symptom diary. It can get you focused and inspired, and

highlight problem areas. You might find that when you eat a heavy meal after, say, 8pm, you don't sleep soundly, so you need to eat earlier. Or maybe when you eat too many sugary cakes and sweets you actually feel tired very quickly that day, so it would be better to change to healthier snacks. Whatever your eating habits, they can probably be improved by eating a nourishing diet from across the five major food groups (see pp42–43).

Taking exercise is important, too. Adults aged 19–64 should do muscle-strengthening exercise that works all major muscle groups at least twice a week, such as yoga, or press-ups and sit-ups. You should also do at least 2½ hours a week of moderate aerobic (or "cardio") exercise, such as cycling or fast walking. See also pp114–115, for more about eating and exercise.

Check your cholesterol

Don't wait until routine health tests are done later in life to check if you are accumulating too much bad LDL cholesterol in your bloodstream (see pp174–175). If this is the case, the sooner you do something about it, the less likely you are to develop significant health problems. It's the LDL cholesterol that furs up the arteries, leading to strokes and heart disease. The culprits that stimulate the body to produce more LDL are saturated fats (see pp24–25) in butter, cream, cheese, fatty meats, and processed meats, such as sausages and salami, so lower your intake.

Look at fibre

Your digestive system plays a huge role in your wellbeing, too. Often the gut is where stress and life's worries have an impact, causing constipation, bloating,

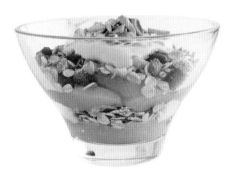

diarrhoea, and other classic symptoms of irritable bowel syndrome (IBS). You should be eating about 18g of fibre a day (see pp22–23), which will help your gut to function well and without the muscle spasms that lead to the discomfort of IBS.

A lack of fibre also makes you far less likely to feel satisfied after eating, so weight can start piling on as you eat more to feel full, increasing the risk of heart disease and many types of cancer. You need both insoluble fibre, found in wholegrains, the skin of fruit and vegetables, and in pulses, and soluble fibre, found in oats and some other grains, fruit, and vegetables. So ditch the white bread, pasta, and rice wherever you can, and go for the delicious, nutty, wholegrain varieties instead. Snack on fresh and dried fruit, nuts, and seeds instead of cakes and biscuits, and at mealtimes have plenty of fresh,

frozen or canned (in water) vegetables with your meal.

Boost water intake

You must drink lots of water – 8–10 glasses a day – to help fibre to swell and perform its magic. Water is also vital for all other bodily functions. See pp38–39 for plenty of ideas to liven water up if you aren't a fan.

Don't skimp on iron

Women in particular need to watch that their regular monthly cycle doesn't leave their body deficient in iron. This is becoming increasingly common as more of us shy away from red meat to cut down on saturated fat. Lean red meat and liver are great sources, but you can also get your iron from non-meat sources such as fortified breakfast cereal, seeds, dried fruit, and pulses (see p30). A diet low in iron exposes your body to hair loss but also to developing iron-deficiency anaemia, which can cause fatigue, depression, and inability to sleep well. To make sure you can

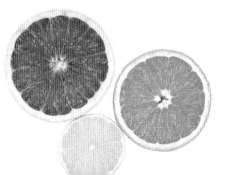

absorb the iron in your diet, have plenty of vitamin C (see p29), preferably at or around the same time as your iron-rich foods. Don't drink too much strong tea or coffee, as the tannin and polyphenol levels inhibit iron absorption (see pp98–99). So do phytates in bran and oxalates in spinach, nuts, chocolate, rhubarb, and parsley – they're all good, but don't rely too heavily on them.

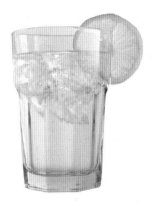

Watch your alcohol

Take care that your alcohol intake isn't too much for your body and lifestyle (see pp100–101). While there are guidelines about the amount we shouldn't exceed (14 units a week for women, 21 a week for men), only you can judge whether you feel well if you reach those limits. While there may be health benefits from drinking a little alcohol, it's good to have at least two alcohol-free days a week to give your liver a chance to rest.

Eating well
during pregnancy

Switching to a delicious, healthy diet will give you and your baby the best of everything throughout your pregnancy and get you in good shape to be a new mum. While you should avoid some foods you might usually enjoy, there are still plenty of options for eating wisely and well.

Eating for two

This doesn't mean eating twice as much, but you do need slightly more of the key nutrients, such as protein, calcium, iron, folic acid, vitamins D and C, plenty of fibre, and 2 litres (3½ pints) of fluid.

How much should I eat?

For the first trimester, you need the same as any other healthy woman – around 2,000 calories a day. In the second and third trimester, increase your daily intake by about 200 calories. That's not very much – just a wholegrain sandwich filled with lean ham, for example, or a large apple and a banana. The average woman should aim to gain 11–16kg (24–35lb). If you are underweight for your height, you should gain a little more: 12.5–18kg (27–40lb). If overweight, it should be less: 7–11.5kg (15–25lb).

Coping with morning sickness

Many women feel queasy in the mornings (or beyond) from early pregnancy until about the twelfth week. Others don't suffer at all. One tip is to have a dry biscuit before you get up – ginger is good, as is ginger tea. Nibbling breadsticks or crackers can help, or raw fruit and vegetables. Some find sipping hot water with a squeeze of fresh lemon works well. Preparing food can make things worse; get your family to help, or make meals simple, with little or no cooking.

Extra minerals and vitamins

A balanced diet – rich in fruit and veg (especially leafy greens), wholegrains, dairy and other calcium-rich foods, some red meat, poultry, and fish (unless you're vegetarian), cooked eggs, pulses, nuts, and seeds – will set you up in pregnancy and beyond. Spend at least 10 minutes a day in sunlight so your body makes enough vitamin D to help absorb calcium. Eat plenty of citrus to help absorb iron, too.

During pregnancy, your baby draws heavily on your iron stores, so include plenty of iron-rich foods to reduce the likelihood of iron-deficiency anaemia. Your GP or health visitor will check for that and see if you also need a prenatal multivitamin and mineral supplement. When trying for a baby, and until the twelfth week of pregnancy, take a 400mcg folic acid

Dealing with constipation

A sluggish gut is very common, particularly later in pregnancy. Have plenty of water and other fluids, along with high-fibre foods, such as wholegrains, fruit and vegetables, and dried fruits, such as prunes. Hot water and lemon are good, too. Being rushed and stressed isn't conducive to keeping the gut moving; sometimes a warm bath can help, as can reflexology.

Keeping safe

When pregnant, you are more susceptible to infection, often because of hormonal imbalances. Your baby, although remarkably resilient, is also vulnerable to bacteria and other outside influences. Good food, and good food hygiene, are essential for keeping both of you as safe and healthy as possible.

Gestational diabetes

This most typically occurs in the third trimester when your body struggles to produce enough insulin to meet your baby's demands and yours. Avoid high-GI foods and choose slow-release energy ones (see p91). Gentle, regular exercise can also help.

Foods to avoid

Listeria, salmonella, and toxoplasmosis are very serious for you both if contracted during pregnancy. Don't have unpasteurized milk, yogurt, or cheese, and avoid mould-ripened soft cheeses, such as Brie and Camembert, and soft, blue-veined ones, such as Stilton and Gorgonzola. Don't eat any type of pâté, even vegetable ones. Avoid raw or soft-cooked eggs, all products containing them, and raw or rare-cooked meat. There's no confirmed advice on cold cured meats such as salami, or smoked fish, but both carry a small risk of listeria or toxoplasmosis, so you may prefer to avoid them. Too much vitamin A can harm your baby, so don't eat liver or liver products. It's also best to avoid raw fish. For peanut allergies, see p134.

Food hygiene is a must

To avoid those same risks, always wash your hands after handling raw meat and poultry. Wrap and store them carefully to avoid drips onto other food in your fridge and cook them right through. Wash all raw fruit and vegetables well, including salads.

Is it safe to drink alcohol?

The UK's Chief Medical Officer recommends avoiding alcohol while trying to conceive and during pregnancy. If you can't resist the odd drink, limit it to 1–2 units, once or twice a week (see pp100–101).

Limit your caffeine intake

Drinking a lot of caffeine (see pp98–99) isn't good for you or your baby and can result in a low birth weight, or even miscarriage. Limit to around 200mg a day, which is the equivalent of two mugs of instant coffee (or smaller cups of filter), or three cups of tea. Chocolate counts, too: a 50g bar of dark has around 50mg caffeine; milk chocolate, 25mg.

Food cravings

Cravings can start early on in pregnancy. Hormones may be the cause as they sensitize taste and smell receptors. There is no evidence that eating weird foods harms your baby, but if you are hooked on high sugar, salt, or fatty foods, try healthier alternatives.

During pregnancy, as your body changes and your baby grows, eating well will pay dividends.

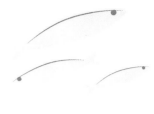

Body-boosters
for new mums

If you are a first-time mum, you may be disappointed that your body hasn't immediately returned to how it was before you were pregnant. It will gradually reccover, so don't starve yourself. Eat regular meals, packed with the nutrients suggested here, and all will be well.

Oily fish

Feeling a bit down and tired? Oily fish, such as salmon, trout, mackerel, sardines, pilchards, and herring, are packed with a fatty acid called docosahexaenoic acid, or DHA, which is essential to get your brain functioning well and to maintain a healthy heart. Research has shown that DHA can lift a low mood and may help prevent postnatal depression. However, if you eat too much oily fish you could expose your body to an unhealthy amount of mercury, so limit your intake to 280 g (10 oz) a week – that's two small portions. You can also buy eggs fortified with omega-3 fatty acids. These are another good source of DHA.

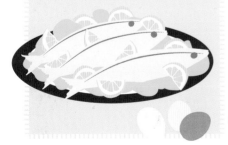

Meat

When you give birth there is inevitably blood loss. This can lead to an iron deficiency and really sap your energy levels. Lean red meat, such as beef, is rich in iron so can help replenish your supply and put you back on track. Meat, eggs, and other proteins, including vegetable sources such as pulses, nuts, and seeds (see pp18–21), are body-builders so they are essential to help your recovery and get you back to full health. Include nuts and seeds in snacks and sprinkle them on cereals, enjoy pulses with meat for main courses, and try baking cooked chickpeas until crisp for a delicious and nutritious snack.

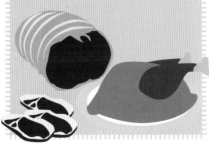

Dairy

While dairy produce should play an important role in everyone's diet (see pp26–27), they are absolutely essential if you are breastfeeding. Your breast milk will be rich in nutrients whatever you eat, because your body directs the right amount of nutrients that are needed by your baby into your milk, even if this leaves your own resources depleted. This means that you have to make sure you consume plenty of calcium from dairy products and green leafy vegetables, so there's enough to keep your bones strong.

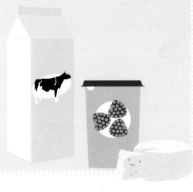

REALITY **CHECK**

 Staying hydrated
Drink plenty of fluid – if you become dehydrated you will feel even more tired. See p39 for tips on how to make plain water taste really refreshing.

 How much?
If you are breastfeeding, drink about 2 litres (3½ pints) of water and other fluids. If you are not, about 1.2 litres (2 pints) will be enough.

Juicy treats

Smoothies and juices are an excellent way of getting a quick fix of nutrients. If you make them yourself you will be able to choose a good balance of ingredients that you may not be able to find in shop-bought ones. Adding milk or yogurt to smoothies will slow down the sugar release, giving you longer-lasting energy. See pp96–97 for more about smoothies and juices and p191 for a great recipe for breakfast-in-a-glass.

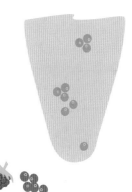

Wholegrain cereals

Lack of sleep goes with the territory of being a new mum, and that can mean it's hard to be alert in the mornings. A bowl of wholegrain cereal for breakfast will give you slow-release energy to help you keep going until lunchtime. Try a home-made bowl of cinnamon and maple granola (see p188) or a bowl of warming porridge, topped with fresh berries or sliced banana, stewed fruits, or compôte and you'll be able to cope with the demands of a new baby. Alternatively, wholegrain toast or bagels with nut butter and a boiled egg, or a protein hit such as the omelette on p190, will do the trick.

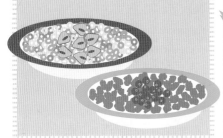

Fruit and vegetables

As they're packed with vitamins, minerals and phytonutrients (see pp28–33) to boost your reserves, fruit and vegetables are the ideal postnatal foods. They also supply fibre to help keep your digestion working properly. Snack on fruit to give yourself a quick boost of energy and to stop you feeling peckish – stewed fruit may suit you best at first as it's easier to digest. You need to eat little and often to maintain your blood sugar levels (see p91), which will help to prevent you feeling tired, particularly if you are breastfeeding. Add salad to your sandwiches and have plenty of green vegetables, roots, and pulses with dinner.

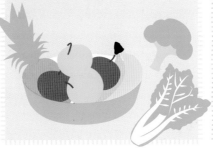

Dark chocolate

Chocolate really does have the feel-good factor. Good-quality dark chocolate, with 70 per cent cocoa solids or higher, increases serotonin levels in the brain, which releases endorphins, the chemicals that genuinely do lift your mood. That doesn't mean that you need to gorge on the stuff, though – a few squares nibbled with a caffeine-free tea or decaffeinated coffee can do wonders. Eat too much and the high sugar and fat levels will delay you getting back your pre-birth figure. Chocolate is high in caffeine, so it's probably best not to eat it just before bed or if you are about to snatch a rest while your baby sleeps.

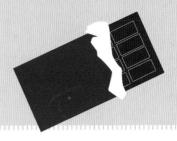

Women at *50 plus*

At this age your oestrogen levels are dropping and after the menopause your body becomes more vulnerable to osteoporosis and heart disease. Taking care of your nutritional needs will help to reduce menopausal symptoms and preserve bone density.

Help with hormones

What is the menopause?

The menopause is a natural stage when the ovaries slow the production of sex hormones, especially oestrogen. Periods stop and there may also be mood swings, anxiety, and hot flushes. The menopause often occurs in the late 40s or early 50s, but it can be earlier or later and affects different women in very different ways.

Can soya help?

Research isn't conclusive, but it could be worth trying to incorporate a small amount of natural phytoestrogens, such as (but not exclusively) soya, to see if some of your symptoms improve. Phytoestrogens resemble oestrogen and may protect against some breast cancers, too. Other sources include dried fruits, pulses (such as beans, lentils, and chickpeas), beansprouts, linseeds, and natural liquorice; all bring benefits.

Time to take stock of how you feel and what you eat – small tweaks can make a big difference.

Opt for omegas

Look to the omega 3 fatty acid-rich foods, too (see p25). Research has shown that they can assist with alleviating mood swings, breast tenderness, and hot flushes. So step up your intake of oily fish, such as mackerel, herrings, sardines, pilchards, salmon, and trout, to four portions a week.

Cut down on caffeine

Caffeine can exacerbate symptoms, so try changing to decaffeinated varieties of tea and coffee. There are also plenty of caffeine-free teas, such as rooibos, all the fruit ones, and camomile. Herbal infusions such as sage tea may also be of benefit. See also pp98–99.

Herbal supplements

Herbs like red clover, black cohosh, dong quai, and ginseng may help to alleviate menopausal symptoms. Consult a medicinal herbalist or your doctor before taking herbal supplements, which should be treated with the same level of respect and care as prescription drugs.

Building strong foundations

Protect your bones

At this stage of life, we lose about 2–3 per cent of our bone density, so we are at a higher risk of developing osteoporosis (brittle bone disease). If you have low weight or are taking regular medication, such as steroids, the risk is higher.

Calcium is key

A diet rich in calcium can help to reduce your risk of osteoporosis (see pp158–159), so be sure you get enough dairy produce or alternatives (see pp26–27) and plenty of leafy greens and other calcium sources (p30). If necessary, your doctor may prescribe a supplement.

Magnesium matters

Bones need magnesium, so try to incorporate some magnesium-rich foods such as brazil nuts and cashews, dried fruits, and seeds (see p30). If you have low bone density, a supplement may be recommended by your doctor.

Careful with salt

Both men and women should keep salt intake down to no more than 6g per day as too much increases the amounts of calcium we lose from our bones (see pp94–95). Season food with pepper, other spices, and herbs instead of salt.

Stop smoking

Smoking affects the bones as well as damaging your health in many other ways. Smokers also have a higher risk of osteomyelitis – an infection of the bones, brought on by poor circulation.

Limit alcohol

Excess alcohol causes calcium to be leached from the bones and may lead to osteoporosis. For more about alcohol, see pp100–101.

Boost activity

Load-bearing exercise, such as brisk walking, jogging, running, aerobics, dance, or boxing, stimulates the bones to produce new bone cells. Passive exercise, such as yoga or pilates, is great for posture and flexibility, which also helps. See pp114–115 for more about daily exercise.

Reducing the risk of disease

Eating well and managing stress (p142) are the best ways of ensuring your diet plays its part in reducing the likelihood of being affected by heart disease (pp174–175), diabetes (pp172–173), cancer (pp176–177), and dementia (pp180–181).

Anti-ageing antioxidants

The powerful antioxidants in vitamin C (see p29) and phytonutrients (pp32–33) help the skin to regenerate and stay supple (pp164–165). So eat plenty of wholegrains, colourful fruit and vegetables, and herbs and spices, all of which are loaded with phytonutrients.

Prioritize fibre

For both sexes, food high in fibre (see pp22–23) and plenty of water (pp38–39) keep the gut healthy. Fibre also helps to prevent constipation, which in turn prevents our body cells being adversely affected by waste products and toxins.

Men at 50 plus

The fifties are a time when many people look at their lifestyle and decide to take better care of their health. Men in particular can be highly focused in achieving their goals, whether these be lowering their cholesterol or reducing an expanding waistline.

Tackling middle-age spread

Fat makes fat

If you eat too much of any fat (not just saturated fat), your body stores it as fat (see pp24–25), increasing your risk of heart disease (see pp174–175). Cut down on all fatty foods, with the exception of two portions a week of oily fish for the omega 3 it contains (see pp24–25).

Watch high GI foods

Food with a high Glycaemic Index (see p91), such as sugars, honey, cakes, biscuits, fruit juices, and ice creams, will also increase fat in your body if eaten in excess. Some fruits are also high-GI, including bananas – it's best to go for citrus, stone fruits, apples, pears, and berries. Higher GI vegetables are baked and mashed potato, cooked squash and pumpkin, cooked carrots, and swede. Wholegrain bread has the same GI as white bread, but offers greater nutritional advantages.

Ditch the junk food

Junk fast foods such as burgers and chips are high in fat, sugar, and salt, and should be kept for treats, not everyday meals. When you're having a takeaway, consider choosing a more healthy stir-fry, sushi, noodles, or a veggie pizza with salad instead of high-fat meat toppings and fries.

Beware the beer gut

Excessive alcohol, particularly beer, will expand the waistline and can lead to fatty liver (see right). Limit your intake to no more than 2–3 units a day (such as 1–1½ pints ordinary strength beer, which some research shows may help strengthen bones).

Take regular exercise

Even if you are not someone who has always enjoyed sport, remember that moderate, regular exercise helps to preserve muscle mass, which would otherwise reduce, leading to an increase in body fat. Walking, cycling, and cross-training are particularly good.

Quit smoking

It's never too late to quit smoking, and the sooner you do so the lower your risk of developing the classic smoking-related diseases, which are more prevalent the older you get.

Common issues and positive changes

Diabetes

Type 2 diabetes (see pp172–173) often affects both men and women in middle age. Always follow the advice given by your doctor, eat healthily, and shed any excess body fat through a combination of nourishing food and exercise.

Male menopause

The male menopause is all too real and isn't just down to hormonal changes. Not only low levels of testosterone, but also poor diet, smoking, and too much alcohol can exacerbate the symptoms, as can stress caused by work or difficult relationships. There is now a male hormone replacement therapy, which doctors prescribe for men who are struggling with low energy levels and reduced libido. Eating a nutritious diet and getting plenty of exercise will improve mood and physical health.

Low testosterone

As men get older, testosterone levels fall. This doesn't affect everyone but if you feel tired or out of shape, or lose interest in sex, it may be the cause. The phytonutrients (see pp32–33) in garlic and cruciferous vegetables may help.

Gout

More common in men than women, gout is painful inflammation of the joints caused by the presence of crystals of monosodium urate monohydrate, a by-product of uric acid. If susceptible, avoid purine-rich foods: game, offal, meat and oily fish, especially sardines. Look for omega 3 in vegetable sources instead.

High cholesterol

Poor diet and lack of exercise can lead to high levels of cholesterol in the blood, which in turn can lead to strokes and heart disease (see pp174–175). Eat plenty of vegetables, salads, and fruit, and reduce saturated fats.

Fatty liver

Fatty liver occurs when your liver is infiltrated with fatty deposits. Even though it is serious, and can lead to liver disease, it responds positively to a reduced fat and alcohol diet, one rich in fruit, vegetables, wholegrains, and low-GI foods.

Prostate cancer

Prostate cancer is highest in men over 50. While there is no absolute proof that diet helps, many doctors believe that one low in saturated fat and high in vegetables, oily fish, and wholegrains is your best nutritional defence.

Stress management

Whether it's because of a demanding job, money worries, family problems, or just life in general, stress can play a huge role in making us ill. See pp144–145 for food strategies that can make all the difference to your health and wellbeing.

Fibre foremost

As with women, it's vital that men have plenty of fibre (see pp22–23) and water (see pp38–39) in order to keep the bowel working properly, avoid the build-up of toxins, and help to prevent colon cancer.

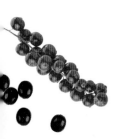

Eating for the
over seventies

Ageing is incredibly variable. Some people reach their older years light in step and lively of mind. Others are afflicted by a range of medical conditions, which might make preparing fresh food seem too much trouble – but now it's even more valuable to help optimize their health.

While we know that certain habits, such as eating poorly, smoking, drinking too much, and not being physically active aren't the best way forward, you may have older relatives or neighbours who have ill-treated their bodies for decades yet are healthy and seemingly thriving in their twilight years. And the opposite exists – those who have been doing everything feasible to look after themselves, living healthily and well, and yet suffer from tiredness, digestive problems, and slow recovery from minor illnesses. The advice below, though, should pay dividends for all.

Enjoying eating

Many older people live alone and come to rely on others for support. Although some people cope very well, it's easy for them to become less motivated about food, feeling it's not worth the effort just for themselves. The sharing of meals both brings back the pleasure of the social side of eating and ensures that older relatives and friends are getting some good nutrition. If you're helping to stock their fridge and cupboards for meals on their own, choose foods you know they love and think about meals that are simple to prepare or just to heat up if you have cooked them in advance. A bowl of tasty lentil soup with fresh bread, then fruit is easy and really good. Consider good-quality frozen ready-meals, too.

Changes to the senses

If you're helping someone elderly with their meals, it's important to realize that the taste buds tend to deteriorate, leading people to add more salt (which may increase blood pressure) or sugar (empty calories, leading to unwanted weight gain) to their meals to compensate. It's better to season foods with herbs, spices (if they are tolerated), and pepper instead of salt and use fruit or occasionally, honey to sweeten. The senses of smell and sight may be impaired, too, which can lead to a loss of appetite, since smelling and seeing food stimulates the desire to eat. It helps, therefore, to make small, colourful, tasty, richly fragrant meals, which will entice them to take an interest in what's on their plate.

Getting enough fibre

An older gut can become sluggish, because, like all parts of the body, it gets tired as we get older. Also, leading a less active life can slow it down. Fibre is really important to keep everything moving (see pp22–23). Because chewing can be difficult if there are dental problems, it's best to choose porridge or wholewheat cereals that soften in milk for breakfast. Ready-to-eat dried fruit, such as apricots or prunes, are soft (and lovely and sweet), and try cooked apple purée or grating an unpeeled apple to mix with yogurt and a little cinnamon for pudding. Scrub potatoes for boiling instead of peeling, and provide plenty of dark green leafy vegetables such as steamed or wilted spinach and kale.

Protecting against disease

Over the age of 70, people tend to become more susceptible to developing health problems such as heart disease, diabetes, and arthritis, as well as more minor conditions that are often alleviated by an improved diet. Although they need a similar balance of nutrients to other adults (pp12–13), the provision of vitamins, minerals, and phytonutrients (pp28–33) becomes even more important since their absorption is not so efficient as it is in the young. Some health problems mean having to follow special diets, or having to avoid, or limit, certain foods because of blood-thinning or other medication. Whatever you provide, make each food count towards maximum nourishment and variety.

Watch the sugars and sweet things

The occasional slice of delicious cake or a melt-in-the-mouth biscuit are wonderful pleasures but they still need to be in moderation. It can be tempting to take a whole cake when visiting an elderly person, and that's fine as long as it contains healthy ingredients (see p236 and pp242–247 for some yummy recipes). Too much sweet food can pile on unwanted weight, which can make moving much more difficult – especially if there is arthritis or other joint problems – and increase the risk of heart disease, diabetes, and certain cancers. It can also lead to tooth decay and play havoc with moods and energy levels. Offer something naturally sweet for delicious nibbles, such as a bunch of grapes, or a dish of dried fruit, such as raisins. Suggest stocking up the cupboard with canned fruit in natural juice, such as pears, too.

Vitamin and mineral supplements

The older we get, the less efficiently our bodies absorb or manufacture nutrients, so in the later years it may be necessary to take some supplements. The skin is less adept at manufacturing vitamin D and this is exacerbated by the fact that some older people spend less time outside in the sun, so a daily supplement of 10mcg vitamin D is a good precaution – but do always check with the doctor before considering any supplements. If there are low levels of calcium in the blood (which could lead to osteoporosis), a daily dose of calcium phosphate/cholecalciferol, which is a mixture of calcium and vitamin D, will help to maintain bone health. Tiredness may indicate that iron tablets are needed, but a visit to the doctor should be made to test for pernicious anaemia, which can then be treated with vitamin B_{12} injections.

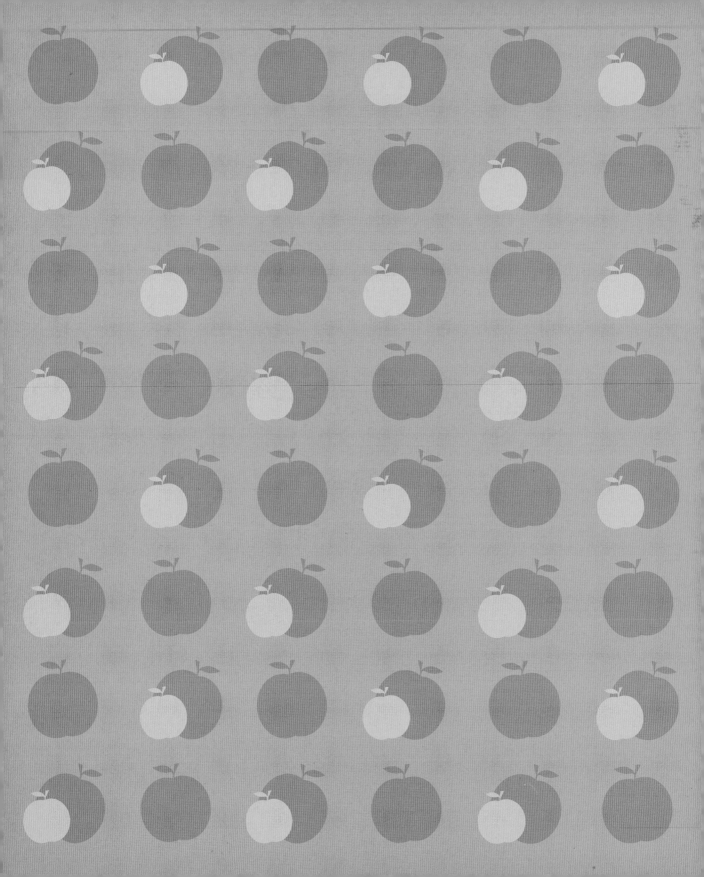

3

Simple steps
to a healthier you

Keeping food *at its best*

Careful storage is a cornerstone of good nutrition – it keeps food at its best, reduces waste, and can decrease the impact of food-spoiling bacteria. Always check the "use by" and "best before" dates given on packaging – the time spans given here for keeping food are only guidelines and individual foods may differ.

Shelf life

Don't leave bags of cereals, flour, grains, nuts, and seeds open to the elements. They all contain natural oils that will go rancid. Buy in suitable quantities and use within 6 months. Leftovers and decanted canned foods should be stored, covered, in the fridge and used within 2–3 days. Opened jars of condiments and pickles with a high acid content will keep in a cool cupboard for up to 1 month, but 6–12 months in the fridge.

Clever containers

Wrapping and storing properly is key to keeping food fresh. Invest in spring clips for bags and screw-topped jars for dry goods. Once cans are opened, transfer any unused food to a sealed plastic container or covered bowl and store in the fridge. Reusable bags and plastic boxes must be scrupulously clean. To avoid cross-contamination, keep separate bags for raw meat, fish, and ready-to-eat foods, and don't reuse.

Food bags

Try the specially designed salad-preserving bags that can make salad leaves last for days in the fridge, instead of the all-too-common sight of limp leaves only a day after they were purchased. Always wash salad leaves before use, unless the packet says they are ready-washed. Check out banana bags, too, as these allow you to keep bananas in the fridge for weeks without them over-ripening.

Cool and dark

Foods don't last as long in a warm modern kitchen as they used to in a cool, dark larder with shelves, where air could circulate around the fresh produce. Even in containers, food will spoil if the temperature is too warm, and dried herbs and spices deteriorate quickly if stored in the light. For jars, packets, cans, and fruit and vegetables, choose cupboards in the coolest, darkest place in the kitchen, away from the cooker.

Date stamps

"Use by" means you should not eat the food after that date. If you are not going to eat it in time and it is freezable, put it in the freezer (see pp84–85). "Best before" indicates that the food will be at its best before the date stamped on it; if you use it a little later, it will be safe to eat but not at its best. "Sell by" or "display until" dates are there to help shops manage their stock, and you may benefit from prices reduced for a quick sale.

Oldest first

When you are filling up a jar of cereal, flour, or other dry goods, take care that you don't get into the habit of just tipping the new in on top of the old stuff. Always use what's there first, or, if necessary, remove it, put in the new, and put the old back on top so that it is used first. Check "use by" dates, too (see left). If you have several cans or packets of the same food, take a moment to check the dates and use the oldest one first.

Know your fridge

Food lasts longer if it's stored the right way in the fridge. To keep the temperature below 5°C (40°F), avoid overloading your fridge so that air can circulate and make sure that all cooked food is cold before putting it in.

Oils and butters

Keep oils and butters in the fridge as they can go rancid in warmth and light. This affects their taste and may lead to them becoming unstable and producing free radicals (see antioxidants, p32), which can increase the risk of heart disease and cancer. (Some oils start to thicken in the fridge; before use, take out to let them warm up, and then shake.)

Cheese

Wrap cheese in waxed paper rather than cling film, as it allows the cheese to breathe rather than sweat. Place in a sealable container to prevent odours transferring to other foods. Store on the middle or top shelf of the fridge, for no longer than 3–4 weeks.

Jams and spreads

Opened jams, marmalades, and pure fruit spreads with no added sugar are best kept in the fridge to reduce the risk of food poisoning. The spreads are more vulnerable, as the high sugar content of jam acts as a preservative. Jams last 6–9 months, pure fruit spreads somewhat less; always check the "best before" date.

Fruit and vegetables

Most fruit and vegetables are best stored in the salad drawer at the bottom of the fridge, but keep tomatoes at room temperature as this allows them to develop their flavour. Potatoes will go black in the fridge – keep in a cool, dark cupboard or a frost-free shed or garage.

Eggs

Keep eggs in the fridge, but for baking or boiling, let them reach room temperature before you use them: very cold eggs tend to crack when you boil them. If you don't have an egg shelf in the fridge door, store in their original boxes so they don't touch and contaminate other foods.

Cooked foods

Cooked foods, leftovers, and desserts should be kept covered or wrapped, as appropriate, on the top or middle shelf. Pre-packed foods should be eaten by their "use by" date, while home-cooked food should, depending on their ingredients, be eaten within 3 days.

Fish

Leave fresh and smoked fish in their packaging and put in a sealed container to prevent any odour and juices escaping. If vacuum-packed, they will stay fresh longer. Always place on the bottom shelf of the fridge – not only is it the coldest part, but it also prevents the fish from touching or dripping onto other foods.

Meat and poultry

Fresh meat and poultry should be removed from any plastic wrapping and wrapped in greaseproof paper to prevent it becoming slimy. Place it in a sealed container or, if a large joint, on a plate on the bottom shelf of the fridge, to prevent any blood dripping on to other foods. Store cooked meat on the shelf above to avoid cross-contamination from raw meat.

Making the most of your freezer

Freezers make it so much easier to have a constant supply of nourishing food, all year round. By putting small portions in the freezer, you can cook ahead for hungry teens who want to eat at all times of day, or for anyone in the family who needs a bit of encouragement to eat well even when time is short.

Why freeze?

Freezing below –18°C (0°F) slows the deterioration of foods down to the minimum, keeping them almost as fresh as when they were picked or prepared. Commercially frozen vegetables have **optimum nutrients** because they are fast-frozen within a couple of hours of being picked. Be sure to freeze food as soon as you get it home so it is at its best. Vegetables should be **blanched quickly** in boiling water, plunged in iced water to cool, drained, then packed in useable quantities in freezer bags or airtight plastic boxes. Remove the air before tying or sealing firmly as air left will cause oxidation and the food will spoil. Always use food within the **storage times** recommended as food left too long will taste unpleasant and lose texture.

Portions and labels

All food should be **thoroughly wrapped** before freezing or it will get freezer burn. The ice damages the outer cells, causing white, dry patches on the food. Foil, freezer bags, or plastic boxes with sealable lids are all suitable. Freeze food in **useable portions** – individual ones or for as many people as appropriate. Unless you tend to use the whole content of packages of meat such as sausages or bacon in one go, split them first and wrap in suitable portions. For portioning bread, see right. **Always label your food** with what it is, the portion size, and the date frozen, using an indelible freezer marker pen, so that you know what it is and when it should be used by (you may think you will remember, but you won't).

What not to freeze

Most foods can be frozen. The exceptions are cottage **cheese** (it becomes watery); cream or cream cheese with less than 40 per cent fat (it curdles when thawed); **egg-based sauces**, such as real custard and mayonnaise (they curdle); eggs in their shells (they explode – instead, freeze eggs lightly beaten, noting how many eggs are in the batch); hard-boiled eggs (they go rubbery); **jam** (it loses its set, so freeze sponge cakes unfilled); **boiled potatoes** (they go watery – mashed are OK); **raw salad** stuffs, such as cucumber or lettuce (they go limp). **Strawberries** go soft and pale but will taste fine if you want to use them for cooking. As a general rule, **don't refreeze** thawed, raw food unless you **cook it first**.

5 ways to freeze fruit

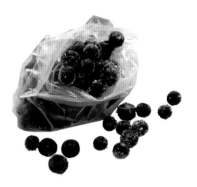

1 Berries, or rhubarb cut in chunks, are best open-frozen first, spread out on trays. Then transfer to freezer bags or sealable plastic containers. Berries can also be frozen in ice cubes to jazz up water.

2 Stone fruits, such as apricots, peaches, plums, damsons, and greengages, can either be frozen whole in freezer bags, or halved, stones removed, open-frozen like berries, and then packed.

3 Citrus fruits for marmalade can be washed and frozen whole or sliced, or peeled with rind and flesh frozen separately, as your recipe requires.

4 The grated or thinly pared zest of lemons, limes, and oranges can be frozen separately, in small plastic boxes. Freeze juice in ice cube trays, then store in freezer bags for making citron pressé later.

5 Fruits such as apples or pears can be peeled, cored, and stewed with or without sweetening and frozen in portions for use as sauce or in pies or desserts. They can also be poached in apple juice.

Tips for bread

Unless you have a large family and eat bread at a rapid rate, it will go stale quickly – and because it doesn't contain the preservatives of a few years ago, it will go mouldy in a warm bread bin. Sliced bread keeps fairly well in the fridge but freezing your bread means you can take it out fresh whenever you need it. Quarter or halve a large, whole loaf (cheaper than buying smaller loaves) and then **individually wrap**. Separate rolls, bagels, and pittas and wrap in useable portions too. **Sliced bread** can be split from frozen if you don't squash it in the freezer. Make stale bread or crusts into **breadcrumbs** and use them for coating fish, chicken, and so on, or for a crisp topping or a stuffing. Crusty bread may shed its crust when thawed.

Flavours to hand

Herbs and spices freeze well, but as they go limp when thawed they're fine for **cooking** but not so great in salads or for garnish. Frozen herbs make great teas, such as mint and lemon verbena (see p98). Make a batch of pesto and freeze it in small amounts that you can use in one go. If you freeze a bunch of **parsley or coriander**, you can crumble it while still frozen, rather than chopping it. Alternatively, chop fresh herbs (after picking off the stalks, if woody, such as thyme or rosemary) and freeze in ice cube trays, then tip into bags when frozen so you can easily take out what you need. Grated fresh **ginger** and chopped **chillies** freeze well in the same way. You can also freeze whole chillies to throw into soups, stews, and curries.

How long?

Food eventually deteriorates in the freezer. It usually won't harm you, but some food poisoning bacteria thrive in the freezer. These times are just a guide, so **check the labels** on packaging.
1 month: milk (thaw then shake).
2 months: bacon, sausages, oily or smoked fish.
3 months: eggs, white fish, minced meat, casseroles, curries, meat or fish pies.
6 months: bread and cakes, cheeses, herbs and spices.
8 months: meat chops or diced.
12 months: fruit, vegetables, meat joints, poultry and game.
Food is best defrosted slowly in the fridge. If thawing at room temperature, **use as soon as possible once thawed**, to prevent bacteria growing. Or use a microwave, following the instructions on the packaging.

Shopping *tips*

Shopping for food is a huge part of our lives, occupying quite a bit of our time and budget. Yet with some straightforward organization so that none of that time and budget is wasted, buying food that you know will contribute to the good health of your family as well as tasting great becomes a pleasure rather than a chore.

Make a list

Making a careful list of what you need before you go shopping can save you a lot of time, effort, and money. Check your cupboards and fridge before you write the list, not least because it's easy to forget that you've got extra packets from "buy one, get one free" deals. It's a good idea to have a thorough sort-out of your freezer every few weeks, too. Even better, keep a note of what's been frozen and when, so you can see at a glance what needs to be eaten and what you need to stock up on. Internet shopping is great for bulky or heavy stuff as it takes away the hassle of lugging it all home, but you can also order from small suppliers who will send you top-quality foods.

Make it fun

If you love food and want your family to love it too, encourage your children to go with you to farmers' markets, farm shops, bakeries, and well-stocked delicatessens so that they will see fresh produce and interesting varieties of food. The more they realize that there are differences in the quality of food you can buy, and that care goes into producing the meat, poultry, cheeses, fruit, vegetables, and other food on your table, the more inclined they will be to develop the habit of eating healthily for life. Let your children help you choose what to buy and talk about how you might cook it. Get them to help in the kitchen, too. It's the best way to learn about food.

Timing is everything

Try to avoid going food shopping when you or your children are ravenously hungry – you will end up buying far more than you intended or needed, because so much of what's on offer will look extra-tempting. Your children will probably be putting pressure on you to buy sweets or crisps and because you're feeling unrelaxed you may be more inclined to give in. It's a good idea to have some fruit or a bowl of soup before you head to the shops, then the whole outing will be much more enjoyable. The same goes for shopping on the Internet – if you're feeling hungry, have a healthy snack before you log on so that you buy only what you need and can eat while it's fresh.

Before you buy, read the label

 + + + + + +

Ingredients
Product packaging must list ingredients clearly, in descending order according to quantity by weight – so the first ingredient is the largest component.

Nutrition values
Most pre-packed foods state the energy value and the amounts of the main nutrients plus salt. Allergy information and vegetarian suitability is also sometimes given.

Date
The "use by" date on perishable goods is when it must be eaten by to be safe. The "best before" date shows when food is at its peak, but it will last longer.

Storage
Frozen and chilled foods state how long they can be kept in the freezer or fridge. Condiments will show if they need to be in the fridge once opened.

Preparation
You may find details about preparation, and sometimes a serving suggestion. Ready-meals give cooking times, often for both oven and microwave.

THE ADVANCE OF ADDITIVES

In 2011, the global market for food additives was worth $28.2bn. Europe was the biggest consumer, using 32 per cent of the total production.

The average UK supermarket stocks around 80,000 options for 25,000 products

WHAT A WASTE

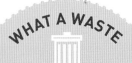

Half the food purchased in the US and Europe is just thrown away. In the UK, the average family wastes £700 of food a year. Check dates on labels so you don't buy food you won't eat.

Online stores make checking ingredients **easy**

Looking at additives

* Some additives are necessary in manufactured foods to prevent them from going off, changing colour, or losing texture. Antioxidants, natural colours, gelling agents, emulsifiers, and thickeners are commonly found and don't affect us.

* A few food colourings have been linked with child behaviour and concentration disorders: tartrazine (E102), quinoline yellow (E104), sunset yellow (E110), carmoisine (E122), ponceau 4R (E124), and allura red (E129). They are best avoided.

* Sulphites (E220–228) and benzoates (E210–219) are used as food preservatives. Both can cause allergic reactions in people with asthma or eczema. Sulphites occur naturally in beer and wine; benzoates in fruit and honey.

* Some flavour enhancers, such as the sweetener aspartame and MSG (monosodium glutamate), can cause allergic reactions in some people. Too much of some other sweeteners, such as sorbitol, can also cause tummy upsets.

* Many everyday foods – such as some breakfast cereals, breads, non-dairy milks, margarine and other bread spreads, and orange juice – are fortified with vitamins and minerals that are lost in the refining process or may be lacking in the diet.

The organic *option*

Many people find themselves in a dilemma as to whether to choose organic produce. They may wonder whether its ethical standards, taste, and health benefits differ enough to be worth what can often be a higher price. Knowing the facts can help in the decision-making.

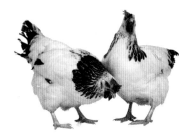

Only you can decide whether buying organic produce is the right choice for you. Organic farmers are **passionate** that it is the best way to farm, even though it is difficult. They have to adhere to **strict regulations** over the use of pesticides, fertilizers, and so on, relying on other plants and wildlife to manage disease and pest infestation instead of using artificial non-organic chemical substances. In the UK, organic regulation is very tight, particularly when it comes to livestock. Animals have to be given organic feed and specific amounts of suitable outdoor space to roam in, and be looked after to defined standards. Because they suffer from **fewer diseases** than intensively farmed animals housed close together in large numbers, there is less need for drugs, which are only allowed in emergency situations. The aim of this way of farming is to produce healthy animals that have a good quality of life and also to protect the consumer from pesticides, fertilizers, antibiotics, and growth hormones.

It is a costly business, but if you believe in the ethos, you will be prepared to pay that bit extra. One way to balance the books is to buy organic meat or poultry and mix it with cheaper vegetable protein, such as pulses, to **make the meal go further**. For instance, if you buy organic sausages, cut them up and make them into a casserole with chickpeas, peppers, tomatoes, and other vegetables. That will make the sausages go a lot further than serving them just grilled with mash and some vegetables.

At present, the UK Department of Health says there is no concrete evidence that organic produce contains **more nutrients** than non-organic produce, but it continues to review research on the subject. However, organic food is likely to contain **no residual pesticides**, and organic meat

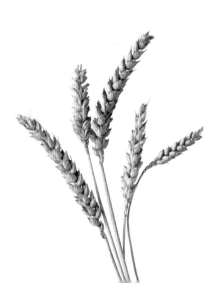

and poultry will not come from animals that have been given growth hormones, or with antibiotics shortly before slaughter. But in deciding whether organic is the right thing for you, don't be swayed into thinking that just because it is organic it must be good for you – an organic packet of sweets can easily contain just as much refined sugar as a non-organic packet, so check the label.

There is debate about whether organic produce **tastes better**, but what tastes good to one person won't necessarily to someone else. It's a matter of **personal choice**. Some people are happy just to buy free-range eggs and meat and don't mind that they aren't organic as long as the animals have had a good quality of life. Others choose to buy organic fruit and vegetables in order to avoid fertilizer and pesticide residues.

Organic fish is a quandary for some, as only farmed fish can be certified organic, and many people object to fish farming. You may prefer to buy **sustainably sourced**, line-caught (rather than dredged) fish from well-managed wild stocks, properly fished to lessen the impact on the environment and avoid over-depletion of the stocks.

Sustainable fish will be clearly marked at the fish counter. Try to **buy local produce** as much as you can, too, in supermarkets and farmers' markets. This helps to reduce the environmental costs of transporting produce (food miles) and you get food at its freshest. Try also to support local shopkeepers, as they can often be a great source of advice on cuts of meat, types of fish, or the best seasonal fruit and vegetables.

Growing your own vegetables brings the pleasure of nurturing plants that provide you with delicious food, and you can do it organically. If you don't have time or space for a garden, try growing herbs, salad leaves, or tomatoes in a window box, or

Many look to organic for fruit and vegetables with reduced fertilizer and pesticide residues, or meat from animals reared on organic feed.

in pots on a balcony. Children love growing plants, particularly if it's a quick process. **Try sprouting some mung beans**, for example. Put a handful of dried mung beans in a jam jar, fill it with cold water, place a piece of muslin over the top, and secure with an elastic band. Leave overnight, then drain off the water through the muslin lid. Rinse the beans with fresh water, then drain again. Repeat every 24 hours for a few days and see them shoot. They're delicious in salads or stir-fries, or as a nibble with other raw vegetables.

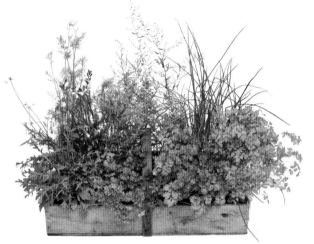

Buzzwords *to look out for*

We constantly see claims about the nutritional value of foods, both in advertisements and on packaging. The terms that are used seem to be offering something that's good for us – however, this may not always be the case, so it's worth taking a closer look.

Low-fat

Products labelled low-fat must have less than 3g per 100g fat in food or 1.5g (100ml) in drinks (or 1.8g/100ml for milk). However, many low-fat products are packed with sugar and thickeners to replicate the pleasant texture that fat provides, so they could be just as high, if not higher, in calories than the normal brand.

Light or lite

This means that the food must be 30 per cent lower in fat or calories than the regular product. It doesn't necessarily signify that it is a healthy option – light crisps could still contain as much as 22g fat per 100g, so are not low-fat.

Low-salt

The product must contain 25 per cent less salt than the standard product – but it may still contain quite a lot, so read the labels.

No added sugar

The product will not have any extra sugar added, but that doesn't mean there isn't any sugar at all – it could still be high in natural sugar from milk, fruit juice, or dried fruit, for instance. If it claims to be unsweetened it may still taste sweet from natural sugar but won't have added sweeteners of any kind. Sugar-free will not contain sugar but may have artificial sweeteners.

Fortified cereals

Many breakfast cereals are fortified with folic acid, vitamins B_1, B_2, B_3, B_6, and vitamin D. But a lot of them contain surprisingly high levels of sugar (more than 12.5 per cent of the total content), especially those aimed at children. The worst are sugar-coated types of cornflakes and own-brand chocolate rice cereals, which can be as high as 36 per cent.

Probiotic yogurt

Most fresh yogurts (but not the long-life ones) are live cultures, which are good for the digestion, but probiotic, or "bio", means that the yogurt contains specific beneficial bacteria such as lactobacillus, which may help maintain a healthy balance of bacteria in the gut (see pp36–37).

High in fibre

A food labelled as high-fibre must contain at least 6g fibre to 100g of the product.

Added omega 3s

Some eggs, bread, yogurts, and milk have omega 3 fats added (see pp24–25), but evidence suggests they may not be as effective as those in fish. For non-fish eaters and vegetarians, they may be worth considering – but check the other ingredients, too, as they won't always be healthier options.

The Glycaemic Index

How high is the GI?

High-GI foods (over 70)
Watermelon, dates, raisins, mashed and jacket potatoes, pumpkin, parsnips, swede, broad beans, white bread, puffed crispbread, rice cakes, cornflakes, sticky rice.

Medium-GI foods (55–70)
Grapes, mangoes, bananas, pineapple, sweetcorn, potatoes (not mashed and jacket-baked), couscous, wholemeal bread and pasta, oats, muesli, wholegrain and fruit breads, long-grain brown, white, and wild rice, bagels, pittas.

Low-GI foods (under 55)
Most other fresh fruits, prunes, dried apricots, avocados, sweet potatoes, tomatoes, green vegetables, peppers, peas, pulses, soya products, white pasta (cooked al dente), pearl barley, nuts, milk.

Watch out for high-GI
Carbohydrates (starches and sugars) are converted by the body into glucose to be absorbed into the bloodstream for energy. This raises the level of sugar in your blood. The Glycaemic Index (GI) of each food measures how quickly this happens compared (usually) with pure glucose, which is absorbed very rapidly. It is rated at 100, while foods with no carbohydrates, such as meat, are rated at 0 because they have little or no impact on blood sugar levels. Foods containing carbs are rated on the scale in between. High-GI foods are absorbed quickly, giving you a spike of energy that is followed by a slump, making you feel tired and often hungry again, so don't eat too many of these. Slow-absorption foods (low- or medium-GI) keep blood sugar levels fairly constant, providing sustained energy.

REALITY **CHECK**

 Some low-GIs are not good
Some foods, such as crisps and chocolate, have low GIs because they are high in fat and protein, which are absorbed more slowly.

 Some high-GIs are good
Jacket potatoes and fruit and veg with higher sugar are nutritionally good. Eat high-GIs with low- or medium-GI foods for balance.

 The sugar rush impact
Not all the glucose from high-GI foods can be used by the body, so insulin converts it to fat.

 The effect of processing food
Grinding grains to flour or cooking, mashing, grating, or puréeing food raises its GI as it is digested faster.

The impact of high-GI foods
The illustration below shows how your blood glucose level might fluctuate over the course of a day depending on your choice of slow-release (low- and medium-GI) and quick-release (high-GI) carbohydrates. Blood sugar slumps make you want to eat more often, leading to weight gain, while spikes of high sugar levels may cause damage to your arteries.

Slow release
Fast release

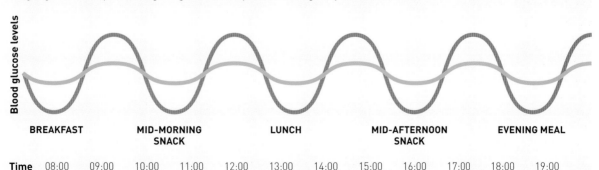

Blood glucose levels

| BREAKFAST | MID-MORNING SNACK | LUNCH | MID-AFTERNOON SNACK | EVENING MEAL |

Time 08:00 09:00 10:00 11:00 12:00 13:00 14:00 15:00 16:00 17:00 18:00 19:00

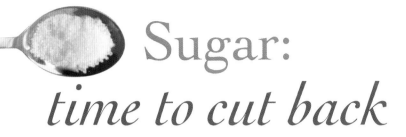

Sugar: time to cut back

Many people are unaware of how much sugar they're eating – not just the amount they add to a bowl of cereal or a hot drink but also the astonishing quantities hidden in processed foods and drinks. From tooth decay to obesity, the health risks are huge. It's time to take stock.

Why does it matter?

Some people seem to get away with eating a lot of sugar-laden foods without gaining weight. You might think this means they are not damaging their health, but appearances can be misleading. Consuming too much sugar potentially leads to high levels of blood fats called triglycerides, which can cause a condition called fatty liver and increase the risk of

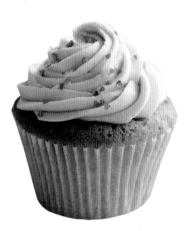

developing heart disease (see pp174–175). Sugar also affects energy levels and moods, and if you eat a lot it will play havoc with your mouth, too. Tooth decay isn't just cosmetic – teeth and gum problems cause mouth infections and may, if untreated, lead to certain cancers and heart disease. A diet high in sugar can also promote resistance to insulin, the hormone that regulates blood sugar levels, which can lead to diabetes (see pp172–173).

Empty calories

Most people who consume a lot of sugar do carry too much weight and are heading for obesity (see pp102–103). Added sugar and sugary foods may afford instant gratification, but this is soon followed by hunger and craving

for something more. Sugar is only 4 calories per gram (the same as protein), but these are known as empty calories because refined sugar doesn't contain any other nutrients. We do need some sugar, for energy, but the processed ones added to our food are just not necessary. We can get all the sugar we need from fruit, vegetables and grains.

Sweet treats

Sugary foods should be just an occasional treat. A square of chocolate with cocoa solids of 70 per cent or more is positively good for you, while a small slice of cake, made with wholesome ingredients (such as the carrot cake on p246), is a joy. Eating packets of biscuits or sweets daily, though, will damage your health.

Did you know?

4g sugar = (1 tsp)  35g of sugar in a can of cola = | | | | | | | | | (1 tsp x 9) =

70% adult limit for added sugar

117% 10-year-old child's limit

15g of sugar per **100g = High Sugar**

5g of sugar per **100g = Low Sugar**

How much is too much?

- The World Health Organization says added sugar (including honey and fruit juice) should not exceed 10% of our daily calories.
- US scientists estimate that we swallow 22 teaspoons of added sugar per day.
- The recommended maximum is about 12 tsp (50g) per day for women, 17 tsp (70g) for men, and 8 tsp (30g) for children.

The more sugar you eat, the more you want!

DIFFERENT NAMES FOR SUGAR

Fructose   **Lactose**
Dextrose   **Glucose**
Sucrose   **Manitol**
Maltose   **Sorbitol**

Hidden sugar

About 80% of all processed food products contain added sugar. Of those, fizzy drinks, fruit juices, and desserts make up 50%. Other culprits include breakfast cereals, tomato ketchup, bread, soup, and ready meals.

Sweet tips

Instead of refined sugar and processed sweet snacks, try these home-made alternatives.

For a **goody bag**, break off a few small pieces of organic chocolate, as opposed to additive-filled dayglo sweets, and add some chopped dried fruits and other little nibbles.

For **cakes and puddings**, replace the sugar with ingredients such as coconut shavings, almond milk, amaranth, agave, carrots, beetroot, or soaked and dried fruits (to name but a few).

Make your own sweets by melting organic, high-cocoa chocolate, dipping slices of fruit such as banana, cherries, dried apricots, or figs into it, then leaving them to set on a sheet of baking parchment.

Buy a bottle of **natural vanilla extract** – the type we use for baking – and take a quick sniff the next time you crave something sweet. This is a traditional remedy for taking away the craving – try it!

There are also some **liquorice teas**, which (if you like this love-it-or-hate-it flavour) can fulfil the desire for something sweet. Alternatively, try **spiced chai tea** (see p98), with milk added, or apple and cinnamon.

Eating *less salt*

We're told that too much salt is bad for us – but most of us think that if we stop adding salt to our food it will taste bland and boring. This need not be the case, since being clever with spices and herbs and cutting back on salt will allow the true flavours of our food to come through.

Why we need some salt

Salt, or sodium chloride, is found naturally in most foods (see p31). It is crucial for controlling the amount of water in our bodies and the acid/alkali balance in the blood. Salt also helps our muscles to contract and expand correctly and transfers nerve signals to the brain.

How much?

It is recommended that adults eat no more than 6g of added salt a day – that's a teaspoonful. Babies under a year old should have less than 1g of salt a day, since larger amounts may cause serious damage to their kidneys. They will get all they need from breast milk or formula, so never add salt when making your baby's food. Children aged 1–3 years need 2g salt a day; 4–6 years, 3g salt; 7–10 years, 5g salt. By not giving them salty foods, you will help to prevent them getting a taste for it, which could lead to high levels of consumption in adulthood.

Health issues

Too much salt raises blood pressure, which puts you at risk of health problems such as certain cancers, heart disease, or strokes (see pp174–175) and, at worst, heart failure. If you lower your salt intake your blood pressure will drop, reducing the risk.

Hidden salt

Some foods are particularly high in salt, including smoked meats and fish and processed meats such as bacon and salami. Other foods may surprise you with their high salt content, such as breads, soups, cheeses, prawns, bought sandwiches, pizzas and other ready meals, and breakfast cereals. But some are obvious as they taste so salty – crisps, yeast extract, canned anchovies, olives, soy sauce, and stock cubes among them. Check the labels: if sodium levels are given in grams, multiply by 2.5 to find the salt content.

Deficiency

Because our intake is so high, deficiency is rare. However, excessive sweating in very hot weather or from extensive exercise, severe vomiting, diarrhoea, or prolonged illness can cause levels to drop rapidly. Rehydrating salts and extra fluids may then be needed.

{ Cutting your daily intake of salt **by 2.5g – that's just ½ teaspoon** – could cut the risk of stroke or heart attack by a quarter. }

5 ways to eat less salt

1
Taste first
When you are cooking, don't reach for the salt automatically – add all the other flavourings you want first, then taste. Only add a few grains if absolutely necessary, and never before you've taken out a portion for your baby. At the table, taste first, too. Often freshly ground black pepper will enhance the meal better than salt.

2
Savour each mouthful
Eat slowly, so that your taste buds can explore all the complex flavours in your mouth, giving you the sensory satisfaction that comes from eating good food. Encourage children to enjoy their food, too, preferably without the distraction of TV or phones – if they hurry their meals now, and automatically add salt, the habit will last into adult life.

3
Use other seasoning
A little crunchy sea salt will give you better flavours than refined sea salt – or try sweet spices or chillies instead. Throw in herbs – plenty if fresh, or a sprinkling if dried. A good olive oil and balsamic vinegar or lemon or lime juice drizzled on a salad is also scrumptious.

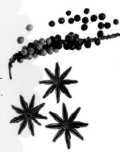

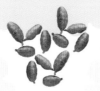

4
Read the labels
Be savvy when buying foods – compare the information on the packaging and consider going for those with less salt. There are now reduced-salt and no-added-salt varieties of items ranging from stock cubes to tomato sauce and cheese. You can also buy canned vegetables and pulses in water with no added salt (or sugar).

5
Eat healthier snacks
If you must have crisps, buy baked unsalted ones. Choose raw or roasted, unsalted nuts, too. Check packs of crackers and bread snacks, and opt for the lowest salt ones. Go for olives in oil, rather than brine, and try sun-dried tomatoes, perhaps with tiny balls of mozzarella, which are packed with flavour and need no seasoning.

Smoothies *and juices*

Glorious blends of fresh fruits and vegetables, smoothies and juices
are easy-to-drink ways of getting one or two of your five-a-day. Some
smoothies are nutritious enough for a meal on the go, now and then,
while juices are perfect for a sweet treat.

Whether you are in a hurry and haven't got time for a full meal, or you want a delicious, soothing concoction, or just a refreshing drink as an occasional alternative to water, smoothies and juices are a wonderful way of getting some great nutrition. If you have a fussy eater in the family, or a child who won't eat breakfast, whizzing up mixtures of fruit or vegetables can make it easy for them to take in a variety of nutrients. They taste delicious too. But they should never replace eating whole fruit and vegetables, and no matter how many you drink they will only count as one of your five-a-day. You need to eat the pulp and sometimes the skin and seeds of fruits and vegetables to get the fibre and full goodness from them. Smoothies are better than juice from this point of view because you use the whole thing, rather than just squeezing out the juice and throwing the pulp and fibres away. Children should also be encouraged to chew whole pieces of fruit or vegetables as soon as they have teeth as this helps develop their muscles and speech.

Crunching and chewing also helps strengthen children's teeth – another reason why smoothies should not act as regular meal replacements.

Watch the sugar

Smoothies and juices shouldn't be considered wonder drinks, as they can still give a sugar-rush (especially if drunk quickly). Even these natural sugars can cause dental erosion, and ultimately trigger tooth decay. Ease this sugar effect by diluting the ready-made smoothies and juices with a little water – babies and toddlers should have them diluted 1 part juice to 10 parts water.

Make your own smoothies

To make smoothies yourself, all you need is a blender. You can ensure that your own blends have good quantities of different fruits, such as berries, apple, banana, melon, orange, mango, or pear – some of the ready-made smoothies have a lot of apple and very little of the other fruits featured on the label. It's good to add some cow's or non-dairy milk (see pp26–27) or yogurt (a way to introduce

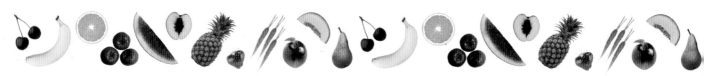

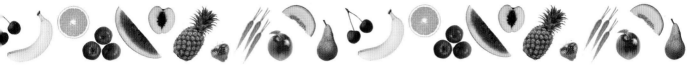

probiotic bacteria, see pp36–37). These add calcium but also a little protein, which slows down the absorption of the sugars from the fruits, so your smoothies won't give the sugar-rush of ready-made ones. Tomatoes, and vegetables such as beetroot, carrots, peppers, celery, and even salad leaves can all be blended together with a little water or apple or tomato juice. You can also add flavourings, such as herbs, fresh ginger, ground almonds, or seeds.

A little of what you fancy

When you whizz up a selection of fruit or vegetables, it makes quite a big glass. You don't need to drink it all at once – store it in the fridge to drink during the day. If it separates, just whisk to combine. For smaller children, serve just a small glassful with a straw. It not only makes smoothies seem fun but sucking through a straw also reduces contact with the teeth, which can help to avoid tooth decay.

Fruit and vegetable juices

To make your own juices you really need to invest in a juicer. This is expensive and only worthwhile if you use it regularly – but it is great for making vegetable juices in particular. If you prefer to buy ready-mades, long-life and non-chilled juices can, surprisingly, contain just as many nutrients as the freshly squeezed juices in the chiller cabinet. Watch out for juice drinks, such as squashes and cordials – they will be next to the pure juices but will be packed with sugar and other additives and may contain only a small percentage of juice. Apple juice has a lower GI value than other juices, so it will give

less of a sugar-rush (see p91). It is also good for soaking muesli or dried fruits overnight, or to use in cakes or fruit salad as a healthy sweetener. Don't forget, though, that juices and smoothies should be part of a meal or snack. Water should always be number one for quenching thirst (see pp38–39).

Breakfast berry boost

SERVES 1

Ingredients
150 g (5¹/₂oz) fresh and/or frozen mixed berries (such as blackberries, blueberries, and raspberries)
1 tbsp porridge oats
1 tbsp plain live yogurt
¹/₂ tsp clear honey (optional, and not for babies under one)
100ml (3¹/₂fl oz) milk, which could be any sort

Method
1 Place all the ingredients, apart from the milk, in a blender and whizz.
2 Add two-thirds of the milk and blend, adding more until you reach your preferred texture (100 ml/3¹/₂ fl oz is only a guide).
3 Pour into a glass, serve with a straw, and enjoy straightaway.

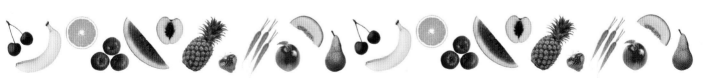

Coffee *and tea*

A cup of tea can be both delicious and restorative, and the same can be said for a cup of good coffee. Drinking tea, whether black, white, or green, is also an easy way to add to the amount of antioxidants and other phytonutrients (see pp32–33) that you get from your food.

Tea and coffee count towards your daily fluid intake, but don't neglect drinking simple, unadulterated water. If you want something warm, a cup of hot water with a slice of lemon is soothing and refreshing. Milky tea or coffee is also a good way to increase your dairy intake and can be a more gentle way to get your body going in the morning rather than drinking them black. But be warned, the caffeine in tea and coffee can prevent the absorption of iron (in breakfast cereals, for example), so it's better not to drink either with your meal.

While caffeine is a stimulant that can temporarily give you a buzz, too much can cause you to feel jittery and anxious. As a mild diuretic, it can also make you need to pass urine more often. Women should limit their intake during pregnancy (see pp70–71)

as high levels of caffeine can cause miscarriage or low birth weight, and when breastfeeding, caffeine in the milk may keep the baby awake. Go for decaffeinated or no-caffeine teas and coffees.

Herbal teas

To make, infuse a big pinch (or a bag) of fresh or dried leaves in a small pot of boiling water for 3–5 minutes, then strain into a cup.

• **Lemon verbena** is thought to help digestion and alleviate stress. It has a refreshing lemon flavour.

• **Rooibos** (red bush) from South Africa is not technically a tea but a legume. It's caffeine-free. Choose good-quality leaves, as some cheaper brands taste musty.

• **Camomile** is a delicious dried flower to infuse in hot water. Although you can buy it in tea bags, the whole dried flowers taste far richer and the sedative and calming effects are more potent.

• **Mint** sipped after a meal, sweetened with a little soothing honey, can ease digestion. Spearmint is gentlest. If you have acid reflux or a stomach ulcer, peppermint can aggravate it.

Chai

Indian chai is a wonderfully spiced, traditionally milky, tea – perfection in the middle of the afternoon, and a great way to get older children to take milk. By making your own you can tailor the spices (adding ginger or star anise, for example) to your taste.

1 Put ½ cinnamon stick, 6 cracked cardamom pods, 4 whole cloves, and 3 black peppercorns in 2 teacups of water in a saucepan. Bring to the boil.
2 Reduce the heat and simmer for 10 minutes. Add 3 cups of milk and bring up to simmer again. Add 3 tsp loose black tea, cover, and turn off the heat.
3 Infuse for 2 minutes, then strain and add sweetener to taste. It is delicious warm, or cooled and served with ice.

Caffeine hit

As coffee has more caffeine than tea, even one cup can have a greater effect (see the Caffeine-o-meter, below right). If the coffee is strong, it will provide a really powerful caffeine hit of the sort provided by energy drinks, which may make you feel more hyped-up than you want. However, you may find that a cup of coffee in the morning is the perfect way to get your body (and a sluggish bowel) going. Some people love an espresso after dinner, but that would keep others awake all night. While it's a personal choice, it's best not have too much (see top right). When you do have coffee, make it a delicious, good-quality one to savour – you'll be more conscious of how much you drink. Sipping a glass of water alongside it helps cushion the caffeine effects, too.

Hot chocolate is low in caffeine but high in theobromine, a mild stimulant that relaxes muscles and lowers blood pressure.

Heart health

A recent study suggested that four or more cups of coffee a day might lower risk of heart failure. Polyphenols in tea and coffee (see pp32–33) may protect against heart disease, but caffeine can increase blood pressure, so moderation is best.

Brain power

Some studies suggest that being a coffee drinker may reduce the risk of developing dementia, but it is not yet known whether drinking more coffee might help further.

Bone density

Although caffeine inhibits calcium absorption, as long as you have a good calcium intake (see p30), drinking coffee and tea in moderation should be fine. But if you need to improve your bone health, think about switching to decaf or caffeine-free varieties.

Children's choices

Full-strength tea, coffee, and cola aren't suitable for young children as they can affect behaviour, sleep patterns, and energy levels. A mug of milk with just a tiny splash of tea or coffee (ideally decaf) is fine, and it's fun for them to share a cup of chai with you.

REALITY **CHECK**

✓ *How much caffeine?*
There is no set limit for healthy adults but general advice of around 400mg caffeine a day is sensible: see the Caffeine-o-meter below.

✓ *Caffeine when pregnant*
Consume no more than 200mg caffeine a day during pregnancy. That is 2 regular mugs of instant coffee, or 2 cups of tea and a small bar of plain chocolate.

Caffeine-o-meter

Mug of filter coffee
140 mg

Mug of instant coffee
100 mg

Can of energy drink
80 mg (can be far higher)

Cup of tea
75 mg

Single espresso
70 mg

Regular latte
40–75 mg

Plain chocolate (50 g / 1³/₄oz)
50 mg

Can of cola
40 mg

Green tea
40 mg

Milk chocolate (50 g / 1³/₄oz)
25 mg

Watch your *alcohol*

For many of us, having a drink or two with friends is one of life's pleasures. However, regularly drinking more than the recommended guidelines can seriously damage your health. You don't have to give up alcohol altogether – just be aware and take steps to keep it in check.

Alcohol and the individual

While there are guidelines as to how many units of alcohol women and men can drink without risk to their health (see far right), these don't allow for how alcohol affects you individually. We don't all have the same metabolism, and only you can judge how you feel drinking the amount you do – even if it's within the guidelines. Women in particular find that once they have the responsibility of children, or are experiencing any period of unusual stress, even the smallest amount of alcohol makes them feel below par, less likely to sleep well, and more likely to wake up shattered.

What is a unit?

A unit equals 10ml (or 8g) of pure alcohol, which is what an average adult's liver can process in one hour. Because we now tend to have bigger wine glasses, and

{ Up to **17 million working days** are lost in the UK each year due to the **effects of alcohol**. But drinking in **moderation** should have no adverse health risks. }

stronger drinks (with a higher ABV, or alcohol by volume), it's hard to know just what a unit is.
• **Spirits:** single pub measure (25ml) = 1 unit.
• **Alcopop:** small (275ml) bottle (5% ABV) = 1.4 units.
• **Wine:** small (125ml) glass (12% ABV) = 1.5 units. Large (250ml) glass (12% ABV) = 3 units.
• **Beer/lager/cider:** 1 pint lower-strength (3.6% ABV) = 2 units; higher-strength (5.2% ABV) = 3 units.

Red wine: truth or myth?

Red wine has been found to contain antioxidants, such as resveratrol, thought to have

several health benefits, including lowering the impact of a high-fat diet. However, the studies were done in a laboratory, using the chemical resveratrol rather than red wine. So although one or two glasses may be fine, we can't assume that drinking plenty of red wine will reduce the risk of heart disease. The harmful effects of too much alcohol – including liver problems, reduced fertility, high blood pressure, and the risk of several cancers – far outweigh any benefits. Rather than choosing an alcoholic drink based on the antioxidants it contains, go for the one you enjoy and keep the quantity down.

Nutritious nibbles

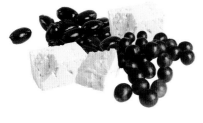

* **Stuffed cherry tomatoes** Cut the tops off the tomatoes and scoop out the seeds. Add a piece of ripe avocado and fill with tabbouleh. Drizzle with extra virgin oil.

* **Celery with goat's cheese** Trim and wash sticks of green celery. Spread soft goat's cheese all along the groove in each stick, then cut into 2.5cm (1in) lengths.

* **Feta, grapes, and olives** Cut cubes of feta cheese and arrange in a dish with stoned olives and seedless grapes. Spear with cocktail sticks.

* **Cucumber with nut butter** Cut 1cm (½in) chunks of cucumber. Scoop out most of the seeds. Fill with nut butter (see p185) and sprinkle with a little cayenne pepper.

* **Wet walnuts** Available for a short season around Christmas – simply shell and enjoy their creamy freshness. Or serve shelled, raw nuts of your choice with pieces of dried pear or some pieces of crisp apple.

* **Quick avocado dip** Mash a peeled, ripe avocado and flavour with lemon juice, a splash of Worcestershire sauce, and chilli flakes. Serve spooned on oatcakes.

Drink plenty of water

Alcohol acts as a diuretic, causing you to lose water from your body by needing to pass urine more often. Consequently, it's a good idea to alternate your alcoholic drinks with a glass of water or a soft drink so that you don't get dehydrated. If you eat beforehand, alcohol absorption is slowed, too.

Avoid salty snacks

Salty nibbles may be tempting, but they'll make you thirsty and so encourage you to drink more. They also tend to be high in fat. A packet of unsalted nuts and raisins or a sandwich are better snack options at the pub. For a treat at home, try some of the delicious, nutritious nibbles above.

Alcohol and weight

Not only does alcohol have nearly as many calories as fat, but it also increases the appetite. It reduces your willpower to resist unhealthy foods and may make you less inclined to spend time preparing healthy meals instead, which won't help if you're watching your weight. People who are underweight can find that alcohol makes them more anxious. If you have weight worries, it's best to give alcohol a miss for a while.

Easy ways to cut down

Have smaller measures; go for lower-strength drinks (the ABV level is on the bottle); and sip and put your glass down rather than holding onto it and drinking fast.

REALITY **CHECK**

✓ *Men*
UK guidelines are that men should not regularly drink more than 3–4 units a day, with preferably two alcohol-free days a week. They should avoid binge-drinking (more than 8 units in a single session).

✓ *Women*
Alcohol intake should be no more than 2–3 units a day on a regular basis, with preferably two alcohol-free days a week. Women should avoid binge drinking (more than 6 units in a single session).

✓ *Trying for a baby*
Avoid alcohol, as it can cause loss of zinc and folic acid and may damage the sperm, egg, and foetus before you realize you're pregnant.

✓ *Pregnancy*
UK guidelines are to avoid alcohol as it can seriously affect the baby's development. If you choose to drink, have no more than 2 units once or twice a week.

Children's *weight*

Many more children are overweight than was the case a generation ago. If this goes unchecked, they will remain that way as adults, which could mean health problems. To maintain a healthy weight for their height, you can help your child make small but significant changes.

Why are more children becoming overweight?

Many children today lead much less active lives than previous generations, spending more time in front of the computer and TV than playing outside. Eating habits have changed, too. Lots of families have lost the confidence and skill to cook – or simply don't think they have the time – so they may reach for ready-made meals and takeaways, which can be high in fat, salt, and sugar. Snacking on high-calorie foods has also increased, and that's down to the huge and tempting array available.

What is a healthy weight?

You may not be sure whether your child is overweight. Health professionals use the BMI (body mass index) to judge whether someone is obese, overweight, underweight, or a healthy weight. The BMI uses the ratio of a person's weight compared with their height, and takes gender and age into consideration. You can plot your child's BMI on a chart but it's easy to miscalculate, so it's better done by your GP or health visitor. Alternatively, you can use the BMI calculator on a reputable website, such as the NHS, and continue to check it every few months to see whether your child is making progress if they do need to lose weight.

Why does it matter?

Studies have shown that children within the healthy weight range tend to be fitter and more self-confident, suffer from fewer illnesses, are better able to learn, and are less likely to be bullied at school. Overweight children who remain overweight as adults risk serious health problems, including heart disease, type 2 diabetes, osteoarthritis, and some cancers.

Time to talk

If your child is starting to gain too much weight, take a moment to look at the reasons why. Is it because he or she is eating the wrong things when they're not at home, and getting too little exercise? Or could it be that something has changed at home or school that is causing them to comfort eat because they're feeling upset? Try to talk to them about it so that you can work things through together.

Lead by example

Maybe you are serving take-aways and ready-meals more than you used to, or you may have become more sedentary. Think about any such habits that have crept into your own routine and cut them out, so that you can get back on track together. Try to take exercise as a family, making it enjoyable for all (see p105).

What to do

Eat together

It might not be possible to share every meal with your child every day if you're a working parent, but when you are at home, try always to at least sit with them while they have their meal to support them in good eating practices, such as eating slowly and enjoying their food. Ask carers to do the same in your absence.

Look at your meal patterns

Every child differs, with some more hungry in the morning, others preferring to eat more later on. Bearing in mind their habits, it's a good idea to get a structured eating pattern going, with three meals a day and a small, healthy snack mid-morning and afternoon.

Avoid distractions

If children have their meal while watching TV or playing a game, their brain doesn't recognize that they are eating and they'll continue to take far more than they need or really want. Make eating a social thing to enjoy, so that they notice and appreciate the food they are having rather than just satisfy their hunger.

Child portions

We tend to judge portion sizes from habit. We can guess how much a child needs, but we may be giving them too much (see portion sizes on p61). A small plate is better than an adult one. If your child wants seconds, suggest they wait a few minutes for the food to go down. If they are still hungry, give them some more.

Going shopping

Many children are bored by everyday shopping trips, but if you involve them in choosing the family food they're going to share, they'll be more likely to take an interest. Encourage them to watch and join in as you cook, too, so they can see that food is a sensory and fun thing and should be treated with respect.

Make it yummy

Children aren't going to enjoy a bland skinless chicken breast and a salad without a dressing. Try to make the main proteins and ingredients interesting and delicious, perhaps with a sauce or relish, but balance them with vibrant and fresh-tasting vegetables that are cooked simply, so that not everything is saucy and fatty.

Make it colourful

Try to present a colourful plate that entices your child to eat and at the same time gives them lots of different, satisfying colours and textures of nutritious foods to help them lose weight. Use pp12–13 and pp34–35 to explain to your child what the food groups are and why everyone needs to eat them.

Have you finished?

Don't always insist that your child finishes everything on the plate before they leave the table. But when they say they've had enough, explain that once they've left the table, the meal is finished. Otherwise they just get into the habit of coming back to the kitchen for too many unhealthy snacks.

Helping an *overweight child*

Children who are overweight are usually aware of it, but need your support to help them lose weight. Let them know how much you love them, whatever they weigh, that you want them to be fit and happy, and that you'll take action together.

Little changes, big results

Weight control can be hard for anyone, but it's especially so for children, who don't have as much experience of actions in the present producing good results in the future. They do often respond well to incentive charts with rewards for meeting targets (though of course you should find non-food ways of rewarding success). You shouldn't put your child on a slimming diet – it's all about changing eating habits to healthy, balanced meals that incorporate all the food groups (see pages 12–13). Swap out high-calorie, fat, salt, and sugar foods for healthier alternatives, including plenty of fruit and vegetables – even little changes can make a big difference. There will always be situations when children want, or need, to veer off course – birthday parties and school trips, for example. They should still be able to enjoy themselves with all the other children and then, the day after, return to the healthy eating habit.

Speak to relatives

Grandparents often like to hand out sweets and other treats. That's fine now and then, but plead with them not to overdo it. Explain what you're trying to achieve as a family, and lay down some simple ground rules about what can and cannot be given. This can ruffle feathers initially, but it's worth it in the end if they can find non-food ways to show their love for their grandchild.

School food

Despite the efforts made by some schools to provide nourishing lunches, many children are still coming home ravenously hungry, grumpy, and tired, having eaten something unsuitable for a child's nutritional needs, such as just a plate of chips. It's a hard nut to crack, as school meals aren't an easy subject for negotiation. If necessary, express your concerns to your child's teacher or the head of the school and, as a back-up plan, request that you can send in your own food. Some schools may be reluctant to let you do this, but if you do have concerns, hold your ground and insist that you provide the food for your child's lunch. See pp62–63 for tips on easy and nutritious packed lunches.

"I'm starving"

Pre-empt your child coming out of school famished by packing a little bag of nourishing goodies – a selection of dried fruits, little rice cakes, a couple of cubes of cheese, and some apple slices, for example – and have a little bottle of water for them to drink alongside, as the combination usually hits the mark. Some raw veggies, such as cherry tomatoes, carrots, and cucumber, can also be good, especially if the journey home takes a while. It sounds like a lot of organization, but once you get into the habit it's easy and all these little things will soon add up to big changes in your child's weight. With healthy snacks to hand, you can resist the pressure to call at shops for sweet or fatty stopgaps on the way home.

Exercise is essential

Exercise is not only effective for burning excess calories – it also produces endorphins, the so-called "happy hormones", which can help your child feel energized and positive about his or her body. It provides a distraction from eating through boredom, too. Your child should have a minimum of an hour's exercise of at least moderate intensity every day to improve their muscle strength, flexibility, and bone health. Pre-adolescent girls in particular may feel self-conscious about their body and regard sport as unfeminine. Encourage other activities such as brisk walking, cycling, dancing, or skating, and make a point of taking exercise as a family, so that it becomes an enjoyable shared activity.

Weight-control tips

✳ Cut out all sugary, fizzy drinks. Dilute fruit juices with plenty of sparkling water to give as a treat instead.

✳ Make sure your child drinks 6–8 small glasses of water or other non-sugary fluid a day. It takes the edge off hunger, too. See p39 for ways to jazz up water.

✳ Instead of whole milk on cereal, provide semi-skimmed milk for two-year-olds onwards or skimmed milk from the age of five. Up to the age of two, children need whole milk.

✳ Grill more and fry less. When you do fry, use a non-stick pan, keep the oil to a minimum, and drain food well on kitchen paper.

✳ Choose lean meat and high-quality sausages with maximum levels of meat. Cheap sausages contain a lot of fat and rusk.

✳ It's not necessary to reach for the low-fat cheeses; just use a cheese slice instead of cutting large chunks, so you serve less.

✳ Grate hard cheese to put in sandwiches and use a strong one for sauces, as a little then goes a long way.

✳ Children's flavoured yogurts and fromage frais often have high sugar levels – go for plain and add your own compôte.

✳ Low-fat yogurt isn't always best: a full-fat plain Greek yogurt is very satisfying. Add fresh fruit for some sweetness, or a little honey (if over one).

✳ Steer your child away from cakes and biscuits, and other high-fat and sugary snacks, except as a once-a-week treat.

✳ Home-made soups, packed with vegetables, can be a real lifeline, filling an "I'm hungry" stomach in no time.

✳ Vegetables are great fillers. As long as your child is eating enough daily carbs, protein, and dairy, allow them as many vegetables as they want.

✳ If your child won't eat salads without a dressing, use just a little – the plus of eating the veg outweighs the added fat.

✳ Include pasta, rice, potatoes, and other starchy foods in your child's diet, as they need them for energy, but also serve a plentiful array of vegetables.

✳ You don't need to add butter or olive oil before serving starchy carbs, though, as this piles on unnecessary calories.

✳ Think of eggs as your ally, as they're a wonderful source of protein and can make a quick breakfast, lunch, or tea.

Teenage *weight gain*

In the teenage years, hormonal changes mean emotions can be in turmoil, which sometimes causes weight issues. One of the ways you can show your support is to have a fridge stocked with foods that will help your teenager find a healthy body weight they're happier with.

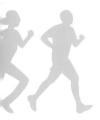

Parents have a far greater degree of influence over young children, from what they eat to how they lead their lives. Once children become teenagers, some of that good work can be temporarily lost if they feel peer pressure or start to struggle with body and life changes. If eating habits become erratic and unhealthy, for some the weight can start piling on. Take comfort that the good foundations you laid will eventually come back to help them – it just might be a few years before they thank you!

Care and share

Keep trying to talk to, and eat with, your teenager. Comfort eating during this tumultuous time is quite common, so try to keep a stock of nourishing snacks in the house. Baking some, too, will reinforce the message of your love and support, with enticing aromas in the warmth of a familiar kitchen encouraging your teenager to sit with you to eat and to talk, so that you can keep the communication channels open. (Turn to pp240–247 for some delicious home-baking recipes.)

Finding the balance

Overplaying any weight issue doesn't help, as it can make your teenager feel uncomfortable talking to you about the subject. Equally, if they have plucked up the courage to ask you for help, it's not a great idea to tell them they look fine if they are clearly carrying too much body fat.

Sensitivity and support

If a mum – or dad – obsesses over their own weight, it can rub off on their children. If your teenager tells you that they feel fat, try to step out of your own shoes and listen to them. Provide as much support as you can, and put great, nutritious meals on the table, which will help them to achieve their goals as far as weight goes.

Ditch the junk foods

Even if the rest of the family are not overweight, it's best not to have crisps, chocolates, junk food, and sugary, fizzy drinks in the house as they'll be hard to resist. Instead, stock up on healthy snacks (see p43 and p62 for some quick tips) and drinks (see pp38–39), and the whole family will benefit.

Family meals

The best thing you can do is to eat nourishing food together as a family and encourage everyone to sit around the table to eat without the distractions of mobile phones or television. By eating slowly and savouring the food, your teenager is more likely to feel nicely satisfied after the meal and more likely to notice that they don't need unhealthy snacks and nibbles in between. It's also a good time to talk together and maybe find out a little about what's going on in their lives.

Everyone together

It's not a good idea to isolate your teenager by giving them a piece of chicken and a salad when the rest of the family is tucking into something they'd much rather be eating. Cook healthy, nutritious meals that work for everyone, and just keep an eye on portion sizes (see pp64–65).

Get them involved

By planning recipes, going shopping, helping you to cook, or doing some of the cooking themselves, teeenagers will see how nourishing, healthy food can help them to feel good about themselves and look good, too.

Teach them some dishes

Make time to show your teenager how to rustle up a few quick healthy dishes – something as simple as an omelette, say, or chunky soups, or great, big satisfying salads with extra ingredients such as pulses or roasted vegetables. They particularly enjoy making something that they can then tuck into in a big bowl.

Insist on breakfast

Breakfast helps to get moods and energy levels off on a good note, even if it's sometimes just a home-made smoothie with fruit or oats added (see pp97 and 191). Have eggs, wholegrain cereals, and interesting breads to hand, and a big bowl of fresh fruit so at least your teen can grab a couple of pieces to eat on their way out.

Eating out

Choose restaurants with a wide variety of healthy, interesting choices that your teenager will enjoy – steaming bowls of Japanese-style noodles in a fresh broth, for example, or dishes of grilled meat, poultry, or fish with temptingly fresh and colourful vegetables or a salad.

Getting some exercise

Your teenager may like the idea of team sports, but feel too anxious about how they'll look in sports gear. If so, look for alternatives such as dance or swimming – anything they'll enjoy – so that exercise isn't something to avoid (see pp114–115).

More about boys' bodies

It's not just girls who may worry about their body shape – boys, too, can feel under pressure. In an age when extremely fit, muscular models, actors, and sports stars air their torsos in advertising and the media, a young boy on his way to becoming a young man can start to have problems working out what he should be doing to gain a torso he's proud to show.

Confusion as to what to eat in order to achieve this so-called perfect male body is rife among teenage boys, especially when they see so many protein shakes on the shelves. They may easily get the impression that they need to start drinking these and eating whole chickens to bulk up. In fact, a muscular male body comes from eating an all-round healthy diet and exercising.

If your son is struggling to lose weight, perhaps having filled out more than he's comfortable with, give him just as much support as you would a daughter in a society where she is bombarded with pictures of skinny models and celebrities. Boys and young men can be affected just as much by what they see in the media, but you can give them the confidence and good health to negotiate their own path.

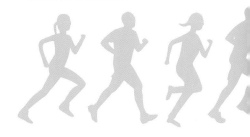

Is my child *too light?*

Having a preteen or teenager who has got into a place where they are
not eating enough, starting to lose too much weight, and struggling
with their body image, can be an anxious time. Emotional eating issues
are not easy to tackle, but a few things can make a big difference.

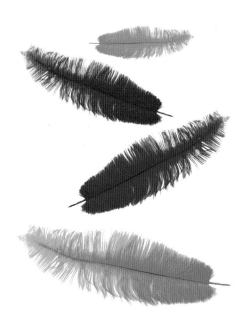

I f your older child or teenager, whether a boy or a girl, has got
themselves on an emotional roller-coaster where food is an issue
and they risk losing too much weight, it's clearly a matter of some
concern – but the suggestions here may help you all to get through this
problem and come out the other side without the situation developing
into anything more serious. They may also limit the effect that having
someone in your family with eating problems has on the rest of you, as
this can often become a pretty miserable time for everyone involved.
We are not talking here about serious eating disorders, as they need
specialist professional help, but instead about **taking early steps** to come
to the aid of a teenager or preteen who has got into a difficult unhappy-
with-eating space.

The classic advice used to be to persuade a child who has lost weight
and is clearly struggling with body image to start eating high-calorie
foods to get their weight back up. Mums often worry that perhaps they're
not serving enough food, or food that is too low-calorie, or that they've
been passing on their own issues about weight to their child. It's easy to
overreact and start to make cakes and and an array of substantial,
feeding-them-up foods, but in fact **offering light meals is the best way
forward**, since it's rarely a lack of fattening foods that makes someone
lose weight this way. It's more likely that for a variety of reasons your
child is not feeling comfortable about eating fatty – what they perceive to
be "fattening" – foods. You may notice that they leave them on the plate
or skip meals, finding reasons not to join you. The worst-case scenario is
that they just stop eating with you altogether. To prevent this from
happening, **persuade them to stay at the table** but give them simple,

nutritious foods as part of your family meals. They may not eat as much of the carbohydrate-rich starchy foods as the rest of the family or tuck into the sauces or desserts, but rather than worrying about this it's usually more constructive to think of the bigger picture of getting them to **eat regular, if light, nourishing meals** with ingredients such as roast chicken, or a joint of lean, honey-roast ham, thinly sliced, with a selection of different salads or vegetables.

> Puberty and the teenage years can be a tough time, and a child trying to exert some control over what they will and won't eat is one of many ways for them to experiment with boundary-pushing.

Have some delicious wholegrain bread, steamed new potatoes, or brown rice to fill up the rest of the family and also there on the table just in case your child feels comfortable having a little – but don't force it. The key is for you to be **calm and supportive**, not stressed. It's not a good idea to pile up plates. You may find it better to have serving dishes on the table so everyone helps themselves (or you help them) to the amount they wish to eat.

Your child will gradually become more comfortable about joining you at the table, especially if mealtimes are not a source of pressure. **Sitting together, eating and chatting in a relaxed way** as a family, may give you an insight into what's leading your child to feel insecure about their body or making them unhappy; something significant may be just dropped into the conversation as a throwaway comment. Even if they eat a limited diet for months, as long as they still have their meals with you, their anxiety about food is likely to pass as a phase rather than develop into a full-blown eating disorder.

As with any teenager, if you're eating out together, choose places where you know your child will find food they're comfortable with. Avoid having a battle in public at all costs, as this will only make things worse and ruin what was intended to be an enjoyable occasion. If you know that eating out is going to be a source of distress, find something else to share as a family instead.

Always keep in mind that not all teenage issues lead to a serious eating disorder, such as anorexia or bulimia. The more laid-back you can be and the more you can **keep the avenues of communication open** and share meals together, the less likely it will be that a serious problem follows. Stock up the fridge and cupboards with plenty of **nutritious things your child feels comfortable eating**, such as skimmed milk, low-fat yogurts, lean proteins such as chicken, lots of salad, and fruit. A tempting vat of home-made soup that they can quickly heat up, to have with a slice of wholegrain bread, is also a good idea. Ask your child to **make a list of foods** that they are happy to eat so that you can accommodate as many of these as possible in your family meals. If you suspect that despite your best efforts your child is still struggling to eat much at all, or that they have been binge-eating and making themselves sick, then **seek professional advice** right away. You may need to go and see your GP on your own first to discuss your concern, as your child may not yet accept that there is a problem. If professional intervention is necessary, some short-term therapy early on can help to nip the problem in the bud.

Weight issues *in adults*

Some of us may feel that we have always struggled with carrying too much weight, while for others it may happen as the body ages. Being overweight has many pitfalls for both health and self-esteem, yet even something as simple as a food and exercise diary could really help.

Excess weight has a habit of creeping up on us. All of a sudden, our clothes don't fit well any more and our body shape makes us miserable. This may be due to poor diet and lifestyle choices or, in mid-life, to hormonal changes. Women experience a fall in the production of oestrogen, and testosterone levels in men also drop – both of which can lead to middle-age spread (see pp74–77).

Apples and pears

When we put on body fat it tends to go either on the hips (pear-shaped) or on the waist (apple-shaped). Too much weight makes any of us more likely to be at risk of heart disease, diabetes, certain cancers, or arthritis, to name but a few. If, however, you are becoming fuller around the middle, you may be more likely to suffer from any of the above. So, if you look in the mirror or see from your tape-measure that an apple shape is forming, it's worth thinking about what you can do to get back in shape.

Keep a diary

A good start is to keep a food and activity diary, recording when and what and how much you eat, and how much exercise you're doing. After 7–10 days you will be able to see what kind of habits you have been adopting. If you can, work out why you've eaten or drunk something extra – was it for comfort, or de-stressing, or just because everyone else in the office has an afternoon biscuit? Genuine hunger is seldom the reason we eat many of the things we do, so we need to get back to trying to eat only when we're genuinely hungry. Your diary can be a very powerful tool in helping you to achieve a new, healthier regime, and even to say no when offered those biscuits or cakes in

Don't delay, fill in your diary today

Date and time	Food and drink consumed	Quantity	Exercise
Remember to fill in your diary every day, and not just main meals but any nibbles, too.	Give as much detail as possible about ingredients, too. Add specifics if you made it yourself, but even descriptions such as "oozing with butter" or "thickly filled" will remind you of exactly what you ate.	Be honest. Put "large" (or small) slice, for example, or "heaped" (or level) teaspoon.	Note all activity – for example, "walked to the corner shop", or "played tennis" – and how it made you feel.

the office or at home. It will really make you mindful of everything that you are eating and drinking, which can be amazingly effective.

Exercise is vital

Many of us just don't exercise enough. Your diary will tell you if you are one of those people. If so, you'll need to try to remedy this. See pp114–115 for lots of tips on how much you should be doing, and ways to achieve it that don't necessarily involve a hefty membership fee (although a gym can be hugely motivating).

Watch the fats and sugars

Look at your diary and see if you can cut down on the most calorie-dense foods – those highest in fats and sugar. Within a week of avoiding sweet things, other than fresh fruit, you'll probably crack the sugar desire. If you happen to be passionate about chocolate, you can still enjoy a couple of good-quality high-cocoa pieces once a week. You'll find more tips on cutting sugar on pp92–93. For fat, put only a scraping of butter, or similar, on bread. Don't butter toast when it's hot – you'll spread on more. Grill, bake, or poach rather than fry. To make mayonnaise lighter in calories, mix it with natural yogurt.

Portion control

Your diary will give you great insight into how much you really eat. Although you don't need to weigh foods all the time, it can be revealing to compare what you call a normal portion with the examples of the recommended quantities on pp40–41. Try using a smaller plate, so that you feel as if you are eating more than you actually are, and you should still feel satisfied. Cut your food into smaller pieces and take little mouthfuls. Eat slowly, chew well, and enjoy savouring the tastes and textures. Your brain will then get the right signals to register when you're full.

Check your water intake

Make sure you drink plenty of water (see pp38–39) to hydrate you and to help the fibre in your food swell in your stomach, which will give you the right fullness signals. We often think we're hungry when in fact we're thirsty.

Think ahead of the curve

Avoid the "I'm starving" moment by having a piece of fresh fruit mid-afternoon. As soon as you get home from work, picking up the kids, or whatever you were doing, make yourself a cup of tea – be this a milky black tea (chai can be

wonderful) or a herbal one (see p98 for ideas) – or a mug of miso or thin vegetable soup. Sit down and savour each mouthful.

Watch the alcohol

Alcohol is high in calories, so try to find other activities to share with your friends rather than going to the pub. The calorie count goes up if you factor in the nibbles you pick at with your drink, increase in appetite, and carelessness about what you eat that usually follows a few drinks. Even at home, depending on the size of your wine glass and the quantity in it, you can easily drink 200 calories per glass. Aim to have alcohol only with your meals, to digest with your food, and have a small amount of what you really enjoy, not more of a lower-calorie alternative. (For more about alcohol, see pp100–101).

Empower yourself

Make a list of positive reasons why you want to lose excess body fat, such as to feel fantastic in your body, to have more energy, or to feel more self-confident. Look at the list often to boost your willpower, and don't beat yourself up if you have a bad food day – this is a long-term strategy, so forget your lapse and move on.

Carrying too much *weight in later years*

If you have an elderly relative or close neighbour who is gaining too much weight and needs some support to help them reduce it, see what you can do to lend a hand. Maybe you could make them some satisfying meals, or help them shop for healthier options. There are other positive things you can do, too.

Cupboard check

Look at the store cupboard together and suggest suitable changes. Minimize unhealthy snacks and sweets. Hearty snacks between meals aren't necessary, but if grazing has become the norm, make sure there is a bowl of grapes or berries on the side to nibble between meals.

Sugar check

Cakes and biscuits are often favourite comfort foods, but a biscuit with a cuppa can be just a habit. Try suggesting a small serving of cut-up fresh fruit, which provides a natural sweetness plus added fibre and other important nutrients. Check sugar in drinks, too. If necessary, get a natural sugar substitute for sweetening.

Why lose weight?

Weight gain in the later years happens because the body digests food more slowly, often compounded by taking less exercise and eating too much. Carrying excess body fat will affect health, and could lead to diabetes, high blood pressure, strokes, and problems with mobility.

Home-cooked

Suggest simple meals, such as pasta with a tomato sauce, grilled salmon steak with potatoes and peas, or chicken breast simmered with veg in a little stock. Perhaps you could make some individual meals such as fish pie or slow-cooked vegetable casserole, to be eaten fresh or put in the freezer. Ensure they're labelled, with date and reheating instructions.

Light meals

If lunch is the main meal, healthy options for the evening could include poached or scrambled egg, baked beans, or sardines on toast with thinly sliced, deep red tomatoes, or a toasted lean ham and cheese sandwich with wholemeal bread. A nutritious soup is also easy – frozen veg such as peas can be added to ready-made soup to boost the fibre content.

Dessert dilemma

When it comes to puddings, creamy, often highly calorific desserts may have been a favourite choice. Encourage scrumptious but healthy alternatives, such as yogurt with some sliced banana, berries, dried fruit or fruit compôte, baked fruit with a simple custard, or canned fruit in its own juice.

Frozen meals

Providing you check the labels for ingredients, there are some excellent, nutritious, frozen ready meals that can be delivered to the door – some supermarket ranges are pretty good and relatively low in calories, too. Make sure freezer food is clearly organized, so that you keep on top of what needs eating and when. Check that meals are being reheated correctly, too.

Exercise

Exercise is important. On days when there's no particular outing planned, it's still good to take a stroll down the road and back. If it's not possible to go out, even walking round the home or doing some gentle exercises is better than sitting in a chair all day. It gets the heart going, blood circulating, and muscles working better.

Fruit and veg

For some, these can seem too much trouble, so it's good to have a colourful array of easy-to-handle, easy-to-eat fruit and vegetables, such as cherry tomatoes, salad leaves, grapes, berries, and ready-to-eat soft dried fruits. Make the most of frozen veg too, such as peas, broccoli, cauliflower, or mixed veg that can be cooked straight from the bag.

Daily *exercise*

For both adults and children, taking regular exercise goes hand-in-hand with eating a good diet when it comes to maintaining a healthy weight. Not only does exercising keep you fit, but many also find it one of the best stress-busters of all.

Which type of exercise?

UK guidelines recommend that, along with a healthy diet, we all need two types of exercise: aerobic activities, such as brisk walking, cycling, swimming, and jogging, plus muscle-toning/strengthening exercise, such as yoga, weight training, or pilates. Moderate aerobic exercise raises your heart rate, you'll breathe more quickly, and feel warmer, but you should still be able to talk at the same time. Vigorous exercise is more intense and you shouldn't be able to talk much at the same time. As well as reducing body fat and keeping you at a healthy weight, aerobic exercise produces endorphins in the brain (which give you the

feel-good factor); it can also lower your risk of developing diabetes, heart disease, and certain cancers. Muscle-strengthening exercise also increases bone density and improves your posture and body shape, which in turn boosts your confidence. If a workout at the gym isn't your thing, think about something more sociable, such as dancing or martial arts.

How much exercise?

A healthy adult should try to be active every day and do at least 1¼–2½ hours of aerobic exercise (depending on intensity) each week, plus a muscle-strengthening workout twice a week. Children should be encouraged to be active every day and, particularly if they

are under five, to minimize time spent watching TV or playing computer games. Young people aged 5–18 need at least an hour a day of vigorous and/or moderate physical exercise plus muscle-strengthening activities three times a week.

What should I eat?

If you are trying to reduce fat, a 30-minute workout before breakfast is good, provided you eat afterwards to ensure muscle recovery and to support your metabolism. If weight isn't an issue, have easy-to-digest carbs before exercise, such as porridge or a banana, for energy and vital antioxidants, which will all help your body to recover later.

Eating for energy

Is carb-loading helpful for long-distance athletes?

Athletes need a sufficient amount of stored energy (glycogen) in the muscles and liver to maintain a steady supply of energy for endurance events such as marathons. Eating plenty of starchy carbs beforehand (along with fibre, protein, essential fats, minerals and vitamins) is vital, since the sugars in carbs that aren't immediately used are stored as glycogen.

What about sports drinks and gels when exercising?

Sports drinks contain glucose and electrolytes. For short workouts and for recreational athletes neither of these is necessary – just sip water. If exercising for longer than 45 minutes, the use of a sports drink or gel can help you sustain your intensity and pace. However, if you are trying to lose weight, using sugary drinks is a bad idea as excess sugar is stored as fat.

Can eating a high-protein diet help bulk up muscles?

Protein builds muscle, provided you also do exercise to work the muscles – one without the other won't work. As a guide, if you want to bulk up, aim to eat around 1.5g protein per 1kg (2¼lb) body weight a day. Combine this with a diet rich in fruit and veg, essential fats, and slow-release carbs to ensure muscle repair and growth.

Why do you need protein after exercising?

You need protein to restore your muscles, ideally within 30 minutes of exercising. A natural smoothie, made perhaps from banana, oats, and almond milk, is best to give your muscles the fuel and amino acids needed, or you could use a commercial protein shake. If you don't stock up on protein, your muscles will start to break down – the opposite of what you want to achieve.

Early-morning exercise

If you are exercising first thing, have a snack such as a banana, a small pot of yogurt, or a home-made smoothie before your workout and eat your breakfast afterwards. You may find it easiest to take it with you in a plastic box, so that you can guarantee getting the nourishment you need straight afterwards when you're ravenous.

Exercising in the evening

If you prefer to exercise in the evening, have a substantial snack a couple of hours before starting – perhaps a bowl of soup, or a wholegrain sandwich and some sustaining fruit, such as a banana or some dried figs, or a slice of wholegrain bread spread with pure-fruit jam or a good nut butter (see p185). Afterwards, have a light meal such as a simple pasta dish or a salad niçoise with some steamed new potatoes.

Keeping hydrated

* Remember to keep your body hydrated by taking regular small sips of water from a bottle. While you're actually exercising, you need about 1 litre (1¾ pints) per hour.

* Unless you're training very hard, don't waste your money on sports drinks, which contain sugar, salt, and carbohydrates designed to cope with high-energy demands on the body. For normal exercising, you need only water.

* If you prefer flavoured water, infuse it with lime, lemon, peppermint, or cinnamon, or add a dash of pure fruit cordial, ideally with no added sugar. Coconut water is also very hydrating.

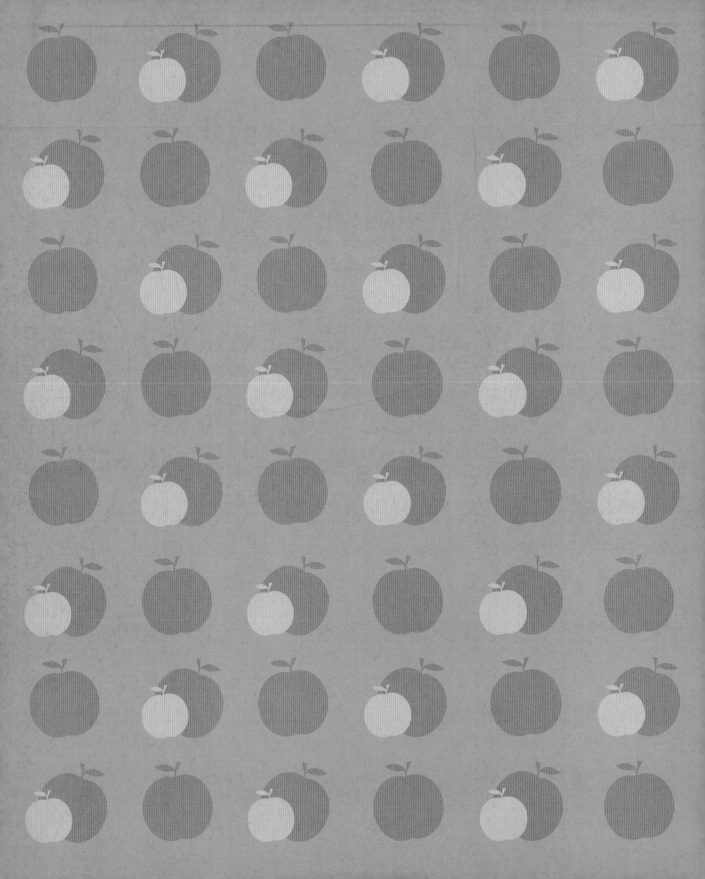

Different needs,
different diets

Feeding *vegetarians*

Many more people are veering towards a vegetarian diet. There are those who just prefer not to eat meat very often, and others who want to avoid any trace of meat, fish, and poultry, for all kinds of reasons. It's important for both that they have the right balance of nutrients.

Both children and adults can thrive as vegetarians as long as their diet is rich in all the essential nutrients. Some studies show that children brought up as vegetarians are particularly inclined to eat plenty of fruit and vegetables as adults, which makes them less likely to develop some types of cancer, heart disease, and excess weight. You should be especially careful, though, that children get the nutrients needed for their growth and development (see pp120–121).

Variety is vital

We all need protein for a strong immune system, for growth and repair of tissues, and for other essential functions. Animal proteins contain all the essential amino acids the body needs, and are known as complete proteins.

Most vegetable proteins lack a few of the essential amino acids, so you need to eat a mix of sources (see the chart opposite) – and, of course, you can get protein from dairy products.

Rich in protein

Good protein sources include lentils, chickpeas, and beans such as kidney, borlotti, and haricot – the type used to make baked beans (see p121 for a recipe). Seeds such as sunflower and sesame are ideal for sprinkling into salads, and there are many ways to get protein from nuts in your diet. Raw nuts (or roasted unsalted) are good staple foods to have in the house for snacks, to make nut butter (see recipe on p185), and to toast and scatter over salads, throw into stews, casseroles and stir-fries, add to smoothies and

crumbles, or sprinkle on natural yogurt with a drizzle of honey. Some grains – buckwheat, quinoa and amaranth – are complete proteins, so you don't have to mix them with other vegetable sources to get the protein you need. While only a small part of your diet, soya products are also complete. Tofu, for example, absorbs flavours well, so marinating it before cooking makes it tasty – try it sliced and grilled, or diced and fried in a herb-infused oil. You can also buy silken or soft tofu, which is indeed softer and can be eaten raw – it's useful for veggie bakes, dips, smoothies, and puddings, and has less salt than regular tofu.

Vitamins and minerals

A diet rich in pulses, wholegrains, nuts, seeds, vegetables, fruits, and dairy will give you a good range of

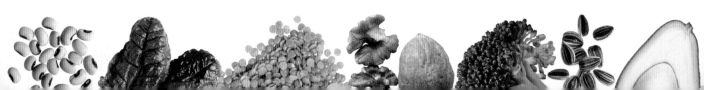

vitamins and minerals, but watch the calcium, iron, and vitamin B$_{12}$ levels in your food. If you eat dairy, eggs, yeast extract, fortified breakfast cereals, and soya milk, you will probably get enough vitamin B$_{12}$. If not, a supplement may be needed (see pp28–29).

Mighty minerals

Calcium is essential for strong bones and teeth (see pp30–31). If you eat dairy, you'll be fine. If not, you can get calcium from fortified soya, rice and oat milks, nut milks (especially those with added calcium), sesame seeds, pulses, dried fruit, almonds, and brown and white bread. You also need vitamin D (see p29) in order to absorb the calcium, so ask your GP about a supplement, especially in winter, when there's less of the sunlight that gives us vitamin D.

Without red meat, liver, and fish, in order to get enough iron you need at least two portions a day of iron-rich foods such as wholemeal bread, pulses, fortified breakfast cereals, dried fruits, and dark green vegetables. Have some vitamin C at the same meal, such as a lemon juice-based dressing or a small glass of pure fruit juice, to help with the absorption of iron.

Fine-tuning your fibre

Too little fibre is unlikely to be a problem for vegetarians, but too much may be. Excessive amounts of bran, from wholegrain husks, can put a lot of a substance called phytate in the body, which inhibits the absorption of iron. Plenty of water will help but, if struggling, substitute some white bread, pasta, or rice for brown, and don't add extra bran to food. A very high-

fibre diet can cause constipation, too. Always have a couple of glasses of water with every meal and snack (see also pp38–39 for how much water to drink daily).

Fats for health

Fats are vital for energy, warmth, heart health, and other benefits (see pp24–25). So eat fats from a variety of sources – dairy, nuts, seeds, avocado, and olives, for example – and watch that your diet doesn't become too dairy-heavy as this risks high levels of bad LDL cholesterol (see p174).

Ready-made

It's not good to rely on vegetarian ready meals as they can be high in fat, sugar, and salt. Try the recipes on pp212–231. If now and then you resort to ready-mades for speed, check the labels first.

5 winning ways to mix protein sources			
Recipes	**Pulses**	**Grains**	**Seeds and nuts**
Hummus with flatbread crisps (p224)	chickpeas	wholemeal	sesame (tahini)
Falafel burgers (p212)	chickpeas	wholemeal	—
Orzo risotto with pea pesto (p218)	peas	barley	—
Couscous-stuffed roast peppers (p226)	—	couscous (wheat)	hazelnuts
Apple and blackberry crisp (p235)	—	oats	almonds

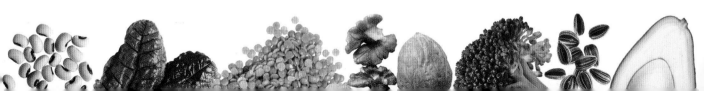

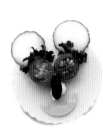

Young vegetarians *and vegans*

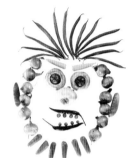

Children need enough energy and nutrients in their diet to grow and develop. This can be difficult on a vegetarian or vegan diet, but it can be done. If your child doesn't seem to be thriving and is grumpy and tired, action may be needed.

What they need

Vegan children have the same potential dietary deficiencies as vegetarians, but as they cannot eat dairy produce or eggs, they have more difficulty in getting enough calcium. Protein choices are more limited, too, so you need to be vigilant to ensure they get enough of both.

Eating little and often

Vegetarian and vegan children often eat plenty of fruit and veg, but you need to make sure they get the right balance of other foods, too. Plenty of variety across their three meals a day is the key to making sure your child gets enough nutrients. Remember to include a couple of nutritious snacks in between, too (see p43 and p62 for some ideas).

Too little iron?

Because the richest sources of easily absorbed iron are liver and lean red meat, your child needs to eat a plentiful mix of green leafy vegetables, bananas, nuts (not given whole to under-fives), wholegrains, pulses, sunflower seeds, and fortified breakfast cereals instead. Egg yolks are another good source for vegetarian children over one.

Calcium sources

Vegan children need vegetable sources of calcium (see p30): fortified soya, rice and almond milks, nuts, seeds, okra, green leafy vegetables, and dried fruits, such as apricots. Vegetarian children can also get plenty of calcium from cow's milk, yogurt and cheeses. They also need vitamin D to aid the absorption of calcium (see p29 for sources) – a vitamin D supplement may be necessary for vegans in particular.

Too much fibre?

Both vegetarian and vegan diets can be too high in fibre for young children, so they tend to feel full up before they've eaten enough nutrients. Try giving them some white bread, pasta, and rice instead of brown.

Proteins

Pulses, nuts, seeds, and soya products such as tofu are the best sources of protein, but it can be found in fruit and vegetables as well. Vegetarian children can also get protein from dairy products – and Greek yogurt can give them twice as much protein as regular.

Healthy baked beans

Serves 4–6

1 Heat 2 tbsp of olive oil in a medium-sized, heavy-based saucepan. Cook 1 small, finely diced onion in the oil for 5 minutes, until softened, not browned. Add 1 chopped clove of garlic, and cook for a further 1–2 minutes.

2 Add 350 ml (12 fl oz) passata, 1 tbsp tomato paste, 1 tbsp soft, dark brown sugar, 1 tbsp cider vinegar, 1/2 tsp Worcestershire sauce, 350 ml (12 fl oz) water, and season to taste. Reduce to a low simmer, and cook, uncovered, for 25–30 minutes, until the sauce thickens.

3 Use a hand-held blender to purée the tomato sauce to a smooth texture – puréeing the onion will also help to sweeten the sauce.

4 Add 2 x 400g cans of haricot beans, drained and rinsed, and continue to cook over a low heat for 10 minutes, until the beans are very soft. If the sauce reduces too quickly, add a little extra water. Check the seasoning, and garnish with chopped flat-leaf parsley to serve.

Cook's tip: if haricot beans are hard to find, try cannellini or flageolet beans.

Energy boosters

Give children high-calorie and high-protein nut butters, such as peanut, cashew, almond, hazelnut, and walnut on toast or rice cakes, or as a base for cakes. They can also be stirred into salad dressings and casseroles. You can buy nut butters or make them yourself (see p185). Seed pastes, such as tahini, can be added to hummus (see p224), stirred into potato salad, stir-fries, and pasta, or spread on bread and crackers. Bananas can provide a much-needed energy boost, too.

Oils, the good fats

Young vegetarians and vegans need vegetable oils as a source of omega 6 fatty acids, which are essential for growth, cell structure, and boosting the immune system. Olive oil is the classic choice, but avocado, nut, and seed oils are good, too.

Some vegetable oils are also rich in omega 3 fatty acids, but they aren't quite the same as those in oily fish and may not be as effective. Omega 3 fatty acids are vital for health (see p25), so make sure you provide them in the form of oils from linseed (flaxseed), rapeseed, walnuts, soya, and pumpkin seed. Have a little dish of a tasty oil such as walnut on the table for dipping bread in rather than using butter. Vegetarian children can also eat eggs enriched with omega 3.

Vitamin B₁₂

Getting enough vitamin B_{12} without animal produce is tricky. Deficiency can lead to a form of anaemia, which will make your child tired and listless. There is some in fortified soya milk, breakfast cereals, and low-salt yeast extract, but ask your doctor whether a supplement is a good idea.

Avocado – a superfood

Since avocados are high in monounsaturated "good" fats, protein, fibre, vitamins, minerals, and antioxidants, they are valuable as well as delicious. The rough-skinned Hass variety is black, while Fuerte is shiny and bright green. Both are best to eat when they are just ripe enough to give slightly if gently squeezed at each end. Slice the flesh into a salad, or whizz it up in smoothies; alternatively, mash it with a little lime or lemon juice as a dip with crudités or as a topping for jacket potatoes, drizzled with olive oil and sprinkled with toasted pumpkin seeds and just a little seasoning.

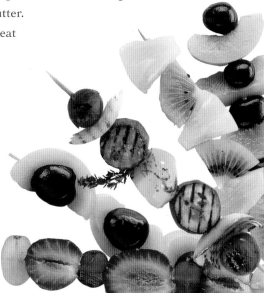

Fish facts

Eating fish offers huge benefits for non-meat eaters. Studies of Inuits, whose diet is based on fish, show they have a low incidence of heart disease compared with other societies. Further research has confirmed that if we too eat more fish – even just once or twice a week – it can help to reduce the risk of heart problems. It is also an excellent source of protein.

Oily or white fish?

Oily fish, such as salmon, mackerel, and sardines, are rich in the omega 3 fatty acids, which are known to be good for the heart and offer other health benefits, too (see pp24–25). However, these sea fish also carry varying levels of pollutants such as mercury, so don't eat more than four 140g (5oz) portions a week – or if you are trying for a baby, pregnant, or breastfeeding, only two portions a week. You can eat as much white fish as you like, except for sea bass, halibut, rock salmon (dogfish), bream, and turbot – these are affected by the same pollutants as oily fish, so the same advice applies.

Shellfish

While shellfish contains a lot of cholesterol, it will have little effect on the cholesterol in your blood (see p174). It is high in iron, both fresh and canned (as is all canned fish), so it's a good choice if you are not eating meat. Brown crab meat does contain pollutants, so it's best not to eat it too often.

Balance of protein

Don't eat fish to the exclusion of eggs, dairy, and vegetable proteins, such as pulses, nuts, seeds, and soya products. Egg yolks have a good iron content, too, and cheese and yogurt will provide calcium as well as protein. As always, a good variety is the key.

Happy to eat *fish*

Many a parent sighs with relief when their child is happy to eat fish, rather than avoiding animal products altogether. It does mean a greater range of food at home, and more choices on the menu when you eat out. Nutritionally, fish is superb, but don't eat it to the exclusion of valuable vegetable and dairy proteins.

Fish is rich in protein and essential fats.

Fish is versatile: steam, grill, bake, or stew rather than fry.

Make the most of canned fish, especially in water, oil, or tomato sauce, rather than in brine (to reduce salt). It is packed with essential nutrients, and if you eat the bones it is a great source of calcium, too.

Cutting out *red meat*

We are all recommended to cut down on red meat because of the high saturated fat content. Although it is a wonderful source of easily absorbed iron, there are compromises you can make in order to provide enough iron in family meals if someone doesn't want to eat red meat, or just doesn't like large amounts.

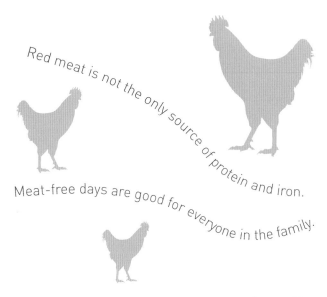

Red meat is not the only source of protein and iron.

Meat-free days are good for everyone in the family.

{ A diet without red meat is fine, provided you still get enough **protein** and **iron** from the other delicious sources available. }

Mixing it up

If you or your child don't eat red meat because you don't want to tackle a slab of juicy, possibly bloody meat, or you find it hard to digest, you could try using top-quality lean mince and mixing it with other ingredients instead. For instance, consider a home-made shepherd's pie with lots of wonderful vegetables and a rich, savoury sauce as the dominant ingredients, or a chilli con carne packed with red kidney beans, tomatoes, herbs, and spices, and only a small quantity of steak mince.

Enjoy poultry

Eaten without the skin, chicken, turkey, and other birds are wonderful low-fat alternatives to red meat. Although lower in iron, they are packed with protein and other nutrients the body needs, so eat them in conjunction with the iron sources suggested below.

Alternative iron sources

Lack of iron can be a problem in anyone's diet if they don't eat red meat, as this is the most easily absorbed form of the mineral (see p30). However, you can still get enough iron if you're careful to eat plenty of egg yolks, fortified breakfast cereals, fish, dried fruit such as prunes and figs, nuts, seeds, dark leafy greens, soya, and other pulses. The iron is absorbed better if you eat food rich in vitamin C at the same time (see p29 for sources).

Soya protein

For those who like the texture of meat but don't want to eat it, use soya mince instead of minced meat in any recipe. Often referred to as TVP (textured vegetable protein), this versatile substitute is high in protein and fibre, low in fat, and available as chunks, mince, sausages, burgers, or steaks.

Food allergies
and intolerances

In our society, the incidence of food allergies and intolerances is rising. As a result, daycare nurseries, schools, restaurants, food manufacturers, and the medical profession take the issue seriously, and it is now much easier to identify problems and find alternatives.

What is an allergy?

True food allergy affects about 2 per cent of the population in the UK, 8 per cent of them children under three. It is caused by the body's immune system mistaking the protein in a food for something harmful. It releases chemicals, especially histamine, to fight it, which triggers an allergic reaction.

What are the symptoms?

Typical reactions include swelling of the lips and around the eyes; itchy mouth, throat, or ears; hives (a raised, itchy skin rash); red, itchy eyes; vomiting; eczema; diarrhoea; runny nose; wheezing; coughing; or headache. Symptoms range from mild to severe, even life-threatening (see panel, right).

When does it start?

A food allergy can appear at any time but often begins early in life. As babies' immune systems are immature, they may overreact to certain substances. This is why some foods are avoided for first solids (see pp54–55) – and during pregnancy, if there is a family history of certain allergies, as babies are then more likely to develop them. Many, but not all, children outgrow their allergy.

Which foods are worst?

In children, the most frequent allergies are to milk (including standard formulas), peanuts, tree nuts, eggs, gluten (a protein in some cereals), soya, fish, and some additives (see p87). In adults, other culprits are fruits such as kiwi, apples, and peaches, celery, some roots and tubers such as parsnips or potatoes, sesame seeds, and yeast.

Seeking advice

Anyone with a food allergy, and particularly children, should receive specialist nutritional support, as it's far too easy to miss out on essential nutrients when you find specific foods are off limits. Your GP is the starting point for further advice.

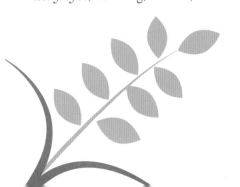

What is an intolerance?

A food intolerance is different from an allergy in that it is not linked with the immune system – it mainly involves the digestion. Unlike an allergy, where even a tiny bit of the allergen can trigger a reaction, an intolerance usually builds up more slowly and a problem food can be eaten in small, infrequent amounts without causing symptoms – though ultra-sensitive people may not be able to tolerate any, or only a little.

What are the symptoms?

Food intolerances can have some similar symptoms to food allergies and may often trigger symptoms of IBS (irritable bowel syndrome), with stomach cramps, tummy ache, constipation or diarrhoea, bloating, and wind. But intolerances are never life-threatening, and won't cause the symptoms of anaphylaxis (see right). You may be intolerant of several foods, which makes identifying the culprits very difficult, and it's often the case that people with food intolerances crave the offending food.

When does it start?

A food intolerance can appear at any time, so if your baby is unwell, check with your health visitor or GP. However, most intolerances don't appear until mixed feeding (see weaning, pp54–55) is well established, and they may set in at any time right up to, and through, adulthood.

Which foods are worst?

The most common offenders are wheat (pp130–131) and lactose (see pp126–127), but certain chemicals in other foods, and food additives, may also cause a reaction.

What should I do?

See your GP first of all. If major problems are ruled out, keep a food diary for a couple of weeks. Record everything that you eat and drink, including snacks, making a note of the approximate quantities and as many details as possible. List your reactions alongside. If you can identify a possible culprit, try removing it from your diet for a couple of weeks – always substituting a similar, nutritious food to ensure a healthy diet – then check again. Food intolerances may be short-lived, or they may stay with you. If the symptoms are mild, you can try reintroducing a little of the food at a later date, when you feel totally fit and healthy, to check if you can now eat it.

What is anaphylaxis?

Anaphylaxis is a life-threatening allergic reaction to a food or drink (or anything from a drug to an insect bite). Symptoms usually develop within minutes or up to an hour after eating, or even touching, the allergen. Initially, symptoms may be any of those listed left but they can lead to rapid swelling of the throat and breathing problems, the heart racing, a sense of impending doom, and a rapid drop in blood pressure, causing confusion and ultimately unconsciousness. The situation is very serious and frightening. The first time it happens, call an ambulance immediately and say you think it is anaphylaxis. Once that is diagnosed, an adrenaline injector will be given to carry at all times.

Be vigilant.
Read labels and look for the "hidden" allergen in everything you eat or drink.

Convince everyone you know.
Some people are still sceptical about food allergies. Convince them to take it seriously – anaphylaxis can be life or death.

Show them what to do.
Make sure that everyone you know can administer the adrenaline kit.

Don't hesitate.
If you see any sign of a severe reaction, use the the adrenaline injector and get to hospital fast.

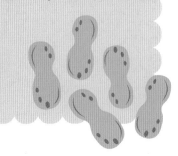

Cow's milk allergy or lactose intolerance?

The range of different milks in supermarkets shows just how many people are seeking alternatives to cow's milk. If you feel that you or someone in your family may be suffering from an allergy or intolerance to milk, it's important to know which of those conditions it might be.

Cow's milk allergy

Full-blown cow's milk allergy is caused by the immune system attacking the protein in milk. The allergy is most likely in babies and young children, but it can occur at any age. The good news is that it's uncommon, affecting only around 2 per cent of infants in the UK, and is much rarer in adults. Children usually grow out of it by the age of five. Reaction usually occurs within minutes of drinking milk. Particularly sensitive babies may develop the allergy through their mother's breastmilk, from the milk she has digested, but it's more common in families with a history of eczema or asthma.

There is another milk protein allergy that is sometimes called cow's milk protein intolerance, because it does not affect the immune system. Symptoms of that can take hours or even days to appear, and although they may be similar (see below), they will not include breathing problems.

What are the symptoms?

Symptoms are usually fairly mild but can be severe (see p125). They may include vomiting, diarrhoea, skin rashes (hives) or eczema, stomach cramps (a baby will draw its knees tightly up to its chest and cry), and, in severe cases, difficulty with breathing.

How do I find out?

Tell your health visitor or GP as soon as you suspect that cow's milk might be a problem. An allergy is often quickly diagnosed.

What to drink instead

If you are breastfeeding your baby, you will need to avoid dairy products. Fully hydrolyzed formula milk will be prescribed if your baby is formula-fed. At a year old, instead of graduating from formula to cow's milk, your baby will need a range of non-dairy substitutes (see p27).

{ **Cow's milk allergy** affects about **1 in 50 infants** but only 1 in 1,000 adults in the UK. **Lactose intolerance** is much more prevalent, affecting up to **1 in 5 people**. }

Lactose intolerance

Lactose intolerance occurs when the body does not have enough of an enzyme called lactase that breaks down lactose, a sugar present in milk. Instead of being digested in the gut, milk moves into the colon where bacteria ferment it, making fatty acids and gases which cause the unpleasant symptoms. It is rare in under-fives, and more likely in 20–40-year-olds. It is often, but not always, genetic, and may be lifelong, or temporary, due to illness. The condition is most prevalent in countries where milk is not part of the adult diet – for instance in China, where most people are lactose intolerant.

What are the symptoms?

The most common reactions are nausea, vomiting, diarrhoea, bloating, stomach pain, excessive wind, and stomach rumbling.

How do I find out?

For adults, lactose intolerance can be diagnosed with a blood or breath hydrogen test. But before you go to see your doctor, keep a food diary (see p110) for a couple of weeks to see if dairy could be the issue.

Apart from considering milk, look at whether your diet was as nourishing and healthy as you thought it was. It's often the case that bloating and the other symptoms blamed on milk and milk products can be due to an imbalance in diet – for example, too many fatty or sugary foods, or not enough water, fruit, and vegetables. Your diary might show you that you just need to redress the balance across the food groups (see pp12–13) to cure your symptoms. But if it appears that milk, and so lactose intolerance, is a possible culprit, make an appointment with your GP and get tested.

What you need to avoid

Some lactose-intolerant people can cope with yogurt and cheese but not milk, or are fine on goat's or sheep's milk. Lactase drops in milk can be effective, as can lactose-free milk. With milk allergy, cut out all animal milks, cheese, yogurt, butter, cream, and any foods made with milk. Soya, almond, oat, rice, hemp, and coconut milks are fine.

In either case, check labels for hidden milk such as cow's milk protein, dried milk, milk-derivative fat/solids, non-fat milk/milk solids, skimmed milk powder, hydrolyzed milk protein, whey, curds, rennet, high-protein flour (which may contain milk), casein, caseinates, lactalbumin, lactoglobulin, lactoferrin, lactose, and lactate.

REALITY **CHECK**

 Milk allergy in children
A milk allergy is more likely to affect a baby or young child than an adult and they usually grow out of it by the time they are five.

 Lactose intolerance in adults
A person aged between 20 and 40 is most likely to become lactose intolerant, but it can affect children or older people too.

 Reactions to dairy
Symptoms may be mild, if rather unpleasant, but can be severe in a few cases, leading to anaphylaxis (see p125 for more details).

 Calcium supplement
Dairy is the most important source of calcium. If you can't have it, you may need calcium and vitamin D supplements. Check with your GP.

What about calcium?

You need to look to non-dairy sources of calcium, such as fortified soya and rice milks, green leafy vegetables, pulses, seeds, such as sesame, and small-boned or canned fish where you eat the bones. A supplement should not be needed while you're investigating, but if staying off dairy, see your doctor or dietitian to discuss whether perhaps you need a calcium supplement, which includes vitamin D to aid its absorption.

Egg allergy

An allergy to egg is one of the most common food allergies in children. For this reason, children under the age of one should be given only hard-boiled or other well-cooked eggs – the cooking of the egg changes the way that the body copes with it, avoiding allergic reaction.

By the time they are 12 months old, most babies have an immune system that's mature enough not to react badly to eggs. However, some children will develop an allergy, usually the first time an egg that isn't well-cooked is introduced into the diet. Egg allergy affects up to five in every 200 preschool-age children and is often linked with eczema. Although 70–90 per cent of **children will grow out of it by the age of five,** for the rest, this allergy can persist in adult life. Adult sufferers are often allergic to birds and feathers, too, as they contain similar proteins. It's unusual to develop an egg allergy for the first time as an adult.

Reaction is usually mild and immediate. The first indication is that your child may refuse a second taste of a food containing egg, and then develop redness or a rash around the mouth, followed by vomiting. Tummy ache and diarrhoea may also occur, and a longer-lasting eczema skin reaction can also be troublesome. A few children develop other reactions, such as wheezing, sneezing, or a cough, but although development of an egg allergy can be dramatic, it **rarely causes the severe anaphylactic reaction** common in nut allergy, for instance (see p125). However, that can happen, so if your child reacts at all, tell your GP or health visitor.

It's comforting to know that an allergy to egg is likely to be resolved by school age. Also, if the reaction is fairly mild, it may only be raw or soft-cooked eggs that remain a problem after a while. As your child grows, she may well be able to tolerate eggs baked in cakes or biscuits, or as glazes on pies and pastries. Later, just-cooked eggs such as in omelettes or fully cooked scrambled eggs may be fine, then soft-boiled ones, with only raw eggs (in home-made mayonnaise, mousses, or ice cream) remaining a stumbling block for a while. The best way forward is to **avoid eggs altogether for 1–2 years after the initial reaction.** Then, with medical advice, gradually include small amounts of cakes and biscuits and check for any reaction. If all is fine, you can try hard-boiled egg and then take it slowly from there. You will also need to **check labels,** because eggs are used in many processed foods, often in the form of albumen (egg white).

Children who have a more severe reaction, such as wheezing, may take longer to grow out of the allergy or never do so – these children are more likely to suffer from other food allergies, too. If this is the case, you can use egg replacers in baking, and potato flour makes a great binder for things like home-made meatballs. Egg-free pasta and other products such as omelette mix and mayonnaise are also on the market.

What to avoid

Consult a paediatric dietitian to help you through the quagmire of products that you will need to avoid. Two key words to look out for are egg and albumen.

Make sure your GP and health visitor know that your child has an egg allergy, to ensure that the medications and vaccines they provide are egg-free and safe for your child.

While the presence of eggs in custard, mayonnaise, soufflés, and cakes is well known, their use in bread, in the glazes added to buns or pies, in pastas, and in sweets may not be so obvious. Always check the labels.

Since heat can alter egg proteins, small quantities of egg in a cooked food may cause no reaction in a child with a mild egg allergy. Severely allergic kids need to take particular care, especially over foods that may have a hidden egg content – such as processed meats, pâté, sausages, some meat substitutes, royal icing, doughnuts, and chocolate with fillings, like chocolate cream eggs.

Foods manufactured within the EU must clearly list any form of egg (and any other major food allergen) in the ingredients, but foods sold loose – at a deli or bakery, for example – don't have to, so ask about egg before buying.

Wheat intolerance

Increasing numbers of people want to take wheat out of their diet because they worry they may have an intolerance. But if you notice that you or your child have any symptoms after eating wheat, it's always best to go to the doctor before you start changing anyone's diet.

What are the symptoms?

True wheat allergy is rare – an intolerance, which does not involve the immune system, is far more common. The symptoms come on slowly, often hours after consuming the food, and it can even take years for an intolerance to build up enough to bother you. Symptoms include:

- a general feeling of being unwell and tired a lot of the time;
- wheezing and coughing;
- stomach cramps and bloating – these can be mistaken for IBS (irritable bowel syndrome) or other, more serious, bowel or stomach diseases.

If the symptoms are weight loss or failure to gain weight, muscle spasms, or very pale, floating or frothy, foul-smelling stools, the cause may be coeliac disease – see pp132–133 for more advice.

How do I find out?

First, see your doctor to check you don't have coeliac disease. If that is ruled out, your doctor may do skin or blood tests for allergy. If you get the all-clear medically, you may still want to look at the issue of wheat intolerance if you feel that wheat is causing some of the symptoms listed here. Start by keeping a food diary for a couple of weeks (see page 110). If it's apparent that your body doesn't feel right after eating wheat, it's relatively easy to exclude major wheat products for two more weeks, then assess again. If you are intolerant of wheat, any symptoms should disappear, or at least reduce significantly. There's usually no need to start checking labels for gluten (the protein in wheat and other grains, such as barley and rye, that is usually the cause of the problem) and other ingredients such as wheat starch, because the body can often cope with small amounts. Wheat has a higher proportion of gluten than other grains, which gives the flour more elasticity and makes it ideal for bread, pasta, and many other everyday foods, so it's worth ensuring that you can replace it with nourishing alternatives before changing your diet.

What to avoid

Obvious sources of wheat are most breads, including rye bread (usually a mixture of wheat and rye, except for pumpernickel, which is all rye), most pasta, bulgur, couscous, farro, kamut, seitan, wheat-based breakfast cereals (including muesli), miso, most cakes, pies and biscuits, and flour-based sauces.

Can I eat other cereals?

There are some good wheat-free, gluten-free loaves, or German-style rye breads; oat biscuits; rice, corn, chickpea, and buckwheat pasta; barley couscous; corn tortillas; quinoa; millet; amaranth; and cornmeal. For wheat-free breakfast cereals, porridge is perfect, but cornflakes, puffed rice, and wheat-free mueslis are often delicious, too. Products labelled gluten-free have no wheat, except for a few wheat products with the gluten extracted.

Can I eat other wheats?

You might like to try spelt, as the form of gluten in it is different from that in traditional wheat and it can be eaten by some people with a wheat intolerance. You may also be able to tolerate French wheat flour, such as in a traditional French baguette (not just any white stick bread – it will be clearly marked as made with French flour).

When will I feel better?

Everyone's different – some notice within a day or two that symptoms have gone, others find it takes more than a month or so. If there is a gradual improvement, you may find that a little wheat can be tolerated – pasta once or twice weekly, for example. It will be a matter of trial and error as to how much you can eat before symptoms resurface. Perhaps it's just that you've had an excess of wheat up to now – easily done when starting the day with toast, having a sandwich for lunch, and then rounding off the day with a bowl of spaghetti.

What if we're eating out?

If you find cutting down is sufficient, it might be a good idea to let children have the usual wheat-containing foods when they're in social situations, say at friends' parties, or when they're out at a pizza restaurant, so that they can be totally comfortable. If your child is avoiding wheat altogether, it's better to go to a grill, where they can have meat, salad, and perhaps rice, rather than an Italian or Indian restaurant where the food will contain a lot of wheat. When you have your child's friends round for tea, try to have lots of things that your child can eat and they'll all love, so that they can share the food together.

Do I need supplements?

If you cut out wheat without considering the rest of your diet, there may be insufficient vitamin B_1 (thiamin), B_2 (riboflavin), B_3 (niacin), and folic acid, plus potassium, iron, magnesium, and phosphorus. However, if you replace wheat with other cereals and starches such as rye bread, rice, or potatoes, and make sure you eat plenty of citrus and other fruits, green leafy vegetables, pulses, some poultry and lean meat, and several servings of fish a week, all should be well. See pp28–29 and 30–31 for more sources of these vitamins and minerals. Ask a dietitian or your GP if you're in any doubt.

REALITY **CHECK**

 Wheat intolerance is different from coeliac disease or an allergy and is not dangerous.

 Wheat is a staple food and is best not excluded from a child's diet, in particular, unless really necessary.

 Gluten-free foods are fine if on a wheat-free diet but wheat-free is not always gluten-free.

 Have plenty of other wholegrains in your diet if wheat is excluded, to ensure you have plenty of fibre.

 An exclusion diet is the best way to discover if wheat is the culprit in causing the symptoms.

 Some wheat may be tolerated, in which case, try having it just once or twice a week.

 Some B vitamins and minerals may be lacking without wheat, so eat more greens, fruit, and pulses.

Understanding *gluten and coeliac disease*

In coeliac disease, the body's immune system treats gluten as a threat to health and attacks it, causing damage to the gut. Although coeliac disease can't be cured, it can be very successfully managed by a gluten-free diet so that the gut can fully recover.

Gluten is a protein found in wheat, barley, and rye. Some coeliacs also have problems with the avenin in oats, a protein similar to gluten.

Who gets coeliac disease and why? Coeliac disease is common, with an estimated 1 in 100 people affected worldwide, although only 10–15 per cent are diagnosed. It is an autoimmune disease, meaning that the immune system mistakes harmless substances or healthy tissue for an antigen such as a virus and tries to destroy it. When a coeliac eats wheat, barley, or rye, the gluten triggers an immune reaction, which damages the lining of the small intestine.

What are the symptoms?
Symptoms vary but may include bloating, stomach cramps and pain, nausea and vomiting, diarrhoea and/or constipation, excessive wind, skin rashes, and headaches. A damaged intestine also means problems absorbing essential nutrients. Lack of calcium can cause bones to become brittle, while poor absorption of iron can lead to anaemia, making the sufferer pale, grumpy, and tired, and sometimes stunting a child's growth. Digestion also suffers, so stools may float and become fatty, grey, and foul-smelling.

When does it start? In babies, symptoms may appear when they are first weaned on to cereals containing gluten. However, it may not be until much later, when your child doesn't seem to be thriving, has frequent tummy aches, and is tired and irritable, that the disease is diagnosed. For adults, symptoms can manifest themselves at any age and many coeliacs are diagnosed when they reach their thirties or forties, or even later.

How do I find out? If you suspect coeliac disease, see your GP before you remove gluten from the diet, as your doctor needs to see what's happening in the body when gluten is present. The doctor will probably do blood tests, then, if necessary, make a referral for a gut biopsy (though this isn't always done in the case of children).

What happens next? The good news is that as soon as you remove gluten from the diet, symptoms vanish and the gut usually recovers quickly. But coeliacs need to follow a gluten-free diet for life.

What should I avoid?

The main sources of gluten are breads, pasta, cakes, biscuits, pastries, and ready-made meals that could have flour in them – in a sauce, for instance. The recommendations given here are guidelines only. To make sure you steer clear of gluten in processed foods, you should contact Coeliac UK, who have a helpful website and will provide you with up-to-date lists of gluten-free foods. You need to check their lists regularly rather than relying on old ones, as the ingredients in processed foods may change at any time.

REALITY **CHECK**

Strict adherence
It's non-negotiable. Even a tiny bit of gluten will have an effect, so it is vital to check everything you eat at home and when out.

Eating out
Many restaurants now offer gluten-free (GF) food. It's best to notify them in advance, and to tell your waiter, too.

Cooking at home
Keep flour or anything containing gluten away from your cooking area, and be careful as even a stock cube may contain gluten.

Taking care
Check labels on foods for the GF symbol, and check lists of GF foods on the Coeliac UK website.

Watch out for wheat starch

Ordinary wheat starch is not sufficiently free from protein to be safe for coeliacs, but a specially manufactured one is used in gluten-free (GF) products.

Is wheat-free ok? Wheat-free is fine for people with wheat intolerance, but not if you have coeliac disease as the food could still contain barley or rye. Only eat if the label says gluten-free.

What about oats? As oats are often processed in the same place as wheat, barley, and rye, they may be cross-contaminated during processing. Oats marked GF can be eaten by most coeliacs.

Are gluten-free products good? The quality and variety of gluten-free breads, biscuits, cakes, and processed foods is so much better these days. Some regions offer bread for coeliacs on prescription.

Be vigilant with a coeliac child Make sure that everyone, from nursery and school to carers, sports clubs, and all their friends' parents, knows what your child can and cannot eat.

Explain to your coeliac child For a young child, say something simple, like "These foods will give you tummy ache or make you feel poorly." Always have tasty gluten-free alternatives, so that your child doesn't feel different or left out.

Checking for gluten-free

Pulses (plain-cooked beans and lentils) should be fine, but check labels on processed ones, such as baked beans.

Corn (maize) and rice breakfast cereals are usually OK, but check labels as some contain barley malt extract.

GF grains and flours include corn, arrowroot, amaranth, quinoa, tapioca, rice, soya, chickpea, potato, and millet.

Meat, fish, poultry and game in their natural state but, if buying ready-prepared, there is often gluten in coatings and sauces.

Fruit and vegetables that are fresh, frozen, or canned in juice or water are fine, but check the labels of any prepared dishes.

Potatoes and rice of all kinds are good, including sweet potatoes and yams, and brown, white, red, black, and wild rice.

Milk, cream, cheeses, eggs, and plain yogurt are OK, but flavoured yogurt and some soft cheeses may contain gluten.

Corn tortillas, tacos, and plain tortilla chips should be fine but check labels to confirm if GF.

Pasta made with corn, rice, or quinoa, labelled gluten-free, and rice noodles are great.

Some chocolates, ice cream, mousses, and sweets will be suitable, but check the labels.

Peanuts and *other common allergies*

The most common nut allergy is to peanuts (groundnuts), but most children and adults who are allergic to them are also likely to react to some, or all, tree nuts. If you suffer from this or other allergies, you can still eat a varied and nutritious diet, checking labels as you go.

When should I avoid nuts?

No whole nuts should be given to any child before the age of five because of the risk of choking. Most babies will be fine with smooth nut butters from six months old. If, however, there is a history of allergy in the family, or your baby already has a known allergy, such as eczema or to cow's milk, they have a higher risk of developing a peanut allergy. Check with your GP or health visitor before giving peanuts to your child for the first time. There is no evidence to show that eating peanuts in pregnancy increases the risk of your baby developing a food allergy, so don't avoid them unnecessarily as they're so nutritious. Many people with nut allergy can eat pine nuts – a seed – but some may have a reaction to these instead of, or as well as, nuts. See pp124–125 for allergy symptoms.

Where should I look for hidden nuts?

Common foods that can include tree nuts and/or peanuts include breakfast cereals, biscuits and cereal bars, cakes, desserts, chocolates, sweets, flavoured yogurts, salads and salad dressings, dips, and stuffings. Peanuts and cashews are popular in Asian and Chinese food, so check labels and in restaurants. Other foods include some pestos (although pine nut ones may be OK for many), marzipan, unrefined peanut oil (also called groundnut oil), and other nut oils. A reaction to refined peanut oil is rare. Many products are now labelled "may contain nuts", because manufacturers are aware of the dangers of cross-contamination. Some cosmetics and skin and hair preparations contain peanut oil: look for "arachis" (the name of the genus to which peanuts belong) on labels.

REALITY **CHECK**

 2 per cent of infants
In the Western world an estimated 1 in 50 babies is thought to have a nut allergy, but there seem to be fewer cases in Asia.

 Is nut allergy for life?
Four out of five children will continue their nut allergy into adulthood. For some the allergy will become less severe, but for 20 per cent it will worsen.

 Usually mild but not always
Most sufferers, both children and adults, will have mild symptoms, but anaphylaxis (see p125) is a real possibility for the minority.

 Coconut but not sesame
Most people with a nut allergy can eat coconut safely, but 25 per cent of sufferers will also be allergic to sesame seeds (see chart top right).

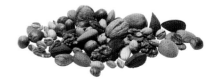

Other common allergies	What to avoid	Where they're hidden
Fish	All types of fish and fish pâté, but you may be able to eat shellfish.	Fish sauce, often used in Thai and Asian foods; furikake, a Japanese seasoning.
Shellfish	Crustaceans (eg shrimp, crab), and/or molluscs (eg mussels, squid, whelks).	Shrimp paste in Asian and Chinese food, even in meat dishes.
Soya	Fresh and dried beans, all soya products, including oil and margarine.	Soya lecithin, isolated soya protein, or soya concentrate in processed foods.
Sesame	Sesame seeds, oil, tahini, tempeh, halva, gomashio, Chinese sauces, furikake.	Many Thai, Japanese, and Chinese dishes and ready-meals.
Fruit	The specific fruit to which you are allergic, such as apple.	Table sauces, condiments, and chutneys; check all the fruit content in smoothies.
Vegetables	The specific vegetable to which you are allergic, such as celery.	Ready meals, soups, and stock cubes, celery salt and seeds, potato flour.
Yeast	Yeast dough, yeast extract, fermented foods and drinks, ripe fruit and cheeses.	Hydrolyzed protein, hydrolyzed vegetable protein, MSG, Quorn, some citric acid.

Allergies around the world

Food allergies are becoming more prevalent worldwide and tend to reflect how commonly the food is eaten in the local cuisine. Here is just a selection of allergies found in some countries.

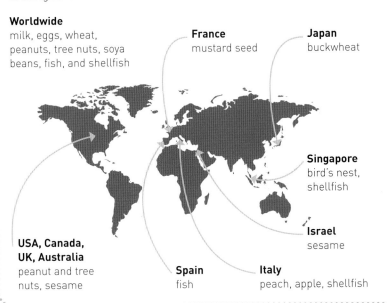

Worldwide
milk, eggs, wheat, peanuts, tree nuts, soya beans, fish, and shellfish

France
mustard seed

Japan
buckwheat

Singapore
bird's nest, shellfish

Israel
sesame

USA, Canada, UK, Australia
peanut and tree nuts, sesame

Spain
fish

Italy
peach, apple, shellfish

Keeping a food diary

✳ If you suspect a food allergy or intolerance, keeping a food diary is a good way of trying to identify the culprit. Put the diary in a prominent place so it's easy to jot down every day all you consume.

✳ Write down everything you eat and drink for two weeks. That includes every snack or nibble as well as main meals. Try to include as much information as possible about ingredients and quantity.

✳ Note, too, how you felt – everything from how full, to symptoms such as bloating, wind, nausea, and rash, as well as mental effects, such as tiredness or irritability.

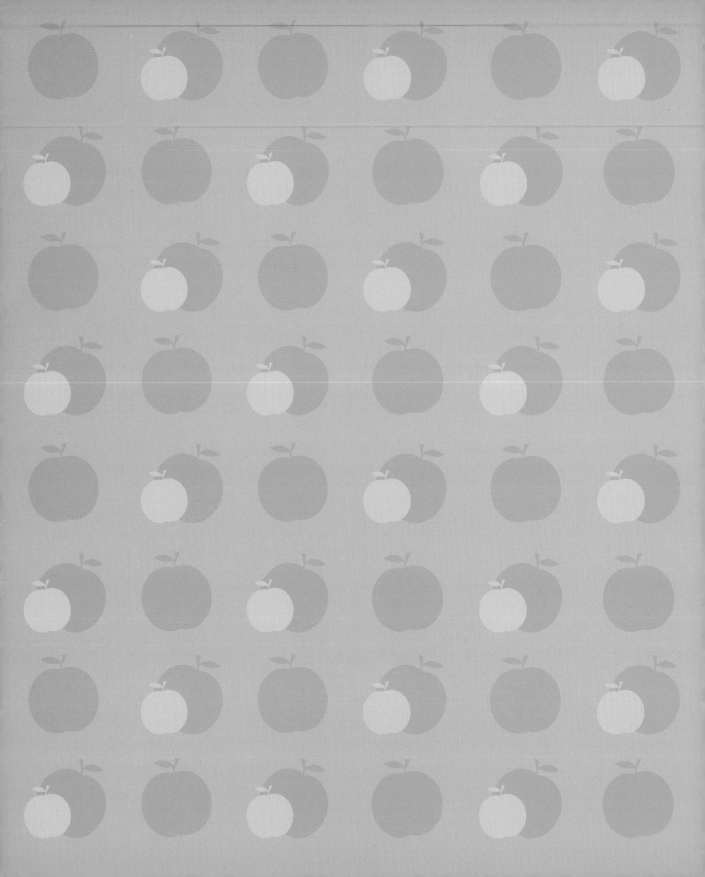

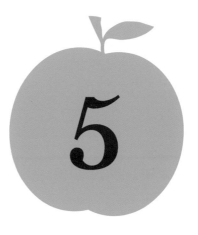

5

Foods that *revive and heal*

Why do I feel tired *all the time?*

"Feeling tired" is often how new and seasoned parents describe themselves as they attempt to juggle childcare with other family responsibilities and with work, too. Adjusting your diet and getting enough sleep to boost energy levels can make all the difference.

Is it your diet?

Off to a good start

Even if you don't feel like eating very much in the early morning, breakfast is important to give you energy to face the day. Some fruit, fresh or stewed, with something simple like a yogurt, or made into a smoothie to which you can add oats, nuts, and yogurt (see p191), can help set you up for the day.

Eat more iron-rich food

If you are lacking in iron, your blood won't have enough red cells to carry oxygen round your body and you will feel tired and listless. This can eventually lead to anaemia. The best sources of iron include liver, lean red meat, egg yolks, canned fish and shellfish, fortified breakfast cereals, nuts, seeds, dark leafy greens, pulses, and dried fruit such as prunes, apricots, and figs.

Have plenty of fibre

An insufficient amount of fibre can cause constipation (see pp152–153), which will make you feel really sluggish. Eat plenty of fruit and vegetables, pulses, nuts, seeds, and wholegrains.

More water, less sugar

Water is vital to energize you. Try to drink at least 8 glasses a day for a woman, 10 glasses for a man, and see pp38–39 for more tips on what fluids to have. Avoid sugary drinks and foods, as their high GI (see p91) gives you a burst of energy and then a slump.

Vitamins and minerals?

Zinc, potassium, phosphorus, and some B vitamins all play a part in making and releasing energy, while magnesium can help to regulate sleep. Provided you eat a healthy, balanced diet, you should get enough of all these, but have a look at pp28–31 to check. Maybe keep a food diary for a couple of weeks (see p110) to see whether you are lacking any vital foods. If you are vegan, make sure you are eating enough protein (see p121).

Rule out medical problems

If you still feel exhausted, have a chat with your GP to rule out any medical conditions that might be causing fatigue, such as anaemia or underactive thyroid.

Is it lack of sleep?

Exercise to sleep well

Exercise is a natural energizer in the mornings and will set you up for the day, but the stimulating hormones that exercise produces in the morning also help to get the body into a better sleep routine at night. If you can't fit in your exercise first thing, try not to leave it until late at night as this tends to get you pumped up, not ready for sleep.

There are lots of things you can do to help improve your energy levels through healthy diet, exercise, and sleep.

Avoid eating too late

Work schedules often force us into eating later than we'd like, but a big meal late at night is harder to digest. Perhaps you could have your main meal at lunchtime and stick to a light supper, say a soup and some wholegrain bread and hummus, or an omelette, or poached eggs on wholegrain toast, followed by some fruit. Alternatively, if you have time at the weekend, cook ahead, making meals that you can take out of the freezer through the week. Putting a meal in a slow cooker in the morning before you go to work is another way of reducing the time spent preparing food in the evening. Many ready meals are high in sugars, fats, additives, and preservatives and can leave you feeling heavy in the stomach, so they are best avoided.

Too much fatty food?

Fatty curries, pies, pizzas, chips, burgers, and creamy dishes are never good for weight and heart health and should particularly be given a miss in the evening, as they tend to lead to night-time indigestion. You may find red meat has the same effect – keep a food diary (see p110) to check.

Try comforting pasta

You may find that a starch-based meal, such as a simple risotto or a pasta dish, lulls your body into feeling ready to sleep well. Watch that you don't serve yourself too big a portion, though, or serve the pasta with something too rich, such as salamis or other sausages, or add too much oil. A simple fresh tomato and seafood sauce may be better. Something very quick to make, such as wholegrain pasta with a splash of olive oil and some frozen or fresh peas, with a little freshly grated Parmesan on top, can also hit the spot.

Coffee and alcohol

Be selective with your night-time drinks, avoiding those laden with caffeine, such as coffee, some teas or cola. Avoid too much alcohol, too. While you may think that alcohol helps you to relax and drop off, it is more likely to cause you to sleep lightly.

Switch off stress

Give your brain the chance to switch off from work by setting cut-off times for checking and writing emails. Make sure you have a milky drink and some "you" time, such as a warm bath, too. If you start to worry about something once you're in bed, try to breathe slowly and deeply. Your heart rate will slow and hopefully you will drift into restful slumber. See pp144–145 for more advice on stress.

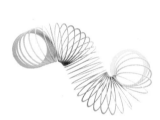

Boosting your *child's energy*

As with adults, children's energy levels fluctuate, particularly once they stop having daytime naps. But if nursery staff say your child seems to be tiring easily, or an older child's energy levels flag consistently, there are several nutritional checks you can make.

Very young children need naps in the day to boost their energy levels, but once they go to school there are many more demands on them and little time to rest. If your child or teenager seems frequently tired, it's worth checking their diet to see if they're getting enough nutrients to fuel both their mental and their physical activity. Check the amount of sleep they are getting, too (see pp142–143).

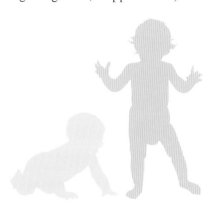

Check water levels

Many children don't drink enough water and become dehydrated, especially in hot weather or when active. Tiredness can be a key symptom. They may also need more water if they've eaten a sugary or salty snack, such as a packet of crisps. See pp38–39 for advice on keeping hydrated and ways of jazzing up water.

Check the amount of food

It's important that your child eats neither too much nor too little; have a look at pp57, 61, and 65 for advice on toddler, schoolchild, and teenage food needs. Even if you think your child is eating well, it's good just to reread the key points to make sure they're getting a varied and balanced diet from across the five food groups

(see pp12–13). If your child is a bit picky as to what they will eat, they can be underweight and lacking in the essential energy-boosting nutrients, such as the B vitamins, starchy carbs, or protein. If they are carrying extra weight that's making them less energetic, you can incorporate wholegrain cereals and bread, which will make them feel satisfied sooner. Rice is also a good source of energy and B vitamins. See pp102–109, depending on your child's age group, for more advice on maintaining a healthy weight.

Check iron levels

Iron-deficiency anaemia is caused by the lack of haemoglobin, of which iron is a major part, to make red blood cells. These carry oxygen in the blood around the body so that our cells can use it to produce energy. If your child is constantly tired, looks pale, has headaches, and is dizzy and generally unwell, see your GP. If they are anaemic, your doctor may suggest an iron supplement, while you focus on giving them more iron-rich foods such as red meat and leafy green vegetables (see p30 for other sources). Give them plenty of vitamin C (see p29 for sources) to help the body absorb iron. To maximize the iron, be careful how much tannin your child drinks, such as in tea. The odd cup is comforting, but made with just a quick dip of a teabag, since tannin reduces the amount of iron that is absorbed.

Check sugar levels

Is your child having too many high-GI foods or juices? These could be sending their sugar levels shooting up and down, leaving them tired long before bedtime. Go for more low- and medium-GI foods (see p91).

Check fibre levels

If your child is getting too much fibre, they might be feeling full before they've eaten enough. If they eat mostly wholegrains, substitute some white rice and pasta, and perhaps go for a white bread with added wheat germ.

Check mealtimes

If your child has a busy schedule, there'll be some days when they don't get time to sit down and eat properly. If so, they're going too long without food and their energy levels dip. Make sure they eat regular, healthy snacks, such as wholegrain cereal with milk and fruit, or wholegrain toast and nut butter, or a nourishing bowl of soup, to keep them going.

If your child is having a growth spurt, they may need nutritious nibbles to keep their energy levels up. Choose from the ideas for simple snacks on pp43 and 62, and do some nutritious baking from the recipes on pp240–247.

Check exercise levels

For maximum energy, your child needs to eat well, drink plenty, run around, and sleep well (see pp142–143). Get them out into the fresh air for some lively exercise to raise their heart rate and give them a boost.

When to see the doctor

If your child seems to be really lethargic and unwell, contact your doctor. Severe tiredness can be a symptom of a food intolerance or allergy or of a more serious illness that needs medical attention.

Eat wisely, *sleep well*

A good night's sleep enables children's bodies and brains to replenish and restore, hormones to settle into a happier rhythm, and growth and development to flourish at the right pace. If your child is not sleeping soundly, a few tweaks to his or her diet and routine may help.

Sleep is a vital part of life for all of us, but for a child it can mean the difference between a happy, well-adjusted individual and a crotchety one. There is no set amount of sleep necessary for any age group, but there are guidelines. Children under four should ideally still have a daytime nap and they can be expected to sleep for about 11 hours a night. By four years, they usually no longer need to nap in the day and sleep for about 11½ hours a night. This gradually decreases to about 8½ hours by the age of 16. Of course, some children seem to thrive on much less, and others need more. You will know your own child's habits – if they are not sleeping as well as usual, some simple dietary changes might help. You should also make sure that the computer, TV, mobile, and other gadgets are turned off well before bedtime.

Avoid stimulants

Discourage your child from having stimulating, caffeine-rich drinks after midday, such as cola, energy drinks, and, in the case of older children, coffee and some teas. Suggest they go for the decaffeinated or caffeine-free options instead (see coffee and tea pp98–99). For other drink ideas, see refreshing ways with water on pp38–39.

Watch the smoothies

As smoothies are made with a large amount of mixed fruit, sometimes sweetened, they can give your child a sugar surge. They are best kept for early in the day, as an occasional treat. Most individual fruit juices have a low GI (see p91), but after midday it's a good idea to dilute them with water (and always dilute for children under five).

Early mealtime

Eat early in the evening so there is plenty of time to digest the meal. Dissuade older children from nibbling fatty and/or sugary foods later on, as these won't help restful sleep. If they are staying up revising for exams, offer a nourishing slice of wholegrain toast with peanut butter, or wholegrain cereal and milk.

Settling suppers

Try to introduce some soporific starchy foods, such as wholegrains, pasta, rice, or couscous, as a large part of the evening meal. These tend to give that lovely, settling, stomach-nicely-full feeling, which can often lull the body into feeling sleepy. Pasta in particular can be incredibly good at helping to calm down a slightly wired, overtired child. Don't have too rich a sauce with it, though. Ever-popular spaghetti with meatballs in tomato sauce (p200) is just one example of a dish that will make everyone happy before bed.

Go easy on the spices

Spicy food can be difficult to digest for some people, so you may be wise to keep them for weekend lunches. It's probably best to avoid curries and other spicy dishes when you want your children to go to sleep early or if they need to be up and raring to go first thing in the morning.

Soothing milk

From the time when your child is a year old right through to teens and adulthood, a glass or mug of milk can have a wonderful, lulling effect. Whether it is warm or cold, cow's, almond, soya, coconut, or oat milk, it is a winner for soothing before bed. They each bring their own blend of nutrients, but oat milk can have a particularly powerful relaxing effect, as it is rich in the sleep-inducing hormone melatonin.

Chocolate dilemma

Chocolate may taste soothing but it contains a small amount of caffeine and a much larger amount of theobromine, a stimulating, caffeine-like substance – so watch that your child doesn't eat much of it in the evening. If they do fancy a hot chocolate before bed, think about making your own – use a chocolate with a higher cocoa solids content, which has very little sugar in it, and melt it in the milk of your choice without adding extra sugar.

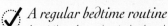

REALITY **CHECK**

✓ **A regular bedtime routine**
A set time for going to bed and light-off moment will soon become an accepted ritual if you stick to it except on special occasions.

✓ **A warm bath**
Older children sometimes prefer a shower after school, but sitting or lying in a warm bath is relaxing. Younger children will want to play with bath toys – try to keep it calm.

✓ **A bedtime story**
Reading aloud to your child at any age can be a great way to wind down. Older ones may enjoy a silent read or just a quiet chat.

✓ **A cool bedroom**
If the room is too warm it exacerbates poor sleeping patterns. It's better (and cheaper) to have a thicker duvet in winter.

Relieving *stress*

We can feel stress at any age, from children coping with exams and rivalries among their school friends to older people dealing with pressurized jobs and keeping family relationships smooth. Here are some tension-busting food and drink tips for adults and children.

Modern life is stressful for many of us, with long working hours and our personal space invaded by emails, texts, and calls to our mobiles demanding our attention. The symptoms of stress include a racing heart, digestive problems, sleeping poorly, fatigue, mood disturbances, and feeling fearful – but by making tweaks to your diet, you could feel a lot better.

1 Breakfast is important, as an empty stomach and low blood sugar will make any anxiety far worse. When you're stressed you may wake up feeling sick, but try to have something small: stewed apple is one of the most settling foods (make a batch once a week and keep it in the fridge); or try fresh fruit, yogurt, or a slice of wholemeal toast with fruit spread or nut butter. Then have a healthy snack (see pp43, 62) to eat mid-morning.

2 Avoid fatty, sugary foods in the morning – such as croissants, filled sweet pastries, sweet cereals, cereal bars, or fatty cooked breakfasts – as these will sit heavily in your gut and, in the case of foods high in refined sugar, will probably make you feel even more out of control. It helps if you eat mostly low- and medium-GI foods to keep your blood sugar levels constant (see p91).

3 Think twice about caffeine-rich drinks, as they can lead to you feeling more wired and on edge. You may think you need a coffee to get you through the day, but many people find they are much calmer and in control if they cut out caffeine – which includes coffee, tea, energy drinks, and cola (see pp98–99) – and drink more water and herbal infusions (see pp38–39).

4 It's best not to look to alcohol for stress-busting. While it may be tempting to pour yourself a glass when you get home after a tough day, it seldom helps after the first few mouthfuls; alcohol is much more likely to make you feel exhausted and less inclined to eat anything nourishing. It's much better to exercise and practise relaxation or meditation, and then eat food that nourishes you. Remember also to keep well hydrated all day as this can help you maintain a steady energy supply and a clear brain.

5 Try to think ahead about food, from what you'll take with you for snacks and lunch to the evening meals, so that you don't have to make big food decisions in a hurry. Ideally, plan and shop once a week, and cook, label, and freeze meals at the weekend, to take out as needed.

Children and stress

1 Make sure children have something nourishing to eat in the morning or they will be too tired to function properly, and become more stressed if they can't keep up at school. If they say they feel sick and don't want anything, offer a small glass of diluted apple juice, or water, and they'll soon feel they can try something more. A high-fibre cereal with milk is full of goodness but can make an unsettled tummy feel worse, so offer a slice of wholegrain toast, spread with an unsweetened pure fruit jam or nut butter, or a small home-made smoothie (see p191) and a sliced banana.

2 Don't overload your child's anxious stomach. Keep the portions small since they are more likely to get tummy ache if they're faced with a plateful. If you're worried they're not eating enough, split the three meals into smaller, more frequent fuellings.

3 Mealtimes are valuable moments to check in with your child as these can be calming times for them to express their worries. Even if you can't eat together every day, try to sit with them at table to help them relax.

4 Sleep can be a problem if your child is stressed. Eat early, so that their tummy has at least an hour to digest the food before bed. An easy-to-eat rice or other starchy carb-rich dish in a bowl can be a soporific meal to help your child get a good night's sleep. Afterwards, ensure they finish homework in time to relax before they go to bed. A less tired child is a happier child, so see also pp142–143 for more advice on sleep.

5 Milk may be an issue. Sometimes a child who is going through a tough time can exhibit lactose intolerance symptoms, such as tummy aches, sickness or diarrhoea. Keep a food diary for a week or so and if you suspect lactose intolerance is the cause, have a look at pp126–127 – it could be that reducing the amount of lactose in their diet temporarily might make them feel more comfortable – but make sure they get enough calcium (p30). If your child isn't eating well at this time, check with your GP that there is no medical problem. Ask about a good child vitamin and mineral supplement, too, as a short-term safeguard.

Stress-busting foods

* Citrus fruits such as oranges are rich in vitamin C, a powerful antioxidant (see p32) that helps to reduce stress-related blood pressure.

* Almonds are high in vitamins B and E, which help to strengthen your nervous and immune systems. They can also play a role in reducing blood pressure.

* Salmon is packed with omega 3 fatty acids. Apart from protecting against heart disease, they also keep adrenaline levels constant.

* Avocados are rich in antioxidant vitamin E, and potassium, which helps to lower blood pressure and regulate your heartbeat.

* Wholegrains such as those found in bread and cereals are packed with starchy carbs, which boost energy and calm the mind.

* Sweet potatoes satisfy the sugar and carbohydrate craving you can get under stress. They're also rich in cleansing fibre.

* Spinach is a great source of magnesium, which can help prevent fatigue and migraines, both of which are associated with stress.

* Turkey contains the amino acid L-tryptophan, which triggers serotonin in the body, giving us the feel-good factor and calming our nerves.

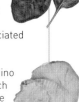

Migraine-type *headaches*

Chronic migraines or other severe headaches are really debilitating. Having a self-help strategy can be incredibly useful – although we don't fully understand what causes them, we do know that certain things we eat, and the way we lead our lives, can trigger them.

What are the symptoms?

Severe headaches may come out of the blue, but migraines have characteristic symptoms and many sufferers get a warning sign known as an aura. This visual disturbance can be flashing lights, zigzags, or blind spots, along with difficulty speaking, disorientation, tingling face and hands, and muscle weakness. About an hour before the pain in the head begins there may be other symptoms, too, including excess or lack of energy, altered sense of taste and smell, anxiety, and mood changes.

The onslaught of the severe headache may be accompanied by vomiting and an aversion to bright or flashing lights or loud noises. There are several ways you can try to prevent and manage migraines and headaches, but see your GP for advice and to rule out more serious conditions.

Keep a food diary

Although severe headaches and migraines can run in families, try keeping a food and symptom diary for a few weeks to see if there are triggers. Take note of not only what you eat and drink but also when you consume it, to see if you can detect any link.

Look at other factors, too, such as lack of sleep, not enough exercise, or hormonal changes – 60 per cent of migraines in women are linked to the menstrual cycle. If it's hormonal, ask your GP about a supplement, which might help prevent migraines and headaches.

Watch out for dehydration

Headaches and migraines can be triggered by not drinking enough fluids. When you dehydrate, the body takes fluid from the bloodstream and body tissues. The blood vessels constrict and a headache starts. Women should drink at least 1.6 litres (2¾ pints) a day, and men 2 litres (3½ pints).

{ Migraine is the most common neurological condition in the world, with more than 8,000,000 sufferers in the UK alone. It affects three times as many women as men. }

Caffeine – friend or foe?

Some people find that caffeine can increase the speed at which migraine medication is absorbed and takes effect, but for others it triggers an attack. Coming off caffeine can cause headaches, too, so if you drink a lot but want to cut down, do so gradually. Taking it with milk instead of drinking it black may be enough, but some people need to avoid coffee, some teas, and colas completely.

Boost your magnesium

Eating foods rich in magnesium may help increase the flow of blood to the brain, and so ease or prevent attacks. Pulses, nuts and seeds, avocados, dairy, meat, and wholegrains are good, but refined foods such as white pasta and rice have lost most of their magnesium. Riboflavin (vitamin B_2) and coenzyme Q10 may also help. Ask your GP about a supplement.

Tyramine the terror

While the amino acid tyramine is naturally in our bodies, migraine sufferers find it hard to process, so it stays in the system and can cause an episode. Foods and drinks high in tyramine are best limited or avoided entirely. It is found in concentrated doses in mature cheese, broad beans, offal, cured sausages such as salamis, and most pickled and fermented products, such as tofu, pickled herring, sauerkraut, yeast, and alcohol – alcohol-free beers and wine may have it, too.

Monitor blood sugars

Eating small meals regularly and avoiding very sweet and high-GI foods so that you keep your blood sugar levels constant can help (see p91). When you've skipped meals your blood sugar levels drop, or if you over-indulge in foods and drinks high in refined sugar they rise and fall rapidly, in each case making a migraine more likely. You're better off reaching for fresh fruits or healthier snacks instead. If you want a sweet treat, have it after a nourishing, protein-rich meal – the protein will slow down the absorption of the sugar, which will make it less likely to cause a problem.

Trigger foods

Some people find specific foods, such as chocolate, citrus, some nuts, or certain additives, cause an attack. A less common, but possible, culprit is wheat and/or gluten. If you've kept a food and symptom diary for a few weeks, you may see a pattern. If a migraine or headache appears after you have eaten bread, pasta, and so on, remove wheat for a few weeks to see if this helps – see pp130–131 on how to do this without losing valuable nutrients. If symptoms persist, remove gluten for a while – see pp132–133 for what to avoid and what to eat instead, and also check with your GP or dietitian.

Stress and sleep

Try not to get stressed, as it can bring on a severe headache or full-blown migraine. So, too, can alcohol on an empty stomach – it's best to save it until you have a good, nourishing meal, but even then alcohol is not an effective way to deal with stress. Switching off emails and other distractions in the evening and getting into a regular sleep routine can reduce the frequency of attacks – see pp139 and 143 for some simple ideas on good practice.

Children and migraines

About 10 per cent of school-age children get migraines, often by not drinking enough fluids, missing meals, and eating sugary snacks. Having plenty of water and frequent nutritious snacks may help. If so, explain to teachers that your child needs to eat at regular intervals.

Fighting off
coughs and colds

While coughs and colds can make you feel very unwell, there's usually
no need to see your doctor unless they last for more than three weeks.
You can help yourself here by eating the right foods and drinking plenty
of fluids to ease symptoms and help build resistance.

The common cold and most coughs are caused by viruses, so your doctor won't want to prescribe antibiotics since they are only effective for bacterial infections. As over-prescribing of antibiotics is leading to resistance to them, the less we take them the better so that they will still be available as a cure for serious illnesses.

Children are especially prone to coughs and colds because their immune system is still developing. Your pharmacist will give you advice on over-the-counter painkillers if needed, while at home, foods rich in certain vitamins and minerals can ease symptoms and help fight the virus.

Zinc

This mineral helps to build a healthy immune system. Zinc is found in all lean meats, poultry, egg yolks, fish, shellfish, oats, rye, buckwheat, brown rice, dairy products, pulses (particularly soya beans), nuts, and seeds. Zinc syrup or lozenges may help, too. See pp30–31 for more on minerals.

Selenium

Working with copper, manganese, and vitamin E in our bodies, selenium helps protect us against viral and bacterial attacks. Good sources are mushrooms, shellfish, fish (especially canned tuna), sunflower and sesame seeds (so tahini and hummus are good),

Brazil and cashew nuts (try the nut butter on p185), offal, egg yolks, garlic (see far right), grain brans, and wheat germ.

Antioxidant vitamins

The antioxidant vitamins A, C, and E really boost the immune system. Go for green, orange, red, and purple fruit and vegetables (soups and smoothies go down well), lean red meat, poultry, eggs, pulses, wholegrains (porridge is soothing), and nuts – see pp28–29 for more sources. A vitamin-C supplement or tailored, immune system booster may be useful if you're surrounded by people with colds and your diet hasn't been ideal lately. Ask your GP to advise.

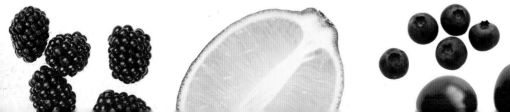
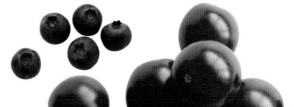

Drink lots

When a cough or cold hits, make sure you drink plenty of fluids to stay hydrated, especially if you're running a temperature – a hot body sweats more and so loses more fluid. Warm drinks rich in vitamin C, such as well diluted blackcurrant or orange juice, may help. If you have a cough or sore throat, try sipping hot water with a spoonful of honey (see below) and some lemon juice to soothe and loosen congestion.

Honey

Honey is great for a sore throat as it not only soothes but also has healing properties. Choose a good-quality honey – opt for organic, or a honey made from a single type of flower, such as lavender or thyme, or manuka, which has particularly powerful properties. But don't give a child under one year old any honey as it could cause infant botulism, a serious type of food poisoning.

Garlic

Garlic has an amazing power to combat bacterial, fungal, and viral infections. One of the easiest, most effective ways to get rid of a sore throat is to chew a fresh garlic clove – although that's not for everyone, so you may prefer to try the remedies in the panel. You need to eat fresh garlic as soon after peeling as possible, as its potency fades the more it is exposed to light. Fresh green garlic, available in summer, has maximum health benefits.

What about dairy?

Some people find that dairy foods make the body create more mucus, though scientific evidence doesn't support this. If you find they have the same effect on you, cut down on dairy when you have a cold or cough but ensure your diet is still rich enough in calcium – see p30 and p127 for non-dairy sources.

Is it serious?

See your GP if there are chronic conditions such as asthma or heart disease; if a high temperature doesn't fall with paracetamol or ibuprofen; if a baby under 3 months has a temperature above 38˚C (100.4˚F), or 39˚C (102.2˚F) at 3–6 months; if your child has a rash, or is vomiting but does not have diarrhoea; or is not drinking, or is very lethargic.

Garlic remedies

Try a garlic hit in the form of a gargle or soothing drink

Crush 5 or 6 garlic cloves, add 6 tsp apple cider vinegar, stir, and refrigerate for 24 hours. Warm in the microwave, add 1 tbsp honey and 4 tsp lemon juice, and leave to cool. Trickle 2 tsp of the remedy down your throat, gargling a little, three times a day.
For a quicker traditional remedy for a sore throat, just crush a garlic clove in a mug of warm milk.

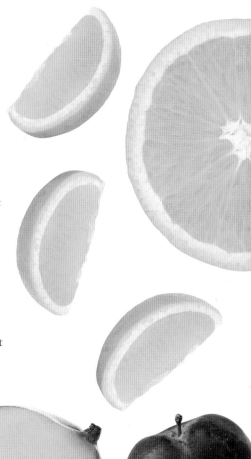

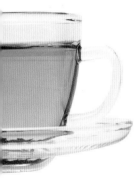

Easing *indigestion*

Indigestion can disrupt sleep at night, can be excruciatingly painful, and all in all is pretty miserable. There is a range of medications to help, but what you eat and drink – and your lifestyle – can have a hugely positive effect on both the frequency and severity of attacks.

There can be many physical causes of indigestion. Anyone, old or young, may find that stress, erratic lifestyle, eating on the go, being sedentary, or being unwell can cause indigestion; it's also common during pregnancy. The foods you eat and how and when you eat them can also exacerbate the problem, while other foods can relieve symptoms.

What are the symptoms?

When food is not digested properly, it causes heartburn (a painful, burning sensation in the chest), an uncomfortably full, bloated feeling, and belching. If you suffer from acid reflux or GORD (gastro-oesophageal reflux disease), the acidic gastric juices are regurgitated into the throat or mouth, leaving an unpleasant sour taste – sometimes undigested food comes back, too. Both indigestion and GORD can also cause nausea, but the following tips can help.

Pace yourself

If you have time to eat slowly, pause between courses, take small bites, and chew well, the gut should be able to cope with the digestive demands placed on it. But if you bolt down your food, it stacks up in the oesophagus – the narrow tube leading to the stomach. The food can't all go down at once, so you feel uncomfortable. It is best to eat little and often rather than have hurried large meals.

Check the temperature

Food that's either very hot or very cold tends to make us gulp air as we try to cool or warm it as we eat. If it's steaming hot, wait a little while before you eat it rather than drawing air into your mouth to try to cool it, or swallowing it whole to avoid a burnt mouth. If you're eating something frozen, such as sorbet, give it time to melt in your mouth before swallowing it.

Foods to avoid

All fatty foods are harder to digest so it's better to eat lean meat, and grill, bake or steam foods rather than fry. Sometimes specific foods – such as peppers, garlic, onions, tomatoes, cucumber, wheat, or too much dairy – can cause indigestion. Keep a food diary for a couple of weeks to identify trigger foods. See pp124–125 for more advice on food allergies.

Plenty of fibre and water

Indigestion is often accompanied by constipation, since they have similar causes. Try to eat more fibre (see pp22–23), but if wholegrains irritate your bowel, eat more fruit and vegetables instead. Drink plenty of fluids to work with the fibre (see pp38–39). For more on tummy troubles, see pp152–153.

Helpful herbs and spices

A mild mint tea can calm the gut, but don't make it too strong if your stomach is feeling acidic or you have a stomach ulcer – infuse the mint leaves or teabag for just 2–3 minutes. Ginger tea, ideally made with finely grated fresh root, is very effective. Parsley, too, settles the stomach. Some people find chillies aid digestion, whereas others cannot tolerate them, nor even mild, sweet spices, such as cumin.

Exploding a few myths

Rounding off a meal with a strong coffee or a shot of alcohol to aid digestion may have the opposite effect. Although some over-the-counter indigestion remedies are sparkling, in general fizzy drinks also make things worse. Along with coffee and alcohol, they can relax the oesophageal sphincter, the valve that should prevent food from returning from the stomach to the oesophagus, and cause acid reflux.

Think about your lifestyle

Smoking and too much alcohol can cause heartburn. Regular exercise (see pp114–115) will help to keep your gut working well, as will maintaining a healthy weight (see pp102–113). Your digestion works best when you are sitting upright, so try to eat a good hour before you go to bed.

When to see the doctor

Persistent indigestion can be a sign of a more serious condition, such as cancer or an ulcer. See your GP if adjusting your diet and lifestyle doesn't swiftly improve matters.

5 foods that help

Parsley and ginger are good, but other foods can also ease digestion and reduce acid reflux. Incorporate them in your diet, and you should get relief from your symptoms.

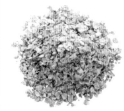

Porridge
Oats, whether oatmeal, rolled, or even as instant cereal, make the ideal breakfast or snack to sustain and soothe.

Chicken
Skinless chicken or turkey is lean protein that is easy to digest. It can help close the stomach valve, stopping food and gastric acids coming back up the oesophagus.

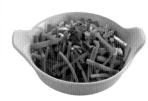

Carrots
Cooked carrots and other vegetables can be easier to digest than raw – ideally lightly steamed, and served without butter or a rich sauce.

Bio yogurt
Probiotics (see pp36–37) are present in some live yogurts and help foster the friendly bacteria in your gut. This will help you digest food properly.

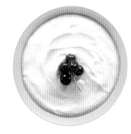

Fennel
Cooked or raw, fennel seems to aid digestion. The seeds in particular, chewed or infused, can help bloating and flatulence. If pregnant, however, ask your midwife or GP whether you should avoid fennel seeds.

Tackling *tummy troubles*

Familiar problems such as diarrhoea, vomiting, or constipation can
make you feel dreadful. Fortunately, for most of us it is no more than
an unpleasant experience, which can be managed with the right fluids
and diet – though the very young or elderly may need extra attention.

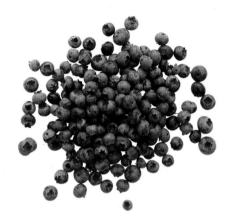

We can be struck down with a stomach problem at any time of life. Even if it is acute and debilitating, it can usually be remedied with the right drinks and foods. **Diarrhoea** (passing stools that are looser or more frequent than is usual for you) may affect you to different degrees and for many different reasons, not all of them physical – it can be caused by anxiety. It may be accompanied by vomiting, and while this is sometimes a result of eating something too spicy or rich or from drinking too much alcohol, it's more often because we've picked up food poisoning. This will be from not cooking or reheating something properly or because either the food or the preparation area was contaminated. As soon as the symptoms start, you need to **replace lost minerals and fluids**. To do this, you can buy rehydration sachets that you dissolve in water or sports drinks. Or make your own by dissolving a pinch of salt and a teaspoon of sugar in 250ml (8fl oz) of boiling water, then letting it cool down – you can also flavour this with a little apple juice or fruit cordial to make it more palatable. You need to **sip at least 500ml (16fl oz) of fluid every two hours** during your illness to prevent dehydration. Avoid drinks that are carbonated, caffeinated, or very hot or cold, since they can irritate the gut even more, whereas **ginger or mint tea** can be soothing (to make, see p151).

As you start to feel a little better and want to eat something, opt for a rice cake or two, some freshly cooked white rice, dry toast, or a little mashed potato, but don't add any oil or butter; keep it light. Although many fresh fruits are hard for an unsettled gut to deal with, **pectin, a form of soluble fibre found in fruits and vegetables**, can help to reduce diarrhoea by absorbing water and important minerals in the bowel. Some people can cope with nibbling pectin-rich raw carrot sticks, or some apple still with its skin on (as the pectin is in the skin of the fruit) or will try grated carrot or apple (skin too). Mashed banana is settling, sweet, and comforting. **Blueberries are also good**, not only for their pectin, but also because they contain anthocyanosides, which have a mild antibiotic action.

When you're recovering from an upset stomach the body can become temporarily lactose-intolerant, so you should avoid all sources of dairy for a few days with the exception of a little live **probiotic yogurt** to replace good bacteria in your tummy, especially if you have had to take antibiotics, which often kill the good bacteria in the gut as well as the bad ones. A bowl of light soup, such as the chicken noodle soup on p210, usually goes down well, but avoid fibre-rich wholegrains for now, as they can be difficult to digest.

> Diarrhoea is quite common. It is only a cause for medical attention if it doesn't clear up within a week, you have other symptoms, or you become dehydrated.

The most common cause of **constipation** (passing stools infrequently, and sometimes with difficulty) is a diet too high in animal fats, such as not-so-lean meat, cheeses, and eggs, or one high in refined sugary foods but low in fibre. This is often compounded by not getting enough exercise and not drinking enough fluids. Constipation is particularly prevalent in older people, who have more sedentary lifestyles (see pp78–79), and also during pregnancy (see pp70–71), but it can affect anyone at any time. To tackle it, gradually increase fibre (see pp22–23), eat plenty of fruit and

vegetables (including **rhubarb and dried fruits**, such as prunes, figs, or dates, which have a natural laxative effect), and drink plenty of fluids – at least 2 litres (3½ pints) of water or other fluids a day (see pp38–39 for more ideas). The dietary fibre absorbs water and softens the stools so they pass more easily. Limit your intake of alcohol and caffeine as they can dehydrate you. Magnesium helps loosen stools, so eat plenty of spinach, nuts, seeds, globe artichokes, raisins, poultry, sweet potatoes, and wholegrains, or consider a daily 300mg supplement. If all else fails, you may need to take a natural laxative for a short while.

Irritable bowel syndrome (IBS) causes repeated diarrhoea, constipation or both, along with flatulence, stomach cramps, bloating, stabbing pain in the bowel, and other unpleasant symptoms. See your doctor for further advice, and to rule out other conditions.

Most tummy troubles are over quickly, but go to your GP if you have blood or pus in your stools; if you can't drink because you can't stop being sick, so you become dehydrated (you will pee just a little dark urine); or if your diarrhoea lasts longer than a week. Contact your GP immediately if your baby or young child has six episodes of diarrhoea in 24 hours, or the diarrhoea is accompanied by vomiting.

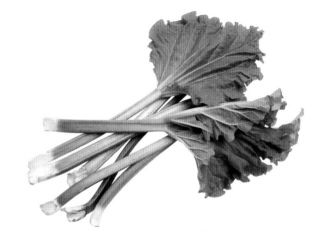

Just for girls:
food for period pains

When girls start their periods, their bodies change in all sorts of ways, as their oestrogen, progesterone, and testosterone levels fluctuate. Lots of TLC is needed and some good, wholesome foods to help with the discomfort, the spots and the moods.

Puberty can be a tricky experience in any girl's life, especially if they're one of the first in their group to start having periods. Many prefer not to talk about it, but they need to be loved and soothed until the period's over, the other symptoms subside, and they can get back to normal . . . until the next month.

Time for TLC

Puberty is also the time when some girls start to feel negative towards their body. They may not understand all the changes that are taking place, so adolescence can throw them off course, and insecurities can start to present problems. Your daughter may begin to eat differently, perhaps restricting specific foods if she feels her body shape is changing

in a way she's not happy with, so it's incredibly important to keep the lines of communication open and to be sympathetic to her anxieties. Make her nourishing, comforting meals (not too big or she might recoil) and have plenty of healthy snacks (see p43) to hand if she feels like grazing rather than eating big meals. Don't put pressure on her to eat a lot. Too much focus on the amount she eats is more likely to risk her trying to gain control of something in this rather confusing time of her life by limiting what she eats to an unhealthy extent – see pp108–109 if you suspect she's heading this way. To give your daughter as much support as you can, ensure she has enough space in her routine for some down time and TLC, with plenty of warm baths,

hugs, and early nights, as this can be one of the best ways to ensure she feels nurtured and able to cope with the changes in her body. Make sure she knows that you understand exactly what this stage of life feels like. Little things like getting her a hot water bottle to hug (or a microwaveable wheat bag) can be very soothing both emotionally and physically for the stomach cramps.

Focus on iron

Once they start their periods, girls need 14.8 mg iron per day to compensate for their monthly blood losses. You should start to include more foods rich in iron in your daughter's diet to ensure she gets enough or she could become anaemic. The best sources are liver, lean red meat, eggs, ready-

{ **Good food** and lots of **sympathy** can help teenage girls through the difficult time of menstruation – coping with the **hormones** and cramping pains is **not easy**. }

to-eat dried apricots (not too many, as they can be a little bloating), and leafy green vegetables such as curly kale and spinach (which makes a lovely, nourishing soup). See pp30–31 for other sources, too. Tea and coffee can inhibit the absorption of iron, so suggest that she drinks them only between meals. Offer her a glass of pure orange juice with an iron-rich meal, as the vitamin C will help her absorb the mineral.

Help her digestion

Bloating (too much gas in the abdomen) can be upsetting for figure-conscious girls, so help your daughter to reduce this by avoiding the worst vegetable offenders – cauliflower, Jerusalem

artichokes, onions, and chickpeas. During menstruation, when any digestive problems often worsen, cooked vegetables and fruits may suit her tummy better than raw as they are easier to digest. To help soothe her digestion and moods, make pots of fruit compôtes and put them in the fridge so she can dip into them to have with some yogurt. Comforting soups are good, too, such as a bowl of chicken noodle soup (see p210). Herbal teas may also help with the bloating (see p98). Keep bottles of still water to hand, so that your daughter can grab one to take with her when she goes out instead of having colas or other sugary drinks that will exacerbate her bloated tummy.

Less salt, more water

Fluid retention, common around menstruation, is often made worse by taking in too much salt and not enough water, so use lots of fresh herbs, black pepper, and juices such as lemon or lime juice to give flavour instead of salt.

Dandelion, nettle, and peppermint teas all help to ease bloating.

Cramp-busting foods

* **Bananas**
This fruit is high in vitamin B$_6$ and potassium, which can help prevent stomach cramps. Potassium also regulates fluid retention.

* **Calcium**
As calcium can ease period pains, give more milk, yogurt, and cheese. If dairy isn't her thing, go for other calcium sources (see p31).

* **Walnuts**
These nuts contain lots of vitamin B$_6$ and some magnesium, which work together with their omega 3 fatty acids to help relieve pain.

* **Parsley**
A traditional remedy, this herb contains apiol, a compound that can help relieve period cramps.

* **Freshly grated ginger**
Not only is ginger warming and soothing when infused as a tisane, but it has also been a Chinese remedy for period pains for centuries.

* **Oats**
Oats contain zinc, which is really important to help ease period pains. They also contain magnesium, another pain reliever.

* **Oily fish for omega 3s**
Sardines and other oily fish are packed with omega fats, which can reduce cramping pains.

* **Camomile tea**
Warm, soothing camomile tea, with a little honey if liked, can relax the muscles and ease stomach cramps.

Boosting *fertility*

For some couples, becoming parents can be the easiest thing in the world to achieve, but others find that things don't go so smoothly. If you're having difficulties, it's reassuring that many fertility specialists say that before you try fertility treatment you should look at your diet.

There is an established relationship between having a well-nourished body and an improved chance of becoming pregnant or fathering a child. Even if you think you both have an ideal diet and lifestyle, there may still be things you can tackle in your diet to help boost your prospects for becoming parents. It's important, too, that you don't get wound up and treat your day's menu planning (and your sex life) as if it's a military operation. If you let all of the spontaneity and pleasure fall by the way, you will both be pretty miserable, and that won't help you achieve your goal.

{ Try to keep **eating and living well** as a positive, **enjoyable**, non-stressful aspect to your lives. It will give you a strong and **empowering** focus for **becoming parents**. }

Folates first

It is now well-recognized that folic acid (or folate) is of critical importance, both pre- and post-conception, in protecting your baby against neural tube defects such as spina bifida. This is why all women, from the time they begin trying to get pregnant, should take 400mcg folic acid every day right up until the end of the first trimester. If you become pregnant unexpectedly, it's not too late – start taking the supplement straight away and continue to take it up until the end of the twelfth week. Try to eat foods rich in folate, too, such as oranges, bananas, asparagus, leafy greens, sprouting broccoli, Brussels sprouts, peas, and fortified cereals and bread.

Assess your size and shape

For both of you, weight and fat distribution matters. For a woman, carrying too much weight or too little can disrupt periods and hinder conception. When you're trying to conceive, you should aim for a body mass index (a measure of how your weight relates to your height) of 20–25. As fertility can be affected by the amount of fat you are carrying, you may want to weigh yourself on bioelectric impedance analysis scales, which calculate your body fat as a percentage of your weight. Most women have a body fat content of 28 per cent, but the ideal for conception is 20–25 per cent. If need be, adjust your diet and exercise to see if you can reduce your body fat content. Look at

{ Trying for a baby should be a **happy time**. Incorporate the advice given here into your life to **help things go well**. }

your shape, too – if you are apple-shaped (more fat around the middle), it has a more negative impact on fertility than age or by how much you are overweight, so work on your waistline with more yoga, or bending and stretching exercises. If you already exercise hard and have a BMI of less than 19, you may have too much muscle and not enough fat to support a healthy pregnancy. You may need to reduce your exercise routine and eat more calorie-intense foods. See pp110–111 for more advice on weight issues.

A healthy, balanced diet

For the best chance of conceiving, make sure you both eat plenty of starchy carbohydrates (such as wholegrains and potatoes); oily fish, nuts, and seeds for essential oils (see below); plenty of fruit and vegetables; some dairy, and proteins (such as poultry, red meat, white fish, and pulses); and increase your fibre (see pp22–23).

Mighty omegas

Omega 3 and omega 6 essential fatty acids are thought to be critical in both male and female fertility as they are essential for cell growth. The best source of omega 3s is in oily fish, such as salmon, mackerel, and sardines. You can also get them from plant sources, particularly linseeds (flaxseeds), pumpkin seeds, nuts, and their oils. It's recommended you don't have more than two 140g (5oz) portions of oily fish a week (or up to 4 medium cans of tuna) before and during pregnancy as they contain pollutants. You should also avoid shark, marlin, and swordfish as they contain more mercury than other fish. Omega 6s are found in vegetable and seed oils. Avoid trans fats found in processed foods (see p24) as they can hamper ovulation.

Alcohol and caffeine

A glass of wine may relax you, but alcohol is a diuretic and can cause valuable fertility nutrients such as zinc (see p31) and folic acid to be excreted. It can also damage the sperm and egg, and the baby once you conceive. Caffeine, too, in tea, coffee, colas, and chocolate (see p99), can have an effect on both sperm health and female fertility. An intake of more than 200mg per day is also a risk factor for early miscarriage.

Non-food tips

If you smoke, it's time to stop – research shows that smoking is linked to early menopause and sperm problems. Take regular exercise (see pp114–115) to improve your fitness and mood. Reduce stress (see pp144–145), and stay positive.

REALITY **CHECK**

Supplements can help
Most people can get enough of the essential vitamins and minerals from food, but the following supplements could help you.

Folic acid
Folic acid is vital. All women need a 400mcg supplement when trying for a baby until 12 weeks pregnant. Men can get enough from a regular, healthy diet (see left).

Vitamin C
Vitamin C can help both male and female fertility. It's vital you eat plenty of fresh fruit and vegetables (see p29 for other sources), but a daily supplement is also advisable if either of you smoke.

Zinc
Zinc is vital for sperm production and the maintenance of male and female sex hormones. Try to get it from food (see p31), or you could take a 15mg supplement.

Stronger *bones*

Our skeletons are very much a living part of us, since bone cells are busy building and maintaining bone all our lives. Although our bones stop growing in length in our late teens, it's crucial that we get the nutrients to keep them strong and healthy right through adulthood.

From the first few weeks after conception, our bones grow and develop healthy, strong bone tissue – as long as the body receives the right nutrients, especially calcium – right up until our late teens. Bone density increases until our late 20s, but from 35 or so, it begins to decrease. Laying down a good, strong matrix of bone when we're young affects how our bones will be in later life and makes us less likely to suffer from bone conditions such as osteoporosis (low bone density). This disease can be hereditary, but you are also more at risk if you are post-menopausal (see pp74–77), a smoker or heavy drinker, or not very active, or if you have a disease such as hypothyroidism, or a lower than ideal body weight. However, it is largely preventable at any age with the right diet and lifestyle.

Dairy calcium

Dairy produce is the best source of calcium. This includes milk, cheese, and yogurt. If you are trying to cut down your intake of saturated fat (see p24), skimmed milk has just as much calcium as whole milk. Low-fat yogurts can be a little insipid (and often have added sugar), so you may prefer to have whole-milk or Greek yogurt for the creamy taste and reduce your fat intake elsewhere. Lower-fat cheeses include mozzarella, cottage cheese, goat's cheese, fromage frais, feta, ricotta, and Edam.

Non-dairy calcium

For people who have an allergy or intolerance to dairy produce (see pp126–127), there are other sources of calcium: fish with small, edible bones, such as whitebait or sardines, and canned fish (if you eat the bones); green leafy vegetables, (though not too much spinach, as it contains oxalates, which hinder calcium absorption); soya products in moderation, such as soya mince, tofu, and fortified soya milk and yogurt; almond milk, nuts, seeds, and tahini; dried fruits such as apricots; okra; and fortified bread and orange juice.

Balance of proteins

There is some evidence that too little or too much protein can reduce bone strength. Too little, so that you are malnourished, can cause bone loss. In that weakened state, you are more likely to fall over and so have more chance of fracturing a bone, too (this particularly applies to the elderly). If you eat too much protein, it may increase the acidity in the blood and other body fluids, causing calcium to be leached from the bones. The recommended amount for adults is 2–3 small servings a day (see p41).

Calcium facts

DID YOU KNOW?

Calcium is key for adolescents, who gain over **20%** of their adult height and **50%** of their adult skeletal mass at this time.

 Adults need 700mg of calcium a day to keep bones healthy – that's the equivalent of a pint of milk. A five-year-old needs 450mg, or two glasses of milk a day. See RDAs on p27.

OSTEOPOROSIS

Around 3 million people in the UK may have osteoporosis. While it's often associated with women over 50, it can affect anyone – younger women, men, and even children – so we all need calcium.

REALITY **CHECK**

 Keep salt intake down
Salt has a negative effect on bones, as it increases the amount of calcium you lose in your urine.

 Watch caffeine and alcohol
Too much caffeine inhibits the absorption of calcium and too much alcohol affects the liver's ability to metabolize it.

Quit smoking
Smoking increases the risk of osteoporosis by inhibiting bone cell growth and the absorption of vitamin C.

Get plenty of exercise
Load-bearing exercise, such as brisk walking or dancing, helps to strengthen bones.

Vitamin D

A deficiency in vitamin D can lead to osteomalacia in adults or rickets in children. Bones become softer, leading to deformity and pain. The body makes vitamin D from our exposure to the sun. About 10 minutes twice a day (not midday) from late spring to early autumn is enough to see you through winter, together with what you eat in oily fish, eggs, and fortified breakfast cereals. Children under five are given vitamin drops. Pregnant and breastfeeding mums and over-65s need a 10mcg supplement daily.

Other vitamins and minerals

Bones need B vitamins (see pp28–29) as they can reduce levels of homocysteine, an amino acid, which may lower the risk of broken hips in later life. Vitamin C is also important, to keep cells healthy. Vitamin K helps to produce osteocalcin, a protein used to build bones – it also helps mend them when broken. Bones also need the minerals magnesium and zinc (see pp30–31) to grow. If you eat a healthy balanced diet (see pp12–13), you should get enough of all these nutrients.

Omegas and phytoestrogens

Omegas 3 and 6 are believed to help calcium absorption, and so help maintain healthy bones. Omega 3 is found in oily fish, linseeds, walnuts, and their oils, and in soya beans; omega 6 is in vegetable oils, nuts, eggs, poultry, and avocados. Phytoestrogens, found mainly in soya products, may help protect women over 50 from bone loss – they behave like a weak form of oestrogen (see p32–33) and so have a similar effect to HRT. But it's best to eat soya in only small amounts (see p74).

Arthritis: *easing the pain*

Around 10 million people suffer from arthritis in the UK, including 12,000 children. Finding ways to reduce its impact on our lives is very important, as there is no cure. Food, drinks, and supplements can have a profound effect on symptoms, so they are worth exploring.

Osteoarthritis

In the UK, osteoarthritis is the most common form of arthritis, with around 8.5 million sufferers. It develops when the cartilage around the joints – often the knees, hips, spine, or hands – wears away, so the bones grind against each other painfully. Over time, the joints may become distorted, causing further agony. You are most likely to get it if you are over 50, if you've had any trauma or injury to a joint or have done repetitive activity (such as competitive sport), or if you are carrying too much weight (which particularly affects the knees).

Rheumatoid arthritis

Less common but more severe, rheumatoid arthritis affects around 580,000 people in the UK. The body's immune system attacks the cells that line the joints, which causes the pain, stiffness, swelling, impaired movement and, often, gradual destruction of the bone and cartilage. You are most likely to get rheumatoid arthritis if you are a woman (a 3:1 chance compared with men) and are aged between 40 and 70, though it can happen to anybody at any time.

Childhood arthritis

Most childhood arthritis is called juvenile idiopathic arthritis (JIA). The causes are unknown, but in many cases the condition improves as children get older so they can often lead normal lives. There are three types of JIA: oligoarticular, affecting four joints or fewer; polyarticular, affecting five or more joints and usually accompanied by a rash and high fever; and systemic onset, which is like polyarticular but also causes lethargy and swollen glands. A fourth type, enthesitis-related arthritis (ERA), affects older and teenage boys more than girls, causing pain to the soles of the feet, knees, and hips.

Gout

The cause of gout, another form of arthritis, is a build-up of uric acid. The acid should be excreted by the kidneys, but if you make too much or excrete too little, crystals build up in the joints. The symptoms are often redness, swelling and pain in the big toe (or in other joints). You are more at risk if you are over 50 and male, carry too much weight, have high blood pressure, diabetes, kidney problems, or a family history of gout, or you drink a lot of alcohol.

Exercise your joints

* **Reap the benefits** if you can control your weight (see pp102–113) and exercise regularly (see pp114–115) – you are likely to be in less pain and feel better than if you are inactive.

* **Regular stretching** exercises will help increase your flexibility. If you keep your joints moving, they are likely to feel less stiff and painful.

* **Strengthening** exercises, if performed regularly, will help increase bone density and muscle strength. Always build up gently – don't overdo it at first or your joints will stiffen even more.

* **Water** exercises, such as aqua-aerobics or swimming, are ideal as your weight is supported by the water, so it doesn't put too much stress on your joints and muscles.

* **Low-impact** exercise, such as gentle walking or Tai Chi, doesn't strain the joints and muscles too much. Walking in particular is easy to include in your daily routine.

Are there foods to avoid?

There are theories that some foods (including potatoes, tomatoes, and aubergines) cause arthritis flare-ups. There is no concrete evidence, but it may be worth keeping a food and symptom diary for two weeks. If you find definite links to any foods, do make sure you are still eating a varied, healthy diet (see pp40–41) before excluding anything. For gout, foods with a high purine content make more uric acid. Avoid offal, meat extracts, oily fish (so you need other sources of anti-inflammatory omega 3s, such as linseeds, pumpkin seeds, nuts and their oils, or consider an omega 3 supplement), and shellfish. It's best to avoid alcohol, too, especially beer.

Eat Mediterranean-style

The classic Mediterranean diet is low in saturated fats and rich in delicious olive oil, fresh fruit and vegetables, oily fish, and lovely cheeses. Olive oil is a "good", monounsaturated fat (see p24), which reduces cholesterol levels, so it could prevent further health problems. Oily fish (unless you have gout) will give you anti-inflammatory omega 3, as well as iron (see p30) to prevent anaemia – people with arthritis are often anaemic. A colourful array of five-a-day fruit and vegetables will give you vitamins, minerals, and antioxidants. Cheese is a good source of calcium (see p159), which is vital for healthy bones – arthritis sufferers are more susceptible to osteoporosis.

Antioxidants

Vitamins A, C, and E, selenium, zinc, copper, manganese, and many phytonutrients in our food are powerful antioxidants, which can fight free radicals that may cause tissue damage (see p32). There is also evidence that a lack of vitamin D (see p29) may cause arthritis to progress more quickly. Before you take any supplements, check with your GP. Other supplements you may want to discuss include:

• **Glucosamine**, with or without **chondroitin**, to build and repair ligaments and joints.
• **Magnesium**, to reduce the pain and fatigue.
• **Evening primrose oil**, which has omega 6s. Taken with omega 3s, it may give some relief.

Eating to ease *angry skin*

Eczema is an incredibly common disorder. It can be triggered in a tiny baby but often – although not always – clears up before school age. Acne, as we all know, is often the bane of the teenager. The right diet can help to ease the symptoms of both.

What causes eczema?

Eczema (also known as atopic eczema or dermatitis) is an inflammatory skin condition which causes itchy, dry, flaky skin that can also lead to the skin becoming broken, with bleeding and sometimes infection. The exact cause of eczema is not known, but it is thought to be an allergic condition that is triggered when the body overreacts to an environmental factor (such as dust or pollen) or a food.

Who gets it?

Eczema usually appears before children are 18 months old, but it can develop at any time, especially if you suffer from asthma, hay fever, or other allergies. Sometimes there is no apparent reason for an outbreak of eczema, but around 10 per cent of cases are caused by trigger foods. If a child has reacted previously to a food, with symptoms appearing quickly, or also has colic, vomiting, or diarrhoea, the eczema is more likely to be caused by a food allergy. The majority of young children grow out of eczema before school age but others can have flare-ups for the rest of their lives.

Prevention in pregnancy

If there is a history of allergy in the family, try eating a diet rich in vitamin E (see p29) as you may then be less likely to give birth to a child who develops an allergy. It's a good idea to avoid the most common food allergens (see far right), but some of them are rich in vitamin E, so you'll need to choose carefully. Some research suggests that taking a probiotic supplement while pregnant or breastfeeding may improve your baby's balance of good versus bad bacteria in the gut, which could reduce the chance of them suffering from eczema. For more information on probiotics, see pp36–37.

Breast and formula

There is some strong evidence that breastfeeding helps to prevent eczema, perhaps because it delays the introduction of cow's milk (in formula), which can be a trigger food. However, it is also thought that vitamin C in breast milk may have protective potential, so try eating foods rich in the vitamin (see p29 for good sources). With formula-fed babies, if your baby shows signs of eczema or if there is a family history of it, discuss with your GP or health visitor whether you should change the formula milk.

Omegas to help

Oily fish, such as mackerel, salmon, and sardines, and other foods rich in omega 3 fatty acids, such as linseed, can help to reduce the inflammation. See p25 for more on omega 3s and p19 on how much oily fish to eat a week. As many children are unlikely to eat enough sardines and the like, if your child has eczema, consider giving an omega 3 supplement suitable for their age group. Be patient, though, as it can take several weeks, or even months, for the skin to calm down.

Vitamins C, D, and E

Skin-healing vitamin C is really important, so offer plenty of fresh fruit and vegetables. For an older child or an adult, consider adding a 10mcg vitamin D supplement, too, as there is some interesting research to show it may give some relief – under-fives are given it in vitamin

drops, along with vitamins A and C. Vitamin E is good at calming irritated skin, so use olive, nut, or seed oils instead of butter and see p29 for more sources.

Trigger foods

If you suspect eczema you should see your GP, who will investigate further and advise on treatments. Keep a food diary for two weeks if you think a food is causing the symptoms. Once the known allergen is excluded from the diet, the skin can return virtually to normal. If the eczema is mild, with just an odd patch here and there, you need to decide whether total exclusion is worth it or if just making your child's diet well-balanced, combined with an omega 3 supplement, is enough. If you and your GP agree that a major food group needs to be excluded, it's important to explain to your child, at a level they can understand, why you're saying no to what may have been their favourite food.

Teen spots

Acne is a common skin reaction to hormonal changes. It's a myth that greasy foods cause spots, but if your teenager eats too many of them in preference to

fruit and vegetables, spots may develop. Try to get them to eat their five a day as part of a healthy, balanced diet. Omega 3s can help, and vitamin C and zinc-rich foods (see pp28–31) can aid the repair of damaged skin. It's good to drink lots of fluids, too – pp38–39 has tips on the healthiest drinks to have.

Common allergens

* Milk – usually cow's milk, but could also be sheep's or goat's (see pp126–127).

* Soya may be a problem as well as dairy, so you will need alternatives (see p27).

* Citrus fruits and tomatoes can cause a reaction from their acidity.

* Eggs are one of the most common allergens linked to eczema (see pp128–129).

* Peanuts and tree nuts can cause severe reactions (see p134).

* Shellfish can cause eczema but the reaction may be limited to certain types.

* Wheat intolerance symptoms (see pp130–131) may include eczema.

* Food preservatives and some colourings are frequent culprits (see p87).

Anti-ageing
foods for your skin

Whether you're worried about dry patches, brown "age spots",
laughter lines, or just generally ageing skin, providing your body
with a range of nutrients will help to keep your skin younger-looking
and give it some protection from damaging ultraviolet rays.

Wrinkle-fighting fats

You need some fat in your diet to build and maintain every cell in the body, especially those in the skin. Without fat, skin cell walls break down so their fluids leak out, leading to dehydration and dryness. However, lashings of butter and lard aren't good for your skin, your waistline, or your health, so focus on oily fish and vegetable oils, such as from olives, seeds, nuts, and avocados. Don't overdo it – a drizzle of good-quality olive oil on salad will do, or a sprinkling of toasted nuts on muesli and yogurt for breakfast.

Fabulous fibre

Fibre-rich foods (see pp22–23) help you to feel nicely satisfied, so you're less inclined to overeat or to snack on foods that you know won't help you or your skin. Not only that, but all the fibre-rich wholegrains, pulses, vegetables, and fruit, are full of vitamins, minerals, and antioxidants (see pp28–33) which help maintain optimum production of collagen and elastin, two proteins that keep skin supple, soft, and young-looking. Antioxidants also protect the skin from ultraviolet rays from the sun, which have a potentially damaging, ageing effect. If too much insoluble fibre from wholegrains makes you feel bloated and heavy, replace half your wholegrains with processed white grains and bread.

Energy boosters

If you are full of energy, you will feel and appear younger. Try to keep your diet based around low- and medium-GI foods, which help to keep your blood sugar levels constant and avoid an energy slump (see p91). If you eat a lot of sugar, it also interacts with collagen in the skin and makes the skin lose flexibility. This in turn affects the skin pigment melanin, causing you to develop brown "age spots". See also pp138–139 for energy-boosting ideas.

Plenty of water

Drink 8–10 glasses a day to keep the skin hydrated and youthful-looking. Water also works with fibre to encourage good digestion, which leads to healthy-looking skin. As caffeine is mildly diuretic and alcohol more so, skip alcohol and reduce your intake of coffee and tea (except herbal, white, or green) to a couple of cups a day.

Top 8 anti-ageing foods

1 Brazil nuts are rich in the mineral selenium, crucial for making an antioxidant called glutathione peroxidase – this helps to protect the skin from the sun's ultraviolet rays, which are a major cause of dryness and lines.

2 Oily fish such as salmon and mackerel are rich in omega 3 fatty acids, which reduce the tendency to dryness (see pp24–25). Fish are also full of protein, which is vital for continually making and repairing skin cells.

3 Lean steak, like oily fish, is a great provider of protein, for the continuous repair and renewal of skin and all other cells in the body. It is also a great source of iron, a mineral that is vital for carrying oxygen to cells.

4 Plums (and all purple fruits) are bursting with anti-ageing anthocyanin nutrients, which keep the walls of the capillaries (tiny blood vessels) in the skin strong, ensuring it receives a good supply of blood and oxygen.

5 Carrots are packed with the antioxidant beta-carotene, which the body converts to vitamin A (see p28). Once ingested, beta-carotene collects in the fat layers of our skin and deflects harmful and ageing ultraviolet radiation.

6 Strawberries are rich in both vitamin C and bioflavonoids. Both help to protect the walls of the fine capillaries in the upper layers of the skin, delaying the appearance of the thread-like veins that often come with age.

7 Shellfish such as oysters and prawns are rich in zinc, which is crucial for making enzymes that help the skin maintain its collagen supply, and in copper, which helps to make collagen and elastin (see pp30–31 for more on minerals).

8 Green and white teas are both rich in antioxidants, which help protect the body from free radicals – unstable molecules that attach themselves to cells and cause damage, which includes speeding up the ageing of skin.

A feast *for your eyes*

Delicious, colourful fruit and vegetables are packed with nutrients that can help your eyes stay healthy day-to-day and also have a role in protecting you from some serious eye diseases. They're so good for you that eating plenty will not only keep you bright-eyed but fit and energetic as well.

Antioxidants

The specific nutrients found in colourful fruit and vegetables include a range of antioxidants, which combat free radicals – unstable molecules that attack cells throughout the body – and prevent them from damaging our eyes. The main antioxidants are the vitamins A, C, and E, found in all dark green, red, orange, and yellow fruit and vegetables (including dried ones, such as apricots). Other sources of antioxidants are red meat, liver, nuts, seeds, dairy produce, and eggs. For more on antioxidants, see p32. Vitamin A also helps to keep the surface of the eye moist.

Carotenoids

Carotenoids are phytonutrients found in the rainbow of fruit and vegetables (see pp34–35). Recent research points to two in particular that may help maintain healthy eyes and reduce the risk of AMD (see right) – lutein and zeaxanthin. Lutein is most plentiful in green leafy vegetables, such as spinach, kale, and chard, and in yellow peppers, mangoes, and blueberries. Zeaxanthin is especially high in orange peppers, sweetcorn, lettuce (but not iceberg), and orange citrus fruits. It is also found in eggs.

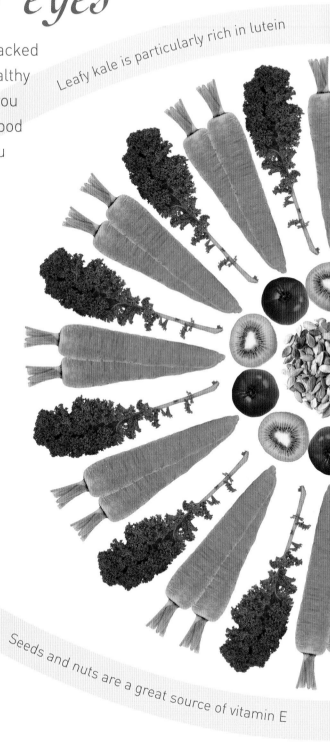

Leafy kale is particularly rich in lutein

Seeds and nuts are a great source of vitamin E

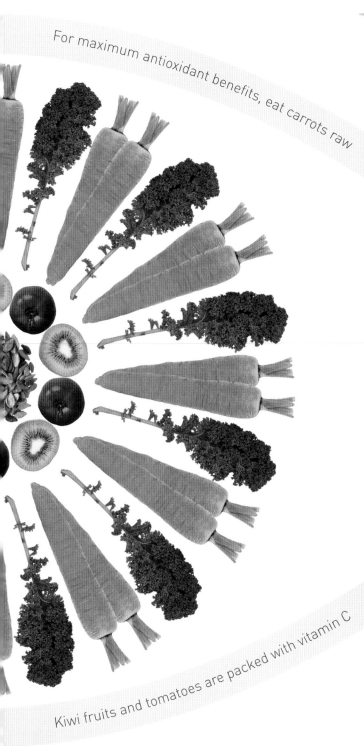

For maximum antioxidant benefits, eat carrots raw

Kiwi fruits and tomatoes are packed with vitamin C

{ More than **115 clinical studies** have shown that **zeaxanthin and lutein** help to keep eyes healthy. }

Vitamins, minerals, and eye diseases

The most common age-related eye conditions are cataracts, glaucoma, and diabetic retinopathy (which often results from poor blood sugar control; see pp172–173). A less common condition, called age-related macular degeneration (AMD), leads to loss of central vision (what you can see when you look straight ahead). Medical opinion is still divided as to whether antioxidant vitamin, selenium, and zinc supplements can prevent or slow down these conditions, but it is generally recognized that if you have a good, balanced diet, including plenty of fruit and vegetables, you won't need supplements. But if you feel your diet may not be adequate, or you're excluding certain things because of a food allergy or intolerance, ask your GP whether a supplement might help. You should have eye tests every two years, but your optician may recommend more frequent checks for a child wearing glasses; for people who have diabetes, or are aged 40 or over and have a family history of glaucoma; and for the over-70s.

Top tips for healthy eyes

• Try to eat at least five portions of different-coloured fruit and vegetables a day (see pp34–35).
• Aim for a healthy, balanced diet, including foods from the five food groups daily (see pp12–13).
• To protect your eyes from strong sunlight's ultraviolet rays, wear sunglasses that meet EU requirements for offering 100% UV protection.
• Don't smoke – it can lead to cataracts and AMD. Passive smoking can also damage the eyes.

Healthy eating
for healthy hair

Everyone wants thick, shining hair, but there are times when hormonal changes, illness, medication, or stress cause dull, thinning locks. Rather than buying a range of hair products to find a cure, it's best to have a look at your diet and lifestyle to see what might help.

Thin, lanky hair can be upsetting at any age, but particularly for women, whose self-esteem may take a bit of a battering during the teenage years or the mid-life menopause. Both are times of major hormonal changes, which can play a part in how hair behaves. Men, too, may be sensitive about hair loss, which can sometimes happen long before they reach middle age. There is no cure for male pattern baldness, but eating healthily can help what hair they do have to look as good as possible.

For girls and women, though, the main cause of hair loss is nutrient-related rather than hormonal. It can take months for the results to show in full, but with the right diet, hair can regain its previous thickness and lustre.

In fact, most people can probably help their hair improve in body and gloss by tweaking what they eat.

Iron levels

Check with your doctor to see whether your hair loss is down to low ferritin levels (the body's store of iron). A simple blood test will show whether your iron stores are depleted, perhaps because you've experienced blood loss during childbirth, surgery, or unusually heavy periods, or you've been lax with your intake of iron-rich foods. If your iron levels are low, a supplement may be prescribed, but it is still important to eat iron-rich foods on a daily basis, to boost your iron levels through your diet.

Iron-rich foods

The richest sources of iron, and the easiest to absorb, are lean beef and liver, although other offal, duck, goose, and game are also good. Ideally, have a portion of these rich sources a couple of times a week, along with a plentiful supply of the other iron-rich foods, such as eggs, dark green leafy vegetables, tofu, and pulses such as chickpeas and even baked beans. Fortified breakfast cereals are good, too, but avoid those high in salt or sugar. Make sure you have plenty of vitamin C at the same meal to aid the absorption of iron, such as a glass of citrus juice with breakfast, or berries with yogurt for your pudding. Vitamin C keeps scalp circulation healthy, too, supporting blood vessels that feed the hair follicles.

Avoid inhibitors

The tannins present in tea inhibit the absorption of iron. Tannins are not to be confused with caffeine – decaffeinated teas contain just as much tannin as normal tea. One option is to go for herbal teas such as fresh mint (see pp98–99); the other is to enjoy a proper cuppa, but not straight after a meal – leave it a couple of hours. Phytates in bran and oxalates in spinach, nuts, chocolate, parsley, and rhubarb can reduce iron uptake too, so make sure that you're choosing other green leafy vegetables as well as spinach and that your diet isn't high in bran.

Vitamins and zinc

If your hair is thinning, it could be from a lack of biotin (vitamin B_7), found in oily fish, liver, nuts, pulses, mushrooms, egg yolks, cauliflower, and yeast extract. Vitamin D is also important. Our body makes most of the vitamin D we need from exposure to sunlight (see p29 for other sources). If you think you may

not be getting enough of this vitamin, consider a supplement – but check with your doctor first. You may also be short of zinc, which you'll get from lean meat, poultry, fish, nuts, seeds, and wholegrains. If your hair is in poor condition, lack of biotin may also be the cause, or you may be short of vitamin B_{12}, which you'll find in red meat, offal, seafood, eggs, and dairy products – the only vegetarian form is yeast extract. If your hair is dull and lanky, you may need to look at riboflavin (vitamin B_2), which comes from the same sources as B_{12} and also from fortified breakfast cereals.

Proteins and fats

If you are not eating enough protein and fat, your hair follicles may not be getting sufficient oils to sustain a strong head of hair. It's common for girls going through the body-conscious teenage years to start experimenting with cutting out foods. If your daughter has started to lose some of her hair, this can be a good moment to help her to work through her worries about eating and body image (see pp108–109 for more advice). To improve things, try to incorporate some "good" fats (see

pp24–25), such as those in olive oil, avocados, nuts, and seeds. Also include some proteins – oily fish such as salmon, seafood, lean red meat, eggs, chicken, or, if vegetarian, a good mixture of pulses, dairy, and a small amount of soya products. It is perfectly possible to maintain a healthy weight while still including nutrients that benefit the hair – see pp102–113 for advice on healthy weight according to your age.

Other factors

In addition to diet and hormones, there are some medical problems that cause hair damage and loss. Conditions such as Crohn's disease (an autoimmune disorder causing inflammation of the lining of the digestive system) and eczema can reduce hair's strength and luxuriance, as can certain contraceptive pills. If you need to undergo chemotherapy, this may also cause temporary hair loss. Periods of stress and anxiety can be a contributing factor, too, so it's worth trying to incorporate some simple de-stressing activities in your life, such as those suggested on pp142–143, to help restore your inner calm.

Alleviating asthma

Asthma is a common but alarming condition, affecting 1 in 11 children and 1 in 12 adults in the UK. Avoiding triggers where possible and eating a diet rich in anti-inflammatory vitamins, minerals, and phytonutrients may help to avoid or alleviate symptoms.

Asthma is a long-term condition caused by inflammation of the airways (small tubes called bronchi) that carry air to and from the lungs. When something irritates them, the muscles around them constrict, the lining of the airways swells, and the production of sticky mucus is increased, causing wheezing, a tight chest, and difficulty breathing. Children with asthma may recover in their teens, while others have it for life; it can also begin at any age. The cause of asthma is not certain, but it is often hereditary. It's also thought that living in overly clean homes or eating foods high in salt and/or additives may have made us more sensitive. Food allergies can also produce an asthmatic reaction, although this is not common. Treatment includes medication, lifestyle changes, and identifying and avoiding triggers that cause an attack. While diet cannot cure asthma, what you eat can have a positive effect.

Possible triggers

Food, drink, and additives are not common triggers, but the most likely suspects are fish, shellfish, eggs, cow's milk, nuts, sesame, yeast products such as bread, and wheat (see pp124–135 for more on food allergies). Acid fruit, such as citrus, and benzoic acid (E210), a preservative in fruit drinks and some fruit products, can also set off an attack, as can foods and wine that contain histamine. If you react badly to tartrazine (E102), you may also react to aspirin. Sulphites (E220–228) may trigger asthma by irritating the airways.

Keep a food diary

Identifying any triggers could help reduce the amount of times an inhaler is needed. To see if there is a link to certain foods or additives, it's worth keeping a food and symptoms diary (see p135) to record what has been eaten and how breathing has been affected. If you're doing this for your child, you'll need to ask their school, friends and parents, and anyone who feeds them to let you know anything they are given to eat. If you do discover certain foods are triggers, always check with your GP before removing food groups from the diet. If it does become necessary to exclude anything, make sure you replace the problem food with suitable alternatives (see top right) to maintain a healthy, balanced diet that all the family can enjoy.

Boost antioxidants

Eating more antioxidant-rich fresh fruits and vegetables can help to relieve symptoms and reduce the chances of developing

Food groups and additives	Possible food triggers to avoid	Foods to increase
Carbohydrates	Wheat (found in baked goods, cereals, sausages, and many other foods)	Gluten allergy is not the issue, so opt for other wholegrains, such as oats and rye
Proteins	Eggs, milk, fish, shellfish, nuts, peanuts, sesame, and soya	Lean meat, chicken, pulses, oily fish, and soya (if fish / soya aren't triggers)
Fats	Nut, peanut, and/or sesame oils, if tree nuts, peanuts, or sesame are triggers	Anti-inflammatory omega 3 fatty acids, found in oily fish (if not a trigger)
Sulphites (additives)	Fizzy drinks, processed meats, ready-made salads, and beer	Water, pure juices (as part of meals), unprocessed meats and salad stuffs

asthma. One antioxidant in particular seems to be effective: vitamin E, found in nuts (but don't give whole nuts to the under-5s, to avoid choking), seeds, vegetable oils, wholegrain cereals, avocados, eggs, and soya products. Onions, garlic, and apples contain quercetin, an antioxidant that inhibits the action of an enzyme responsible for releasing inflammatory chemicals, so these foods can also help to improve lung function; a glass of freshly squeezed apple juice is one of the healthiest ways for an asthmatic to start the day.

Opt for oily fish

Omega 3-rich oily fish, such as salmon and sardines, are thought to have an anti-inflammatory effect, too. Aim for at least one portion a week (or up to four a week for men and boys, up to two a week for girls, and women of childbearing age, as they contain pollutants that could affect foetal development). If fish is a trigger, you can boost your intake of omega 3s by eating nuts, seeds – particularly linseed (flaxseed), and their oils.

Watch the salt

Research has shown that high salt intakes can aggravate asthma, so it's best not to add it when cooking. Try to avoid salty snacks, processed foods, and hidden salt in foods, such as breakfast cereals and bread. See also pp94–95 for ways to reduce salt.

Selenium and magnesium

Unsalted nuts and seeds make great snacks as they are rich in magnesium, which reduces inflammation and relaxes the muscles of the airways. Studies have shown that some asthma sufferers have low blood levels of selenium, and that boosting selenium may help. Brazil nuts are a particularly rich source, along with wheat germ, garlic, and sunflower seeds. Egg yolks are a good source of both minerals.

Keep active

You may have to take powerful steroid medication, which tends to increase appetite and therefore cause weight gain. Exercise keeps the lungs healthy and helps to keep weight in check; losing excess weight often reduces the symptoms of asthma. Check with your doctor as to how much exercise is advisable, depending on the severity of your asthma. It's recommended you use a reliever inhaler 10–15 minutes before exercising, and after, if your exercise has lasted more than 2 hours (though short bursts of activity are often better). Always have an inhaler with you.

Dealing with *diabetes*

Diabetes is known to affect 2.9 million people in the UK, and it's thought that many more are still undiagnosed. Although you need to pay special attention to your diet and lifestyle if you have diabetes, that needn't stop you enjoying your food.

What is diabetes?

Diabetes is a lifelong condition in which the body's blood sugar levels are too high. They are usually regulated by a hormone called insulin, which is made by the pancreas. When you eat food, the body converts carbohydrates into glucose. Normally, insulin moves the glucose from the bloodstream into the body's cells to provide energy – but if you have diabetes, the pancreas doesn't produce enough, or any, insulin, or the insulin that is produced does not work properly (known as insulin resistance). Long term, diabetes can affect the heart, eyes, kidneys, nerves, and feet. The main symptoms of diabetes include:

- feeling very thirsty;
- feeling unusually tired;
- needing to pee a lot, especially at night;
- unexplained weight and muscle loss;
- slow healing of wounds or cuts;
- blurred vision.

If you have these symptoms, see your doctor. Diabetes is easily diagnosed and you will need to start treatment immediately.

Three types

Type 1 is often called insulin-dependent diabetes because it occurs when the immune system attacks and destroys the cells that make insulin, so none is produced. It is also sometimes called juvenile diabetes as it often, but not always, starts in the teenage years. It is treated with insulin injections for life, accompanied by careful management of lifestyle and diet.

Type 2 is more common than Type 1 and mainly appears after the age of 40, though it is now increasing in children and teenagers. It happens when the body does not make enough insulin, or the body has insulin resistance. Excess weight is a major cause and although a careful diet may be sufficient to control your blood sugar levels, you may also need medication, either orally or by injection.

Gestational diabetes occurs in about 5% of pregnancies, often between 14 and 26 weeks. It usually disappears when the baby is born, but women who have it are more likely to develop Type 2 diabetes later in life.

Planning your diet

If you have Type 1 diabetes, consult a specialist dietitian to help you manage your diet and exercise alongside your insulin regime, as careful planning is required to ensure your blood sugar levels remain constant. For type 2s, the advice opposite should help. It's also worth reading about the Glycaemic Index on p91, which explains how some carbohydrates are broken down quickly, giving a surge in blood sugar levels (high GIs), while others take longer to absorb, giving slow-release energy (low and medium GIs). While this is an indication of which foods to choose and which to avoid, it depends how much you consume. One sugary sweet may have a high GI, but it won't give you a huge sugar rush, whereas a whole packet of them would. That said, go for low- and medium-GI foods to keep your blood sugar levels constant, as part of a well balanced diet (see pp12–13). Gestational diabetes can often be controlled by a similar diet, though medication may also be necessary.

Living well with diabetes

Do I need diabetic products?

No, you don't need to resort to eating diabetic products, which are often expensive and, in terms of flavour, usually fall short of delicious home-made food. Your meals and snacks need be no more complicated than simply following a well-balanced, nourishing diet with low- or medium-GI foods.

Can I still eat cake?

You can include some cakes and biscuits in your diet, as long as you eat them in moderation as just an occasional treat. Make your home-baked goodies as nutritious as possible, using ingredients such as wholemeal flour and dried fruits (see pp242–247) so that you're getting valuable nutrients and fibre along with your tasty treat.

What about drinks?

To keep as healthy as possible, drink the recommended amount of water daily (see pp38–39). Remember that fruit juices and smoothies are high in natural sugar and will affect sugar levels. If you take medication to keep your blood sugar levels down, alcohol may bring them down too low, so eat first and if you're drinking in the evening have a carbohydrate snack before bed.

Is it just about sugar?

It's not enough just to watch sugar and other high-GI foods to regulate blood sugar levels – you also need to eat the right type and quantity of fats to reduce LDL cholesterol (see pp174–175), and go easy on salt (see pp94–95), to help to avoid raised blood pressure. With diabetes comes the risk of heart disease and stroke, linked to high cholesterol and high blood pressure.

Which foods can help?

Foods rich in vitamin B$_3$, magnesium, zinc, and chromium all help keep blood sugar levels steady, so eat plenty of wholegrains, nuts, seeds, green vegetables, bananas, pulses, seafood, and low-fat dairy produce. Cinnamon may help to lower blood sugar and LDL "bad" cholesterol levels, so try adding it to spicy food, hot drinks, cakes, and biscuits.

What about my weight?

If you're carrying too much body fat, losing this healthily and steadily can have a very positive effect on your blood sugar levels (see adult weight issues pp110–111). But if you're losing weight and you don't know why, contact your diabetic consultant or GP right away as you may need to be given medication, or to have your present dosage adjusted.

How does exercise help?

It's really important to take regular exercise as this will help you to maintain a healthy weight and good blood sugar levels. See pp114–115 for more advice. Type 1 diabetics should discuss with their specialist or GP how to tailor insulin and food intake to avoid hypoglycaemia (when blood sugar levels go too low) as a result of exercising.

Eating
for your heart

Around 82,000 people in the UK die from heart disease every year. Fortunately, we can drastically reduce the incidence and severity of this disease on so many levels now – not only through medical intervention, but also by adopting a healthy diet and lifestyle.

Heart disease

Coronary heart disease (CHD) occurs when your blood can't pump freely through your blood vessels. There are several contributing factors: high cholesterol (see right), smoking, high blood pressure (when blood presses too strongly against the artery walls as it's pumped around, and damages them), being overweight, or diabetes (see pp172–173). If you have a male relative under 55 or a female relative over 65 with CHD, you are more at risk. We can try to **protect against CHD** by eating a varied, healthy diet that is low in saturated fat, with a little lean protein and dairy, and plenty of fruit, vegetables, and wholegrains; by watching our weight, shape, and body fat (see pp110–111); by being active (see pp114–115); by watching our cholesterol levels; and by not smoking.

Cholesterol facts

Cholesterol is a fatty substance in our blood. The liver produces most of it to make vitamin D, build cells, and perform other vital functions. Some foods contain it, but they're thought to have less effect on our blood cholesterol than saturated fats (see pp24–25). The cholesterol is transported in proteins called lipoproteins. There are two types: LDL (Low Density Lipoprotein), and HDL (High Density Lipoprotein). LDL delivers cholesterol from the liver to cells, but if there is more than is needed, it is deposited in the arteries and can clog them up, causing heart disease and strokes – this is **"bad" cholesterol**. HDL carries unused cholesterol back to the liver to be broken down and excreted, so it can help protect the arteries and is therefore **"good" cholesterol**.

Finding a balance

It's the balance or ratio between the LDL and HDL that's important. Blood cholesterol is measured in millimoles per litre (mmol/l). In the UK we are advised to have a total cholesterol level of 5mmol/l or less. The LDL cholesterol should be 3.0 mmol/l or less, and the HDL cholesterol should be more than 1.0 mmol/l for a man, 1.2 mmol/l for a woman. If the ratio of the total cholesterol figure (the two added together) divided by the figure for your HDL cholesterol is over 6, you are considered high risk – so a **higher HDL is better** as it will give you a lower ratio. If you have been told you have CHD or hardened (clogged) arteries, your **diet is still vital**. It can help to prevent any further blockage and may also reduce any damage that's already been done.

What's the right diet?

It's good to concentrate on the Mediterranean diet. It is low in saturated fat and rich in omega 3 and 6 fatty acids, from oily fish, nuts, and seeds, and from olive oil, which are thought to help reduce the risk of heart disease and boost the immune system. It also contains plenty of vegetables and fruit, packed with vitamins, minerals, and heart-protecting antioxidants (see pp28–33).

What about fats?

Go for unsaturated vegetable fats that can help reduce LDL levels. Olive oil is the Mediterranean choice, but for dressings also try rapeseed, linseed (flaxseed), avocado, and nut oils, such as walnut or hazelnut. They all contain essential omega 3 and 6 fats, which may help reduce the risk of heart disease. Eat plenty of oily fish for omega 3s, too. Go easy on saturated animal fats in butter, cream, fatty meats, and the skin of poultry as these increase LDL (see also pp24–25). While we should eat 2–3 portions of dairy products daily for calcium, they can be high in saturated fat, so choose low-fat options, such as skimmed or semi-skimmed milk and lower-fat cheeses (see on pp26–27 for more about dairy).

Do "butter" spreads help?

Butter-like spreads rich in plant stanols or sterols may help to reduce LDL cholesterol levels, but shouldn't be seen as the only solution to bad cholesterol. Try making your own nut butter, for example (see p185 for the recipe).

Can I still eat red meat?

A small piece of grilled, lean steak can be relatively low in calories while being high in protein and extremely satisfying. It is also a very good supplier of minerals, such as iron and zinc, but try not to undo the benefits by eating it with a rich, creamy sauce. If using cheaper, fatty cuts, trim off all the fat before stewing or casseroling, and spoon off all fat floating on top before serving.

What else should I eat?

It's wise to have lean red meat no more than twice a week. Other protein choices are skinless game and poultry, pulses and a small amount of soya products, eggs, and fish. White fish is good, but try also to have a two portions of oily fish such as mackerel a week (up to four for men), as they're rich in omega 3 fatty acids, which are thought to lower your risk of heart disease. Be clever with the way you eat them, though.

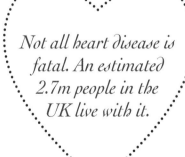

Not all heart disease is fatal. An estimated 2.7m people in the UK live with it.

A smoked mackerel pâté made with butter is full of saturated fat. If you make it with ricotta cheese instead, and serve on wholegrain toast with a big mixed salad, it's a lovely, nourishing meal. Have plenty of fibre, too (see pp22–23). Insoluble fibre in wholegrains and fruit and vegetable skins keeps the gut healthy and may reduce the risk of Type 2 diabetes (see pp172–173), which can lead to heart disease. Soluble fibre in fruit, vegetables, oats, and barley binds with cholesterol in the stools, ready for excretion.

How much salt?

Too much salt increases the water that is retained in the body, which raises blood pressure. This can damage the arteries, causing heart disease. It is recommended we eat no more than 1 level teaspoon of salt a day (6g), but preferably less (see pp94–95).

Cancer and *food*

Research has shown that nutritional factors play a part in about a third of cancers. Some foods are thought to damage body cells, exposing them to precancerous changes, but many others are thought to have a positive, protective effect on our bodies.

Prevention is better than cure, and the more we can tweak our lifestyle to reduce the likelihood of being affected by cancer the better. Of course there are other factors involved: genetics, smoking, pollution, and occupational hazards can all influence whether we are vulnerable to developing cancer. But if we can be confident that we're eating in the best possible way to help reduce the likelihood of any diet factors exacerbating the risk, this must be a good thing. Eating a poor diet doesn't mean that we will get cancer, but it is known that a healthy diet and regular exercise (see pp114–115) can reduce the risk of developing the disease. For those diagnosed with cancer, research has shown that some foods may help fight the disease as part of a healthy, balanced diet (see panel, far right).

Fruit and vegetables are top of the list. Your five – or more – portions a day give your body vitamins, minerals, and phytonutrients to sustain, protect, and restore it. In particular, vitamins A, C, and E, selenium, and many of the phytonutrients, including beta-carotene and lycopene, are all antioxidants. These help reduce the impact that free radicals and pollutants, such as smoking, have on our bodies, which may trigger abnormal cell behaviour and cancer. For more about these valuable nutrients, see pp28–33.

Prioritize fibre in wholegrains, fruit, and vegetables. Insoluble fibre helps prevent a build-up of harmful toxins and waste products in the body. Soluble fibre ferments in the gut, making short chain fatty acids that are thought to protect against bowel cancer.

Red meat should be eaten in moderation. It's high in saturated fat, contributing to weight gain, which can in turn increase the risk of cancer (see right). It's fine to eat a little lean red meat a couple of times a week, as it is a good source of protein, iron, and zinc. Balance it with other proteins, like skinless poultry, eggs, pulses, and plenty of fish – and include oily fish, nuts, and seeds to boost your omega 3 fatty acids (see p25), which may help protect against cancer.

Reduce salt and sugar. Salt may contribute to stomach cancer. Salty pickles in large quantities are thought to be culprits, so go easy on them. Beware of cured meats, too (see carcinogens, right). But you don't need to avoid salty foods such as smoked salmon completely since they can still be a nourishing, if occasional, treat. Have only a little and eat with wholegrains and fresh salad or vegetables for a better balance. Sugary foods raise blood-sugar levels (see pp172–173), which have been linked to increased weight gain and cancer risk. See pp92–95 for ways to cut back on sugar and salt.

Wine, especially red, contains the antioxidant resveratrol but in tiny amounts, so don't see it as a health-protector. Drinking too much alcohol increases the risk of cancer of the mouth, throat, liver, breast, oesophagus, and bowel. The more you drink, the higher your risk, so stay within the guidelines: for women, 2–3 units a day; for men, 3–4 units a day. If you have cancer, your consultant will advise on eliminating alcohol.

Dairy foods are fine to include in your diet, but it's best to avoid whole milk and go for semi-skimmed or skimmed milk and lower-fat cheeses to reduce saturated fat. Try not to exceed 2–3 portions a day (see dairy pp26–27 and portion sizes p41).

Soya beans and certain other foods contain phytoestrogens known as isoflavones, similar to a weak form of the hormone oestrogen. There is a debate whether eating more soya may reduce the risk of some breast cancer and other cancers. But other cancer patients on hormone therapy may be advised not to eat too much soya since there is concern that a high intake of phytoestrogens may have harmful effects. If you are being treated for cancer, consult your GP before changing your diet.

Being overweight increases your risk of developing oesophageal, pancreatic, bowel, endometrial, kidney, gallbladder, and post-menopausal breast cancer. If you're very overweight, the fat tissues in your body produce more growth factors (natural substances that stimulate cell growth) and hormones, and it's the high levels of these, especially oestrogen and insulin, that increase your risk.

Carcinogens are certain chemicals in food that may contribute to cancer. They include polycyclic aromatic hydrocarbons in meat that's burnt, or charred on the barbecue; heterocyclic amines in meat fried or baked a long time at very high temperatures; and nitrosamines in processed meats, such as bacon, and sausages. Eat them in moderation. Aflatoxin in mouldy foods, particularly peanuts, is also carcinogenic.

Foods to fight cancer

If you've been diagnosed with cancer, these are some of the delicious foods that can help you boost your body's defences.

* **Red and yellow peppers** and all other vitamin C-rich foods boost the immune system, heal, and repair.

* **Carrots** and all red, yellow, and dark green fruit and veg are full of beta-carotene, for a strong immune system.

* **Broccoli** and other green cruciferous vegetables contain indoles, thought to help fight several cancers.

* **Pomegranates**, berries, and some nuts have ellagic acid, a detoxifier thought to help fight most main cancers.

* **Almonds** and sunflower seeds are packed with zinc and vitamin E, which work with vitamin C to help heal.

* **Brazil nuts** are high in selenium, an antioxidant that works with vitamin A to boost the immune system.

* **Egg yolks** give you vitamin A, a powerful antioxidant, and B_6 to boost the immune system and fight infection.

* **Mackerel** and other oily fish have anti-inflammatory omega 3s, which may ease some chemo side-effects.

* **Garlic** contains sulphides, thought to have cancer-destroying properties.

Food-boosts for *convalescents*

Whether you have a child getting over a bout of flu or a member of the family recovering from an operation, nutrition is vital when the body is trying to heal itself. As it's also a time when they have little or no appetite, tempting, health-giving little meals are what's needed.

When we've been ill, we are at our most vulnerable. No matter whether we've had surgery or a spell of sickness, our body has been through trauma. Hormonal responses cause us to quickly use up a lot of our nutrient stores – not only vitamins and minerals, but also fat and protein in the muscles. It's important to sip plenty of fluids, especially water, to keep the body hydrated, but as soon as there are signs of appetite returning, you need to focus on replenishing those stores and gradually rebuilding the patient's health. The advice given here is about general principles to boost recovery; some illnesses will have particular nutritional needs, which your GP will explain.

First foods

If your patient is perking up and says they feel like something in particular, give them a very small quantity just to get their tastebuds going. Try to keep it simple and starch-based rather than citrussy or fatty – maybe something from the panel opposite. If they've been vomiting or had diarrhoea, start with just some plain boiled rice, dry toast, plain biscuits, or crackers for them to nibble until the symptoms subside completely. The stomach needs some time to settle. Once that's happened, a comforting bowl of light soup is often a good starting point, like the chicken noodle soup on p210.

The body builders

Once your patient is on the mend, you need to provide plenty of calories for energy, to repair the body, and to fight infections. The food should be appetizing and easy to digest and eat, so give small amounts, nicely presented, little and often. Big portions can turn the appetite off, so serve half-sized portions until they ask for more, which they will. They

{ To **build up** a weakened body, provide the patient with **small meals** or snacks that are full of health-giving **nutrients**, visually **tempting**, and **easy to eat**. }

need lean proteins, such as skinless chicken, white and oily fish (salmon and tuna are good options during convalescence), eggs, and pulses (red meat is too indigestible at first); dairy foods, such as milk, yogurt, and cheese; some fat (see pp24–25); and some starchy carbohydrates, such as bread, rice, pasta, and potatoes.

Fine-tune the fibre

A small amount of fibre will help with constipation, but high-fibre wholegrains tend to fill a depleted stomach before enough valuable nutrients are eaten. So it may be best to make a good-quality white-bread sandwich with a protein-rich filling such as fish, eggs, tender chicken, cheese, avocado, or nut butter (see p185), with a little salad for garnish.

Vital vitamins

Vitamin D is vital for healing, but we get most of it from the sun and your patient may not be ready to go out. Food sources are oily fish, milk, cheese, eggs, and fortified breakfast cereals and spreads, but if it's been a long illness, ask your GP about a supplement. Vitamin C is vital, too, so offer pure, unsweetened fruit juice or a nutrient-packed smoothie (see p97 and p191).

Try giving vitamin C-rich berries with some good-quality ice cream, or bake peaches with yogurt and honey (see p234). Fish pie (p194) or orzo "risotto" (p218) are also good. B vitamins are needed to process energy and boost the immune system – offer a rainbow of fruit and vegetables (in soups, for example, with maybe just a little cream to enrich them), plus oats, other grains, and quinoa, a grain-like food that's also rich in body-building protein.

Top up iron and zinc

Low iron levels are common after illness, especially if there has been blood loss, so provide foods rich in iron and also zinc to boost the appetite. Both are found in dark leafy greens, dried fruits, baked beans, canned fish, shellfish, eggs, cheese, fortified breakfast cereals, and nut and seed butters and milks. If the patient is pale and listless and doesn't rally, ask your GP about an iron supplement.

Plenty of fluids

It is very important to keep hydrated with plenty of fluids (see pp38–39 for drink ideas). Milky drinks (with whole milk or nut milk) will top up the nutrient intake, too. Add a little honey for an extra energy boost.

Ten tempting boosters

* **Grapes**
Probably the best-known treat for convalescents, grapes are full of vital nutrients and have anti-inflammatory properties.

* **Bananas**
Potassium is one of the key minerals lost in a stomach bug; bananas can put it back.

* **Porridge**
Oats contain the phytonutrient beta-glucan, which boosts the body's response to infection.

* **Eggs**
Easy to cook and eat, eggs supply body-building protein, healing vitamin D, and immune system-boosting B vitamins.

* **Salmon**
Offering healing vitamin D and body-building protein, salmon is also easy to eat.

* **Chicken**
Without its skin, chicken is a tender, digestible protein with all the B vitamins to strengthen the immune system.

* **Probiotic yogurt**
This yogurt is good for soothing the gut and has plenty of protein for body repair.

* **Spinach**
Not only does spinach have iron and anti-inflammatory phytonutrients, it's rich in appetite-boosting zinc too.

* **Avocados**
Rich in monounsaturated oil and protein, avocados also have anti-inflammatory properties.

* **Chocolate**
A small square of good, 70 per cent cocoa-content chocolate can help to boost the appetite.

Dementia

As dementia affects about 800,000 people in the UK, it has an impact on many families with ageing relatives. While there is as yet no cure for most forms of dementia, it may be possible to reduce the risk of developing it by eating a healthy diet, including some key nutrients.

What is dementia?

Dementia is a term used to describe a group of symptoms that appear when the brain is damaged. While it mainly affects people over the age of 65, it can strike earlier and sometimes remains undiagnosed for some time, with changes in behaviour blamed on getting old. The most common of the several causes is Alzheimer's disease, where brain cells die as a result of chemical and structural changes. Another is vascular dementia – the result of the oxygen supply to the brain failing, often following a stroke.

What are the signs?

Symptoms of dementia include memory loss (mainly short-term memory, such as failing to recall recent events), trouble finding the right words or remembering names, loss of mental agility and inability to follow conversations or television programmes, confusion about a familiar environment, and changes in mood and personality, often showing as depression and anger or, for some, as a lack of social inhibitions.

Who is at risk?

Anyone can get dementia but the older you get, the more likely you are to develop it. Two-thirds of diagnosed patients are women. This may be due to depletion of the hormone oestrogen, but research has shown that HRT does not lower the risk and may even increase it. Other risk factors that are also more likely to appear from the middle years onwards are high blood pressure, heart or circulation problems, strokes (overweight people are more at risk of developing these, and so dementia, too), the body's weakened ability to repair itself, and changes to the immune system and nerve cell structure. There's also some evidence of a hereditary factor, but this is still not fully understood.

How can food influence the brain?

Having a nourishing, well-rounded diet gives your brain the best chance of not succumbing to dementia. This is because there are strong relationships between eating well and reducing the likelihood of suffering from a stroke or the other causes of dementia. So establishing a well-balanced, Mediterranean-style backdrop of nutrients from the five food groups is the place to start (see pp12–13).

Foods that might help

It's thought that certain nutrients, included as part of a healthy, balanced diet, may help reduce the risk of dementia.

Vitamins B$_6$, B$_{12}$, and folic acid break down an amino acid called homocysteine, which can damage memory when levels are high. Good sources are green leafy vegetables, wholegrains, eggs, fish, dairy produce, and lean red meat.

Anthocyanins are phytonutrients in all purple and red fruit and veg (see p32), such as blueberries, pomegranates, cranberries, red grapes, and red cabbage. They may protect the heart and brain.

Vitamins A, C, and E are antioxidants that help prevent damage to the brain. The main sources are red, green, and yellow fruit and vegetables, eggs, nuts, seeds, wholegrains, lean red meat, and skinless poultry.

Vitamin D deficiency is linked to dementia, so (safe) exposure to the sun is vital, backed up by eggs, oily fish, and fortified breads, spreads, and cereals.

Omega 3 fats in oily fish, linseed (flaxseed), other seeds, nuts, and oils may have a protective effect on the brain and may also slow the development of dementia.

Turmeric, an anti-inflammatory spice, may improve symptoms.

What if you suspect it?

Just because you are forgetful doesn't mean you have dementia. But if you are worried that you, or a member of your family, may have a problem, go to your GP. He or she may carry out a simple cognitive test and discuss other possibilities, such as stress, depression, or other medical conditions. If necessary, you will be referred to a specialist.

Eating problems

When dementia sets in, sufferers can forget to eat, or may not even realize that food in front of them is there to be eaten. Mealtimes can be difficult and frustrating for everyone involved. Try to keep calm as you help to feed a person with dementia or help them to feed themselves. Cut food up small, if necessary, and don't overcrowd the plate. One-pot, easy-to-eat meals, such as beef and butternut squash tagine (p203), lentil and lamb shepherd's pie (p204), or mixed bean soup (p214), could be ideal – and if the dementia isn't too advanced, involve the sufferer in preparing the meal. If eating is a problem, ask your GP or local authority for help, as an occupational therapist can advise on ways to make mealtimes easier.

Weight issues

As dementia progresses, you may have difficulty persuading the sufferer to eat enough of the right foods and loss of appetite and weight can be a problem. Offering tasty, nutritious snacks, perhaps little sandwiches with a protein-rich filling such as egg with some cress, could help. Alternatively, eating too much may become an issue as the sufferer can forget that they've eaten. They may also have difficulty knowing when to stop, as they may not register that they're no longer feeling hungry. It's important to encourage them to get some exercise, not just for weight reasons but also because it can improve cognitive functioning.

Supplements?

When someone is not eating enough of the right nutrients, vitamin and mineral supplements can be invaluable, if you ensure they are taken correctly. Ask your GP about a supplement regime, including multi-vitamins, omega 3s, magnesium, and zinc.

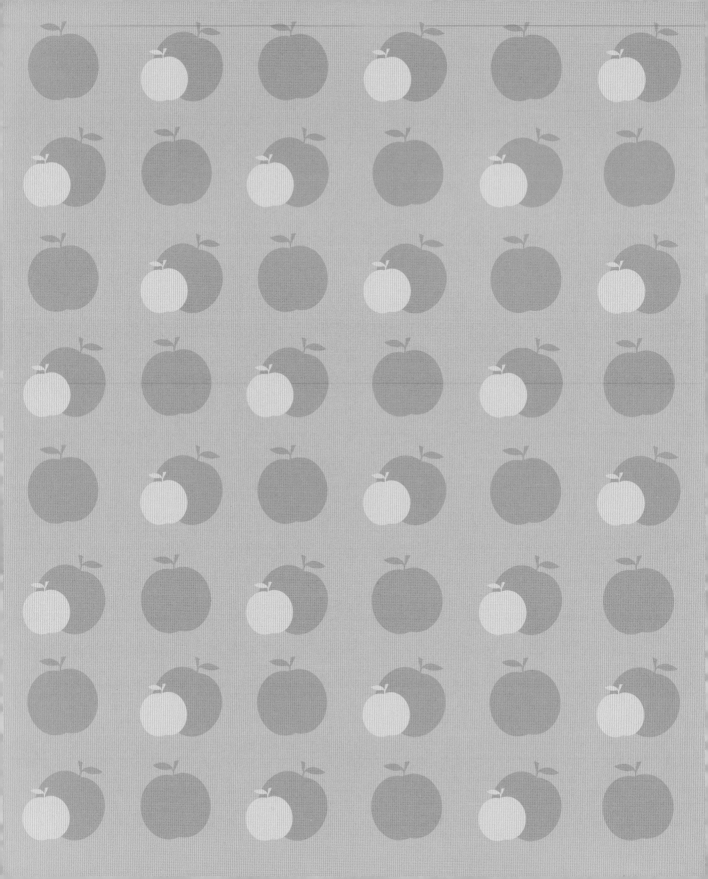

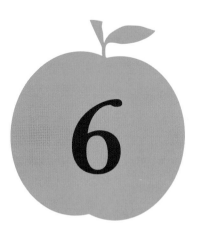

6

Classic recipes
made healthy

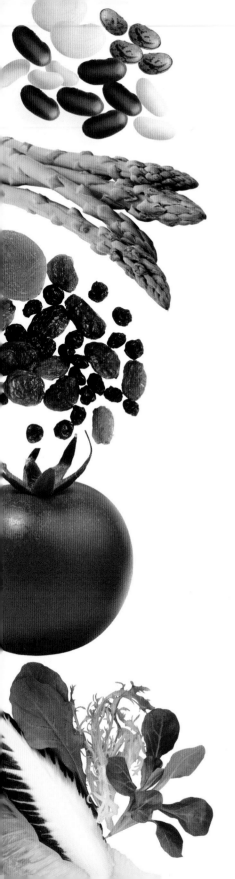

Recipes *for life*

There may be days when time and energy are short and cooking healthy meals for the family seems like extra pressure. However, you'll see from the recipes here that healthy can in fact be easy, enjoyable, and rewarding.

Cooking nutritious meals soon becomes second nature to you once you have the know-how. If you start with a few of the simple but delicious recipes in this chapter, you'll soon want to try some **variations and embellishments** of your own – and you'll find that rather than adding to the list of tasks you have to get through in the day, producing dishes full of goodness is a **satisfying, nurturing**, and often relaxing thing to do.

Although the recipes in this section of the book are divided into suggestions for breakfast, main courses, puddings, and baking, encompassing vegetarian dishes, sides, and starters along the way, don't feel constrained by this – some recipes can work just as well at different times of the day, with different tweaks made to them to **suit you and your family**. Many of them are wonderful, classic recipes, with just little twists to incorporate all the nutritional ideas discussed throughout this book, but you should feel free to play around with them and **make them your own**, tailoring them to suit your family's likes and dislikes. We often need a little encouragement to break out of the routines we tend to follow when shopping and cooking, so start with a few of these delicious basics and branch out from there.

One of the most useful strategies to adopt as a family is to build up some great **store-cupboard staples** which are simple to make and yet a nourishing, healthy version of things we love to dip into. Take the example of the recipe for nut butter (far right). It's the easiest thing to make, and the advantage it has over ready-made

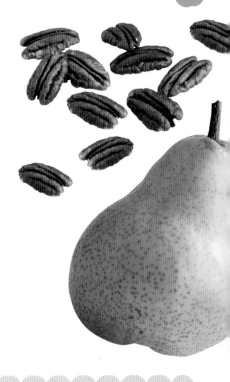

nut butters is that you can choose what goes into it – not only which type of nuts, but maybe the addition of some spices too, tasting as you go. It's also great to **show the family how food is made**, rather than just opening a jar, so that thought and care is associated with every mouthful we eat. A slice of warm, wholegrain toast, topped with some home-made nut butter and sliced banana, can be a perfect start to the day or a late-afternoon booster.

There are no doubts about the benefits of oily fish, but you may have fussy eaters in your family who need a bit of persuading to like it. The tuna teriyaki with stir-fried greens (see p198) and grilled mackerel fillets with coriander, ginger, chilli, and lime (see p199) both taste so vibrant and are completely in tune with the fusion cooking trends we see on the high street. Teenagers in particular enjoy being a little more experimental and fashionable with food, and if you encourage them to **join in with the preparation**, they'll take much more interest in eating food that's really good for their health. If those recipes sound a little too complex for a young cook's first steps, try them with the oat-crusted salmon nuggets (see p195). They're delicious warm and can be scrumptious cold the following day as part of a packed lunch to take to school or college.

For another change from lunchtime sandwiches, especially in the winter, wide-topped flasks are wonderful – you can ladle all sorts of things into them, such as noodle dishes (perhaps soup-based, such as the classic chicken noodle soup on p210) or even spaghetti and meatballs (see p200), for a warming lunch that will **keep your child fuelled for hours**. Snacks such as the cranberry and hazelnut chewy oat cookies (see p242) are heaven in a little mouthful and packed full of all sorts of nourishing ingredients – and so much better than a high-GI chocolate snack bar from the nearest shop to the school gates.

Small changes, simple recipes, and shared moments cooking together can have a major impact on the health of your family. A kitchen full of wonderful aromas soothes the soul, while the food on the table nourishes the body too.

Nut butter recipe

For a 200g (7oz) jar of home-made nut butter, all you need is 200g (7oz) nuts, unroasted and unsalted (almonds, peanuts, hazelnuts, or cashews, or a combination), 1 tbsp extra virgin groundnut or rapeseed oil, ½ tsp sea salt, and ½ tsp honey (optional).

1 Put the nuts in a food processor and pulse until they are quite finely ground.
2 Add the oil and process until you have a creamy paste.
3 Add the salt and honey, if using, and taste. You can also stir in a few chopped nuts at the end, if you prefer a chunky butter.
4 Store in the fridge, in an airtight container, and use within 1 week.

PROVIDES USEFUL IRON AND BETA-CAROTENE

Poached Autumn Fruit Compôte

A marvellous mixture of fresh and dried fruit makes this seasonal compôte easy to put together from a few simple store-cupboard ingredients, and will keep for up to three days in the fridge.

Ingredients

200g (7oz) mixed dried
   fruit, such as figs,
   apricots, and cherries
300ml (10fl oz) apple juice
1 cinnamon stick,
   broken in half
1 star anise
2 tbsp runny honey
2 dessert apples, peeled,
   cored, and roughly chopped
2 pears, peeled, cored,
   and roughly chopped

SERVES 4   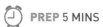 **PREP 5 MINS**   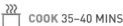 **COOK 35–40 MINS**

1 Roughly chop all the dried fruit to the same size as the dried cherries and set aside. Place the apple juice, cinnamon stick, star anise, and honey in a small, lidded, heavy-based saucepan and bring to the boil.

2 Add the dried fruit to the pan and reduce the heat to a low simmer. Cook, covered, for 15 minutes, until the dried fruit is soft.

3 Add the apple and pear to the pan and cook for 15 minutes, stirring occasionally, until the fresh fruit is soft as well. Increase the heat and cook, uncovered, for 5 more minutes until the sauce has reduced. Serve warm or cold, with yogurt or over muesli.

Nutrition data per serving

Energy	272 kcals
Protein	2 g
Fat	0.5 g
Saturated fat	0
Carbohydrate	66 g
Sugar	66 g
Fibre	6 g
Salt	0.1 g

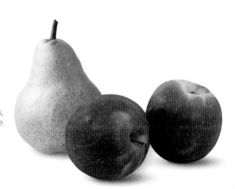

Apples and pears
These fruits are full of vitamins, phytonutrients, and gentle fibre. Try some of the more unusual, seasonal varieties for different textures and flavours.

Buckwheat, Oat, and Apple Pancakes

Buckwheat produces dark, nutty pancakes, which are lightened by the addition of grated apple. Serve them with extra apple slices, fried in just a little butter and sugar, for an indulgent treat.

FULL OF SOLUBLE AND INSOLUBLE FIBRE

Ingredients

50g (1¾oz) rolled oats
50g (1¾oz) buckwheat flour
or spelt flour
2 tbsp caster sugar
1 tsp baking powder
1 tsp cinnamon
125ml (4¼fl oz) buttermilk
or whole milk
1 egg, separated
½ tsp vanilla extract
1 large apple, peeled and roughly
grated (about 100g/3½oz of
grated apple)
1 tbsp butter, plus extra
if needed

MAKES 8   **PREP 10 MINS**   **COOK 10 MINS**

1 Process the oats in a food processor to a fine flour consistency. Transfer to a bowl and add the buckwheat flour, sugar, baking powder, and cinnamon. Mix well to combine.

2 Whisk together the buttermilk, egg yolk, and vanilla extract. In a separate bowl, whisk the egg white to form soft peaks. Make a well in the centre of the flour mixture, and whisk in the milk mixture. Beat until smooth. Fold the grated apple and then the whisked egg white into the pancake batter.

3 Melt the butter in a large, non-stick frying pan over a low-medium heat. Pour small ladlefuls of batter into the pan and then tip the pan to allow the batter to spread. The pancakes should spread to about 7cm (3in) in diameter. Cook each pancake for 2–3 minutes, until the edges start to set and small holes appear on the surface. Turn them over and cook for a further 1–2 minutes, until well browned and cooked through.

4 Set the cooked pancakes aside in a warm oven and continue with the rest of the batch, until all the batter has been used up, adding a little extra butter as needed. Serve with maple syrup or fruit compôte (see left).

Nutrition data per serving

Energy	97 kcals
Protein	3 g
Fat	3 g
Saturated fat	1 g
Carbohydrate	15 g
Sugar	6 g
Fibre	1 g
Salt	0.2 g

Buckwheat
It looks like a grain, but buckwheat is a fruit seed. The flour is gluten-free, high in fibre, protein, and other nutrients, and full of flavour.

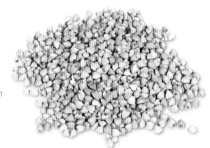

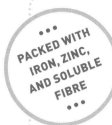

PACKED WITH
IRON, ZINC,
AND SOLUBLE
FIBRE

Cinnamon and Maple Granola

Home-made granola is surprisingly simple to make, and can be easily tailored to include all your family's favourite ingredients. A bowlful is a delicious start to the day.

Ingredients

25g (scant 1oz) unsalted butter
100ml (3½fl oz) maple syrup
¼ tsp fine salt
1 tsp cinnamon
300g (10oz) rolled oats
30g (1oz) pumpkin seeds
30g (1oz) sunflower seeds
75g (2½oz) flaked almonds
75g (2½oz) hazelnuts,
　roughly chopped
100g (3½oz) dried fruit,
　such as raisins, cranberries,
　cherries, and dates,
　roughly chopped

MAKES 650G (1LB 6OZ)

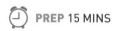 **PREP** 15 MINS

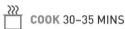 **COOK** 30–35 MINS

1 Preheat the oven to 150°C (300°F/Gas 2). Melt the butter in a small saucepan over a low heat. Take it off the heat and whisk in the maple syrup, salt, and cinnamon.

2 Mix all the remaining ingredients, except the dried fruit, together in a large bowl. Pour the maple syrup mixture over them and toss well to combine.

3 Spread the granola mixture over two large oven trays. Bake in the centre of the oven for 30 minutes, turning the mixture over every 10 minutes and spreading it out again so that it browns evenly. The granola is ready when it is golden brown and crunchy.

4 Cool the granola, mix in the dried fruit, and store in an airtight container for up to 2 weeks.

Nutrition data per serving

Energy	518–390 kcals
Protein	12–9 g
Fat	27–20 g
Saturated fat	5–2.5 g
Carbohydrate	56–42 g
Sugar	23–17 g
Fibre	7–5 g
Salt	0.2–0.15 g

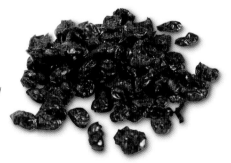

Dried cranberries
Tart yet sweet, cranberries have a deliciously intense flavour, and add a lovely splash of colour to any cereal. They're also a great source of antioxidant vitamins and minerals.

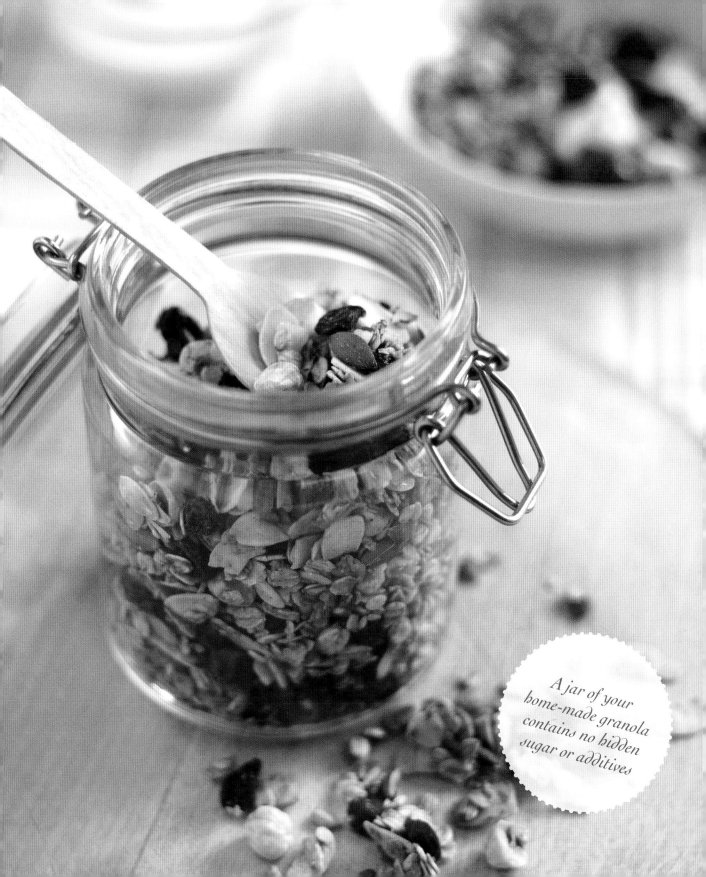

A jar of your
home-made granola
contains no hidden
sugar or additives

• • •
RICH IN
PROTEIN,
RIBOFLAVIN,
AND FIBRE
• • •

Spinach and Mushroom Egg-White Omelette

Egg-white omelettes can often be bland, but this version – full of dark, intensely flavoured mushrooms and spinach – is incredibly tasty and a nourishing start to the day.

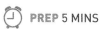

Ingredients

1 tbsp butter
1 tbsp olive oil
1 large Portobello mushroom, cleaned and finely sliced
large handful of baby spinach, about 50g (1¾oz), roughly chopped
small grating of nutmeg, or a pinch of dried nutmeg
salt and freshly ground black pepper
3 egg whites

SERVES 1   **PREP 5 MINS**   **COOK 5–7 MINS**

1 Heat the butter and oil in a large, heavy-based frying pan or an omelette pan over a medium-high heat. Add the sliced mushroom and cook for 5 minutes, stirring frequently, until softened and brown at the edges.

2 Add the chopped spinach to the pan, along with the nutmeg, and season well. Cook for 2 more minutes, until the spinach has wilted, and any excess liquid has evaporated.

3 In a large bowl, whisk the egg whites, using an electric whisk, until light and frothy. Spread the vegetable mixture evenly around the pan and pour the egg whites over. Use a heatproof spatula to smooth the egg over the mixture to incorporate all the ingredients.

4 Cook the omelette over a low heat for 1–2 minutes, until the edges are set and the underside turns brown. Using the spatula, gently fold the omelette in half, so the filling is completely covered. Continue to cook for 1 more minute on each side, pressing down gently with the spatula, until the centre is light and fluffy, but just set.

Nutrition data per serving

Energy	271 kcals
Protein	12 g
Fat	24 g
Saturated fat	9.5 g
Carbohydrate	1 g
Sugar	1 g
Fibre	3 g
Salt	0.9 g

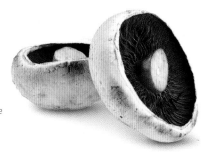

Portobello mushrooms
These mature versions of button mushrooms have a richer texture and flavour and make a tasty alternative to meat in many dishes.

Mango and Banana Breakfast Smoothie

FULL OF FIBRE, POTASSIUM, ANTIOXIDANTS, AND CALCIUM

This simple, nutritious recipe is a great breakfast-in-a-glass, takes hardly any time to prepare, and can be adapted to suit your personal taste. Children love inventing new versions.

Ingredients

2 tbsp rolled oats
1 small ripe banana
50g (1¾oz) frozen
    mango pieces
150ml (16fl oz) almond,
    soy, or cow's milk
pinch of cinnamon, to taste

SERVES 1   **PREP 5 MINS**

1 Place the oats in a food processor and process until reduced to a fine powder. Prepare more than you need and store the remainder in an airtight container or jam jar.

2 Place all the remaining ingredients along with the oats in a blender and blend until smooth.

Boosters: There are so many good things to add to a smoothie to increase its nutritional benefits. These include ground almonds and other nuts, all kind of seeds including flax and hemp seeds, and fresh or frozen berries. If you have a powerful blender it is a good idea to grind up the dried nuts and seeds before adding them to the smoothie, as this will give your drink a better consistency. Try grinding together a few different ingredients, and keep the powder in a jam jar to add to your smoothie a spoonful at a time.

Cook's tip: Bags of frozen fruit, or fruit mixes for smoothies, are a good thing to have available. Not only are they convenient, but they also help to chill and thicken the smoothie as it blends.

Nutrition data per serving

Energy	348 kcals
Protein	11 g
Fat	6 g
Saturated fat	1 g
Carbohydrate	62 g
Sugar	41 g
Fibre	6.5 g
Salt	0

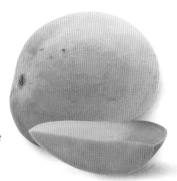

Mangoes
A feast for all the senses, ripe and fragrant mangoes are bursting with antioxidant vitamin C.

RICH IN VITAMIN B6, ANTIOXIDANTS, AND PROTEIN

Mediterranean Baked Fish

This tasty topping is packed full of Mediterranean flavours, and can transform even the mildest of white fish. The brightly coloured vegetables come with an array of antioxidants, too.

Ingredients

3 tbsp olive oil
1 onion, finely sliced
1 red pepper, halved, deseeded, and finely sliced
1 yellow pepper, halved, deseeded, and finely sliced
2 garlic cloves, finely sliced
16 cherry tomatoes, about 100g (3½oz) in total, halved
2 heaped tbsp finely chopped flat-leaf parsley
10 black olives, pitted and roughly chopped
1 tbsp capers, drained
2 tbsp lemon juice
150ml (5fl oz) fish or vegetable stock
salt and freshly ground black pepper
4 skinless and boneless white fish fillets, such as cod or haddock, 150g (5½oz) each

SERVES 4   **PREP 20 MINS**   **COOK 20–25 MINS**

1 Preheat the oven to 200°C (400°F/Gas 6). Heat the oil in a large frying pan over a medium heat. Add the onion and peppers and cook for 10 minutes, stirring occasionally, until the vegetables soften but do not brown. Add the garlic and cook for 1–2 minutes.

2 Take the frying pan off the heat and mix in the tomatoes, parsley, black olives, capers, lemon juice, and stock. Season well with black pepper and a little salt as the capers and olives will be salty.

3 Place the fish fillets in an ovenproof dish that fits them snugly and season well on both sides. Heap a quarter of the vegetable mixture over each fish fillet, pouring any excess around the dish.

4 Cook the fish for 20–25 minutes until it is cooked through and the fish flakes easily when gently pushed with the side of a fork.

Nutrition data per serving

Energy	242 kcals
Protein	29 g
Fat	10.5 g
Saturated fat	1.5 g
Carbohydrate	7.5 g
Sugar	7 g
Fibre	3 g
Salt	0.3 g

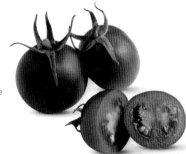

Cherry tomatoes
Bursting with antioxidant lycopene, these pop-in-your-mouth tomatoes taste sweet when raw and even more intensely flavourful when cooked.

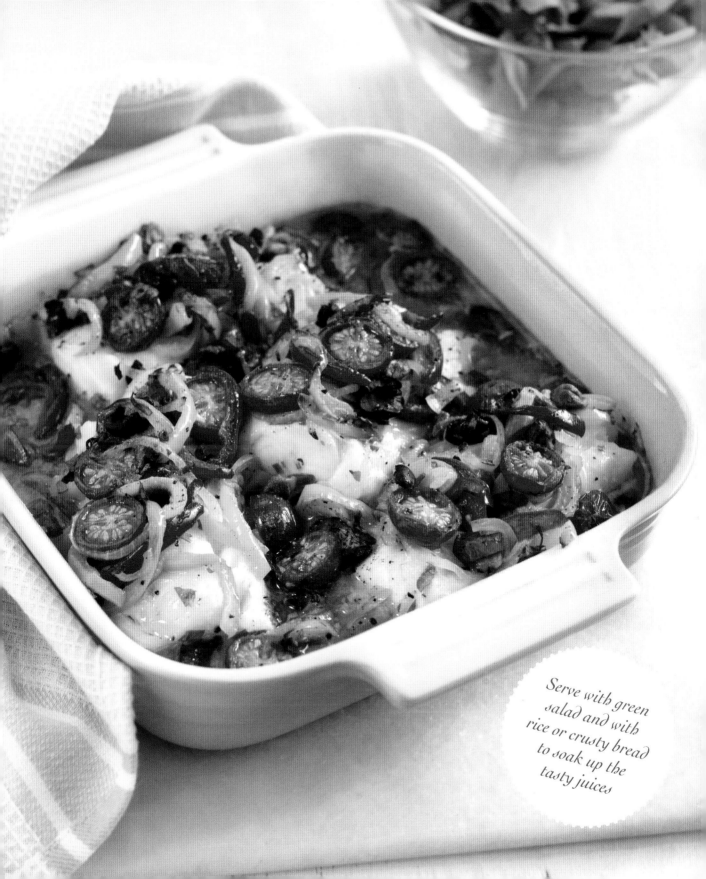

Serve with green salad and with rice or crusty bread to soak up the tasty juices

Herby-Topped Fish Pie

This new twist on an old classic is adorned with a topping that takes minutes to prepare and needs far less time in the oven than a traditional fish pie.

FULL OF PROTEIN, FIBRE, AND IRON

Ingredients

350ml (12fl oz) skimmed milk
1 bay leaf
1 tsp peppercorns
500g (1lb 2oz) mixed skinless and boneless fish, such as salmon, smoked haddock, and cod
125g (4½oz) king prawns, cooked, peeled, and roughly chopped
50g (1¾oz) butter
50g (1¾oz) plain flour
pinch of nutmeg
salt and freshly ground black pepper
50g (1¾oz) baby spinach leaves, roughly chopped

For the topping

4 thick slices of stale wholemeal bread, about 125g (4½oz), crusts removed and chopped into 1cm (½in) cubes
4 tbsp olive oil
2 tbsp finely chopped flat-leaf parsley
1 tbsp finely chopped dill

SERVES 4   **PREP** 30 MINS   **COOK** 30 MINS

1 Preheat the oven to 200°C (400°F/Gas 6). Place the milk, bay leaf, and peppercorns in a medium-sized, heavy-based saucepan. Add the fish and bring to the boil. Reduce to a low simmer and cook for 5 minutes, or until the fish turns opaque. Remove the fish and strain the milk. Discard the seasoning and reserve the milk for the sauce. Cool the fish in a mixing bowl and break into large chunks, then add the chopped prawns and set aside.

2 For the sauce, melt the butter in a small, heavy-based pan over a medium heat. Remove from the heat, whisk in the flour with a small whisk, then gradually whisk in the reserved milk. Cook over a medium heat, stirring constantly, until the sauce thickens. Season with the nutmeg, salt, and pepper, and cook over a low heat for 5 more minutes. Add the spinach to the cooled fish, pour the sauce over, and mix thoroughly, seasoning to taste.

3 For the topping, toss the bread with the oil and herbs and season well. Transfer the fish and spinach mixture to a 20cm (8in) square ovenproof dish. Spread the topping over the fish mixture. Cook in the oven for 15–20 minutes, until the top is golden brown and crispy and the filling is hot. Remove from the oven and cool for 5 minutes before serving with a crisp green salad.

Nutrition data per serving

Energy	520 kcals
Protein	37g
Fat	30g
Saturated fat	10g
Carbohydrate	26g
Sugar	5g
Fibre	3g
Salt	1g

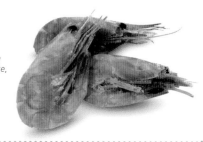

King prawns
These prawns have a distinctive sweet taste, and are surprisingly low in fat as well as rich in protein.

Oat-Crusted Salmon Nuggets

For those with a wheat intolerance, these nourishing oat-crusted salmon pieces are a healthy alternative to shop-bought fish fingers. Everyone will love their fabulous flavours, too.

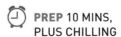

PACKED WITH BENEFICIAL OMEGAS AND PROTEIN

Ingredients

50g (1¾oz) rolled oats
25g (scant 1oz) grated
   Parmesan cheese
grated zest of 1 lemon
8 large basil leaves
salt and freshly ground
   black pepper
600g (1lb 5oz) piece of
   salmon fillet, skinned
1 egg, beaten
2 tbsp olive oil
1 tbsp butter

SERVES 4   **PREP** 10 MINS, PLUS CHILLING   **COOK** 5–7 MINS

1 Process the oats in a food processor until reduced to the texture of fine breadcrumbs. Add the Parmesan, lemon zest, and basil, season well, and process briefly to combine. Transfer the mixture to a shallow bowl.

2 Slice the salmon fillet into 1.5cm (¾in) slices. Place the egg in a separate shallow bowl. Dip each piece of salmon in the egg and then coat in the oat mixture. Place the coated fish on a plate, cover in cling film, and place in the fridge for 30 minutes before cooking. This will help the coating stick to the fish.

3 Heat the oil and the butter in a large, non-stick frying pan over a medium heat. Fry the fish for 2–3 minutes on each side, until they are golden brown and cooked through.

Nutrition data per serving

Energy	440 kcals
Protein	36 g
Fat	30 g
Saturated fat	7 g
Carbohydrate	8 g
Sugar	0.5 g
Fibre	1 g
Salt	0.4 g

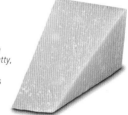

Parmesan
One of Italy's best-known cheeses, Parmesan is nutty, salty, and full of calcium and protein – a little goes a long way.

• • •
FULL OF
PROTEIN AND
NOURISHING
OMEGA 3
• • •

Zesty Fishcakes with Yogurt and Dill Sauce

Canned salmon is an easy and affordable way to get oily fish, which is packed with heart-healthy omega 3, into your family's diet. The herby sauce adds a piquant and creamy finishing touch.

Ingredients

500g (1lb 2oz) white potatoes, peeled weight, cut into large cubes
salt and freshly ground black pepper
105g can skinless and boneless salmon, drained
100g (3½oz) smoked salmon trimmings, chopped
4 spring onions, trimmed and finely chopped
2 tbsp finely chopped dill
1 heaped tbsp capers, drained and finely chopped
zest of 1 lemon
1 small egg, beaten
1 tbsp sunflower oil
1 tbsp butter, plus extra for the mashed potatoes (optional)

For the sauce

200g (7oz) low-fat Greek yogurt
1 heaped tbsp finely chopped dill
1 tbsp Dijon mustard

SERVES 4 **PREP 15 MINS** **COOK 40 MINS**

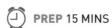

1 Preheat the oven to 200°C (400°F/Gas 6). Place the potatoes in a large saucepan of cold, salted water and bring to the boil. Reduce to a simmer and cook, uncovered, for 15–20 minutes until the potatoes are soft. Drain well and return them to the hot pan. Mash the potatoes to a smooth consistency, without using any extra liquid – this will help the fishcakes hold together later. If they are difficult to mash alone, use a teaspoon or two of butter. Leave to cool.

2 Place the cooled, mashed potato, fish, spring onions, dill, capers, lemon zest, and egg in a large bowl, season well, and mash together with the back of a fork, until well combined. Divide the mixture into 8 equal-sized balls, and press between your palms until they are smooth, with no cracks. Place the balls of fishcake mixture on a chopping board and pat them down on top, and around the edges, to make 8 evenly sized patties.

3 Preheat the oil and butter in a large frying pan and fry 4 of the fishcakes for 2–3 minutes on each side, until they are well browned. Place the browned fishcakes on an oven tray and fry the remaining 4. Bake the browned fishcakes in the centre of the oven for 10 more minutes, until they are hot right through.

4 For the sauce, combine all the ingredients in a bowl, season with salt and pepper, and mix well. Serve the fishcakes hot from the oven with the sauce on the side.

Cook's tip: These fishcakes can also be scrumptious served cold, for summer picnics and packed lunches. Or try serving them with some steamed asparagus and a poached egg on top, for a simple yet sophisticated supper dish.

Nutrition data per serving

Energy	304 kcals
Protein	22g
Fat	14g
Saturated fat	4.5g
Carbohydrate	24g
Sugar	4g
Fibre	2.5g
Salt	1.8g

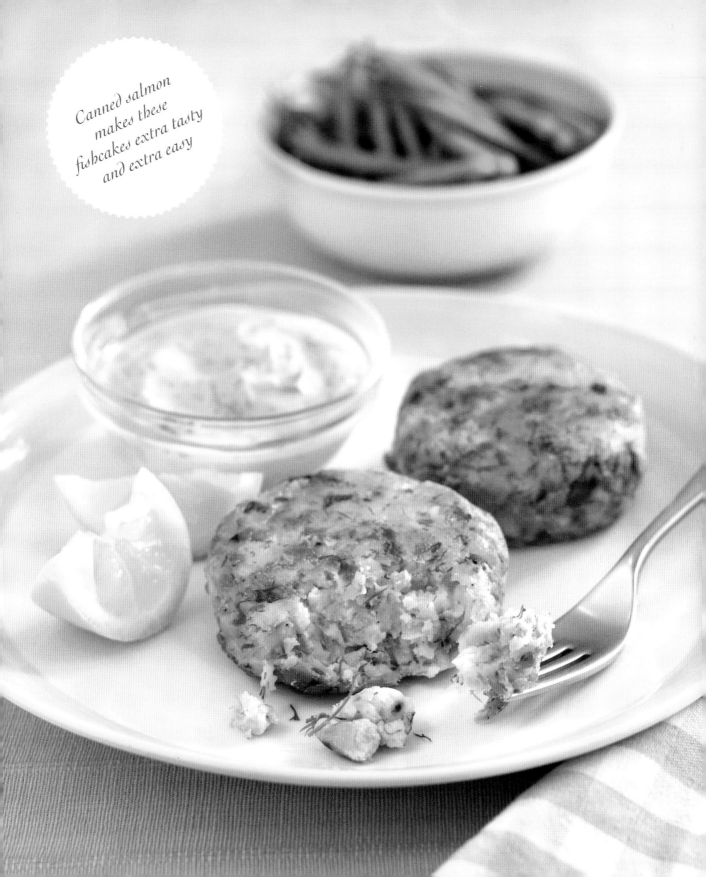

Canned salmon makes these fishcakes extra tasty and extra easy

• • •
PACKED
FULL OF
PROTEIN AND
OMEGA 3
• • •

Tuna Teriyaki with Stir-Fried Greens

Fresh tuna has a mild taste and meaty texture, and and is a good choice for people who don't usually like stronger-tasting fish. Use different seasonal greens as available.

Ingredients

For the tuna marinade
2 tbsp reduced-salt soy sauce
4 tbsp rice wine
2 tsp soft, light brown sugar
1 large garlic clove, crushed
3cm (1¼in) piece of fresh root ginger, finely chopped
4 tuna steaks, about 150g (5½oz) each, 2–3cm (¾–1¼in) in thickness

For the stir-fried greens
bunch of thin asparagus, trimmed and halved lengthways
bunch of tenderstem broccoli, about 200g (7oz), trimmed and halved
1 tbsp sesame oil
1 tbsp sunflower oil
bunch of spring onions, trimmed and cut into thirds
2 tbsp oyster sauce
1 tbsp reduced-salt soy sauce
1 tbsp rice wine or dry sherry

SERVES 4   **PREP** 10 MINS, PLUS MARINATING   **COOK** 10 MINS

1 Place all the marinade ingredients, except the tuna, in a shallow dish and mix well. Place the tuna steaks in a single layer in the marinade, cover with cling film. Chill in the fridge for at least 1 hour, turning once so both sides absorb the marinade.

2 In a large pan of boiling salted water, blanch the asparagus and broccoli for 1 minute. Drain the vegetables. Refresh in cold water, drain well, and set aside.

3 Preheat the grill to high. Grill the tuna on each side – 1 minute for rare, 2 minutes for medium, and 3 minutes for well done.

4 Heat the sesame and sunflower oil in a wok and stir-fry the spring onions for 1 minute. Remove from the heat and add the oyster sauce, soy sauce, and rice wine. Return the wok to the stove and cook until the sauce bubbles.

5 Toss in the blanched vegetables and cook for 1 more minute, until they are warmed through and the sauce has reduced. Serve the grilled tuna on a bed of stir-fried vegetables, with white or brown rice, or noodles.

Nutrition data per serving

Energy	328 kcals
Protein	40 g
Fat	13 g
Saturated fat	3 g
Carbohydrate	8 g
Sugar	6.5 g
Fibre	3 g
Salt	2 g

Asparagus
Fresh asparagus is a real delicacy, but its tender spears don't keep long – use them quickly to make the most of their flavour and many nutrients.

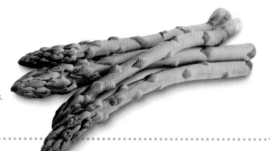

Grilled Mackerel with Ginger, Coriander, Chilli, and Lime

RICH IN OMEGA 3, VITAMIN C, AND PROTEIN

Marinating mackerel in citrus juice helps cut the oiliness of the fish, and softens its strong taste. Removing the skin makes it palatable for people who prefer a milder-tasting fish.

Ingredients

zest of 1 lime
juice of 2 limes, plus extra
    to serve
1 mild red chilli, deseeded
    and finely chopped
3cm (1¼in) piece of fresh
    root ginger, finely chopped
3 tbsp finely chopped
    fresh coriander
1 tsp soft, light brown sugar
4 large or 8 small
    mackerel fillets

SERVES 4

 PREP 10 MINS, PLUS MARINATING

COOK 10 MINS

1 To make the marinade, place all the ingredients, except the fish, in a bowl and whisk to combine well. Place the mackerel fillets, flesh-side up, in a single layer in a large, shallow dish. Spoon the marinade over the fish, spread it out evenly, cover, and chill for 30 minutes.

2 Preheat the grill to its highest setting. Line a large baking tray with tin foil and place the mackerel flesh-side up in a single layer. Grill the fish for 5–7 minutes, until golden brown on top and firm to the touch.

3 Use a fish slice to remove the mackerel from the foil. The skin should come away from the flesh and stick to the foil. Serve the mackerel with rice, a crispy salad, and extra lime squeezed over, if preferred.

Cook's tip: If you prefer to serve the fish with the skin on, as it holds a lot of the essential oils that are beneficial to your diet, grill the fish until it is just cooked on the first side, then flip it over and grill it skin-side up for 1–2 minutes until the skin is crispy.

Nutrition data per serving

Energy	445 kcals
Protein	37 g
Fat	32 g
Saturated fat	6.5 g
Carbohydrate	1 g
Sugar	1 g
Fibre	trace
Salt	0.3 g

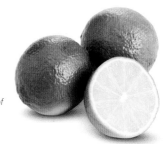

Fresh limes
Zingy in colour and taste, they are an excellent source of antioxidants vitamin C and K.

Spaghetti and Meatballs

Spaghetti and meatballs are a family favourite. Covered in a rich tomato sauce, the lean red meat is a great source of iron, while the wholewheat pasta provides extra fibre.

RICH IN PROTEIN, IRON, AND SELENIUM

Ingredients

For the meatballs

450g (1lb) lean minced beef
1 small onion, finely chopped
1 garlic clove, crushed
50g (1¾oz) fresh
    white breadcrumbs
25g (scant 1oz) grated
    Parmesan cheese
1 tbsp finely chopped thyme
1 tbsp finely chopped oregano
2 tbsp finely chopped
    flat-leaf parsley
1 egg, beaten
salt and freshly ground
    black pepper
2 tbsp olive oil

For the sauce

1 onion, finely chopped
2 garlic cloves, crushed
2 x 400g can tomatoes, chopped
    or crushed
250ml (9fl oz) chicken or
    beef stock
2 tbsp finely chopped
    flat-leaf parsley
300g (10oz) wholewheat spaghetti

SERVES 4 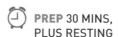 **PREP** 30 MINS, PLUS RESTING   **COOK** 1 HR

1 For the meatballs, place all the ingredients in a large bowl, season well, and mix thoroughly with your fingertips. Form 24 walnut-sized meatballs, cover with cling film, and allow to rest for 30 minutes. This will help them retain their shape on cooking. Heat the oil in a large frying pan with high sides. Fry the meatballs over a medium-high heat for 2–3 minutes on each side until they are browned, but not cooked through. Remove them from the heat and set aside.

2 To prepare the sauce, add the onion to the same pan and cook over a low heat for 5 minutes, until softened but not brown. Scrape up any residue left in the pan from the meatballs, as this will flavour the sauce. Add the garlic and cook for 1–2 minutes. Add the tomatoes, stock, and chopped parsley and season well. Bring the sauce to the boil, reduce the heat to a low simmer, and cook for 30 minutes until reduced and thickened. If the sauce looks too thick, add a little water. You can also make the sauce smoother, if you prefer, by either mashing it with a potato masher or using a hand-held blender.

3 Boil a large pan of salted water for the spaghetti and cook according to packet instructions. Add the meatballs to the sauce 10 minutes before the end of the cooking time. Turn them so that they are well covered in the sauce, reduce the heat to a low simmer, and cook, covered, until the spaghetti is ready. Drain the spaghetti and toss with the meatballs and sauce before serving with extra Parmesan, if you prefer.

Cook's tip: It is easy to make double the meatballs, then open freeze half of them on a tray. Once frozen, pack them into freezer bags for later use.

Nutrition data per serving

Energy	510 kcals
Protein	32 g
Fat	15 g
Saturated fat	5 g
Carbohydrate	60 g
Sugar	8 g
Fibre	10.5 g
Salt	0.9 g

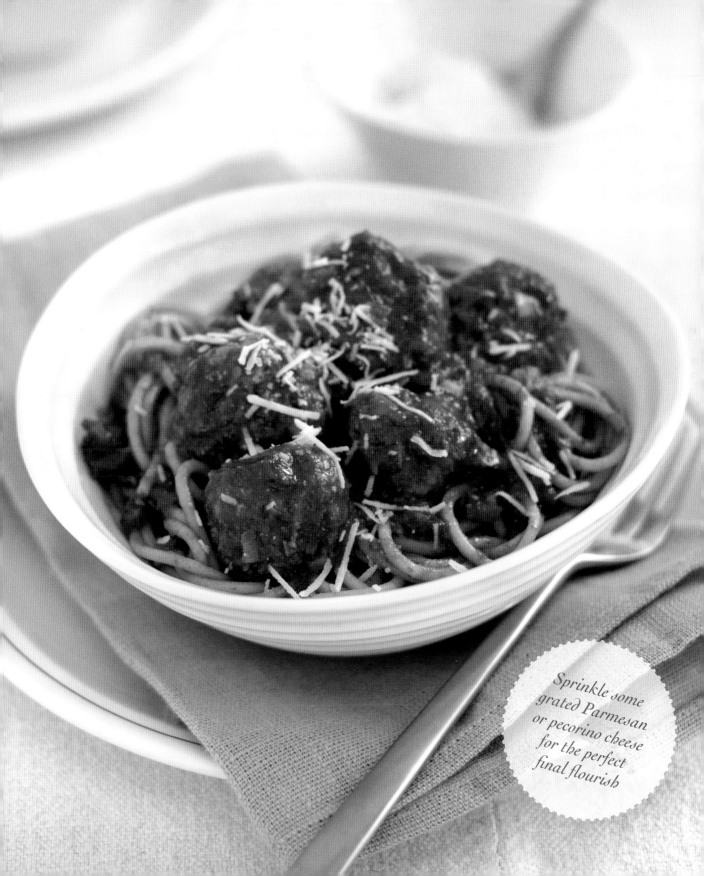

Sprinkle some grated Parmesan or pecorino cheese for the perfect final flourish

Beef, Sweet Potato, and Aubergine Moussaka

RICH IN FIBRE AND EASILY ABSORBED IRON

Sweet potatoes are a great substitute for white potatoes, as they cook more quickly and tend to give us a more consistent source of energy. Children also love their mild, sweet taste.

Ingredients
4–5 tbsp olive oil
1 onion, peeled and finely chopped
2 garlic cloves, peeled and finely chopped
450g (1lb) lean minced beef
400g can chopped tomatoes
200ml beef stock
½ tsp dried thyme
½ tsp dried oregano
2 tbsp finely chopped parsley
¼ tsp cinnamon
salt and freshly ground black pepper
2 sweet potatoes, about 200g (7oz) in total, peeled and thinly sliced
1 large aubergine, about 500g (1lb 2oz), cut lengthways into thin slices

For the white sauce
50g (1¾oz) butter
50g (1¾oz) plain flour
400ml (14fl oz) skimmed milk
pinch of nutmeg
2 eggs, beaten

SERVES 4–6   **PREP 30 MINS**   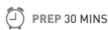 **COOK 2 HRS 30 MINS**

1 Heat 2 tablespoons of the oil in a large, heavy-based saucepan. Add the onion and cook over a medium heat for 5 minutes, until soft, but not brown. Add the garlic and cook for 1 more minute. Increase the heat, add the beef, and fry, moving the meat around continuously, until well browned.

2 Add the chopped tomatoes, stock, herbs and spices, and season well. Bring to the boil, then reduce to a simmer and cook over a low heat for 1–1¼ hours, until the liquid has evaporated and a wooden spoon drawn across the bottom of the pan exposes the surface of the pan.

3 Meanwhile, heat a griddle pan and brush it with a little oil. Chargrill the sweet potato slices, in batches, until charred on both sides, but still firm. Set aside. Do the same with the aubergine slices.

4 Preheat the oven to 180°C (350°F/Gas 4). For the white sauce, melt the butter in a small pan over a medium heat. Remove from the heat, whisk in the flour with a small whisk, then gradually whisk in the milk. Return the pan to the heat, and cook over a medium heat, stirring constantly, until the sauce thickens. Season with the nutmeg, salt, and pepper, and cook over a low heat for 5 more minutes. Remove from the heat and whisk in the beaten eggs.

5 To assemble the moussaka, spread half the meat on the bottom of an ovenproof dish. Cover it with half the aubergine, then half the white sauce. Place the sweet potatoes over the sauce in an overlapping layer, then the rest of the meat, followed by the remaining aubergine. Top with the rest of the white sauce and bake for 45 minutes to 1 hour until golden brown.

Nutrition data per serving

Energy	604–402 kcals
Protein	38–25.5 g
Fat	37–24 g
Saturated fat	14–9 g
Carbohydrate	31–21 g
Sugar	13.5–9 g
Fibre	7–5 g
Salt	1–0.6 g

Beef, Butternut Squash, and Red Pepper Tagine

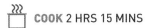

A GOOD SOURCE OF IRON AND BETA-CAROTENE

This heart-warming, mildly spiced stew is a tasty way to introduce a colourful and nourishing variety of vegetables into your family's diet.

Ingredients

4 tbsp olive oil
1 onion, finely chopped
1 red pepper, deseeded and thinly sliced
2 garlic cloves, finely chopped
3cm (1¼in) piece of fresh root ginger, peeled and finely chopped
500g (1lb 2oz) stewing steak, cut into cubes
2 tbsp plain flour
salt and freshly ground black pepper
1 tsp ground cumin
½ tsp smoked paprika
½ tsp cayenne pepper
¼ tsp cinnamon
½ tsp ground coriander
400g can chopped tomatoes
300ml (10fl oz) beef stock
200g (7oz) butternut squash, cut into 1.5cm (¾in) cubes
1 tbsp runny honey
handful of fresh coriander, roughly chopped

SERVES 4   **PREP** 20 MINS   **COOK** 2 HRS 15 MINS

1 Heat 2 tablespoons of the oil in a large, heavy-based saucepan over a medium heat. Cook the onion and red pepper for 5 minutes, until softened, but not browned. Add the garlic and ginger and cook for 2 minutes. Remove the cooked vegetables from the pan and set aside.

2 Toss the beef in the flour and season well. Heat the remaining oil in the pan and fry the beef over a high heat, a few pieces at a time, until well browned on all sides, then reduce the heat to low. Add the spices and ground coriander, stir them into the meat, and cook for 1–2 minutes until fragrant. Add the tomatoes, cooked vegetables, and stock and stir well to combine.

3 Bring the mixture to the boil, reduce to a low simmer, and cook, covered, for 1½ hours. Remove the lid and add the squash and honey. Cook for a further 20–30 minutes, uncovered, until the squash has softened and the sauce is reduced. Sprinkle with the chopped coriander and serve over couscous.

Nutrition data per serving	
Energy	362 kcals
Protein	34g
Fat	16g
Saturated fat	3g
Carbohydrate	21g
Sugar	13g
Fibre	4g
Salt	0.5g

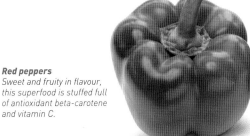

Red peppers
Sweet and fruity in flavour, this superfood is stuffed full of antioxidant beta-carotene and vitamin C.

Lamb and Lentil Shepherd's Pie with a Sweet Potato Crust

••• FULL OF FIBRE, PROTEIN, AND FOLATE •••

Lentils are an easy way to bulk up a favourite meat dish, lowering the fat content and boosting the protein. Here they take on some of the colour and texture of the meat sauce.

Ingredients

100g (3½oz) puy lentils
2 tbsp olive oil
1 onion, finely chopped
1 celery stick, finely chopped
2 carrots, finely chopped
1 small leek, trimmed and
    finely chopped
1 garlic clove, crushed
450g (1lb) minced lamb
1 tbsp plain flour
500ml (16fl oz) chicken,
    beef, or lamb stock
1 tbsp Worcestershire sauce
1 bay leaf
1 tbsp finely chopped rosemary
salt and freshly ground
    black pepper
700g (1½lb) sweet potatoes,
    peeled and cut into chunks
50g (1¾oz) grated
    Parmesan cheese

SERVES 4   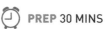 **PREP** 30 MINS   **COOK** 1 HR 30 MINS

1 Place the lentils in a small, heavy-based saucepan. Cover them with cold water, to a depth of at least 3cm (1¼in), and bring to the boil. Cook on a low boil for 5 minutes. Drain and rinse the lentils, and set aside.

2 Heat the oil in a large casserole or heavy-based saucepan. Cook the onion, celery, carrots, and leek for 5 minutes over a medium heat, until they are softened, but not browned. Add the garlic and cook for 1 minute.

3 Turn the heat up to high and add the lamb to the vegetables. Use a wooden spoon to break up the meat and move it around the pan frequently, until well browned. Stir in the flour, and cook for 1 minute. Add the stock, lentils, Worcestershire sauce, and herbs to the pan, and season to taste. Bring to the boil, and then reduce to a low simmer. Cook the lamb, uncovered, for 50 minutes to 1 hour until the sauce has reduced almost completely and the lentils are soft. If the stock evaporates before the end of the cooking time, add a little water.

4 Meanwhile, boil the sweet potatoes for 10–15 minutes, until tender, and drain them well. Transfer to a pan, add the Parmesan, and mash well. Season to taste, cover, and keep warm.

5 Preheat the oven to 200°C (400°F/Gas 6). Remove the rosemary and bay leaf from the lamb and place the lamb in a 20cm (8in) square ovenproof dish. Top with the mashed sweet potato and bake for 30 minutes until the top is golden brown.

Nutrition data per serving

Energy	620 kcals
Protein	36g
Fat	26g
Saturated fat	10.5g
Carbohydrate	56g
Sugar	15g
Fibre	11g
Salt	1.2g

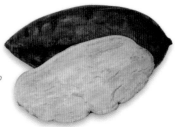

Sweet potatoes
Bursting with colour, flavour, and beta-carotene, sweet potato makes a lovely, nutritious twist on the more traditional mash.

Turkey and White Bean Chilli

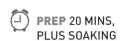
RICH IN PROTEIN AND HIGH IN FIBRE

This tasty and nourishing version of a traditional chilli is fantastic served as a simple lunch with flatbread – or you can serve it over rice, with a shredded salad, for dinner.

Ingredients

200g (7oz) dried haricot beans
4 tbsp olive oil
1 onion, finely chopped
1 celery stick, trimmed and finely chopped
1 large leek, trimmed and finely chopped
2 garlic cloves, finely chopped
1–2 mild green chillies, deseeded and finely chopped
450g (1lb) minced turkey
1 tbsp plain flour
2 tsp ground cumin
1 tsp ground coriander
½ tsp dried oregano
½ tsp cayenne pepper
750ml (1lb 10oz) chicken stock
2 tbsp finely chopped flat-leaf parsley
juice of 1 lime, plus 1 lime quartered, to serve
3 tbsp coriander, finely chopped
4 spring onions, trimmed and finely chopped
sour cream, to serve

SERVES 4–6

PREP 20 MINS, PLUS SOAKING

COOK 1 HR

1 Place the dried beans in a large bowl, cover them well with cold water, and leave to soak overnight. Drain and rinse the beans. Place them in a small, heavy-based saucepan and cover them with water to a depth of at least 3cm (1¼in). Bring them to the boil and cook for 15 minutes, until they are partially softened. Skim the surface of any residue, drain and rinse the beans, and set aside.

2 Meanwhile, to make the chilli, heat 2 tablespoons of the oil in a large, heavy-based saucepan. Cook the onion and celery over a medium heat for 5 minutes, until softened, but not brown. Add the leeks, garlic, and green chillies and cook for 1 minute. Add the remaining oil and the minced turkey to the pan. Use a wooden spoon to break up the meat and move it around the pan frequently, until well browned.

3 Add the flour, cumin, coriander, oregano, and cayenne pepper to the meat, and cook for 1–2 minutes to allow the spices to release their flavour. Add the stock, partially cooked beans, and parsley to the pan and bring to the boil, stirring well to release any residue at the bottom of the pan. Reduce to a low simmer and cook, uncovered, for 40–45 minutes, until the beans are soft and the sauce has thickened and reduced.

4 Remove from the heat and stir in the lime. Stir through most of the coriander and spring onions, reserving a little of each to sprinkle on top. Serve with sour cream, extra lime wedges, and hot sauce on the side.

Cook's tip: Minced chicken can also be used in place of turkey, if you prefer.

Nutrition data per serving

Energy	437–291 kcals
Protein	39–26 g
Fat	13–9 g
Saturated fat	2–1 g
Carbohydrate	30–20 g
Sugar	4.5–3 g
Fibre	13–9 g
Salt	0.8–0.5 g

• • •
A GOOD
SOURCE OF
PROTEIN AND
VITAMIN C
• • •

Spicy Turkey Burgers with Avocado Cream

These Mexican-inspired burgers are a low-fat alternative to the usual beef burgers. The avocado cream makes a tasty replacement for commercially made ketchup or mayonnaise.

Ingredients

For the patties
450g (1lb) minced turkey
50g (1¾oz) fresh
    white breadcrumbs
1 mild red chilli, deseeded
    and finely chopped
2 heaped tbsp finely
    chopped coriander
2 large spring onions, trimmed
    and finely chopped
zest of 1 lime
2 tbsp sunflower oil

For the avocado cream
1 very ripe avocado
1 tsp lime juice
2 heaped tbsp low-fat
    sour cream
salt and freshly ground
    black pepper

To serve
4 burger buns
lettuce leaves, sliced tomatoes,
    cucumber (optional)

SERVES 4 **PREP** 15 MINS **COOK** 12–15 MINS

1 Place all the ingredients for the patties, except the oil, in a large bowl and mix well. Make sure the mixture is thoroughly combined.

2 Form 4 equal-sized balls of burger mixture. Place them on a chopping board and pat them down on top, and around the edges, to make 4 evenly sized patties. Do not compress the mixture too much, or the burgers will be tough when cooked.

3 Heat the oil in a large frying pan over a medium heat. Fry the patties for 5–6 minutes on each side, until they are well browned and cooked through.

4 For the avocado cream, mash the avocado and the lime juice together until smooth. Mix in the sour cream and season well.

5 Assemble the burgers by placing the cooked patties in the buns, along with as many fillings as you like, and add a spoonful of avocado cream on top.

Nutrition data per serving	
Energy	480 kcals
Protein	36 g
Fat	18 g
Saturated fat	4 g
Carbohydrate	43 g
Sugar	3 g
Fibre	3.5 g
Salt	1.4 g

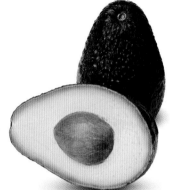

Avocado
Ripe avocado adds a smooth, buttery taste to this recipe, and is packed with good fats, fibre, and vitamins.

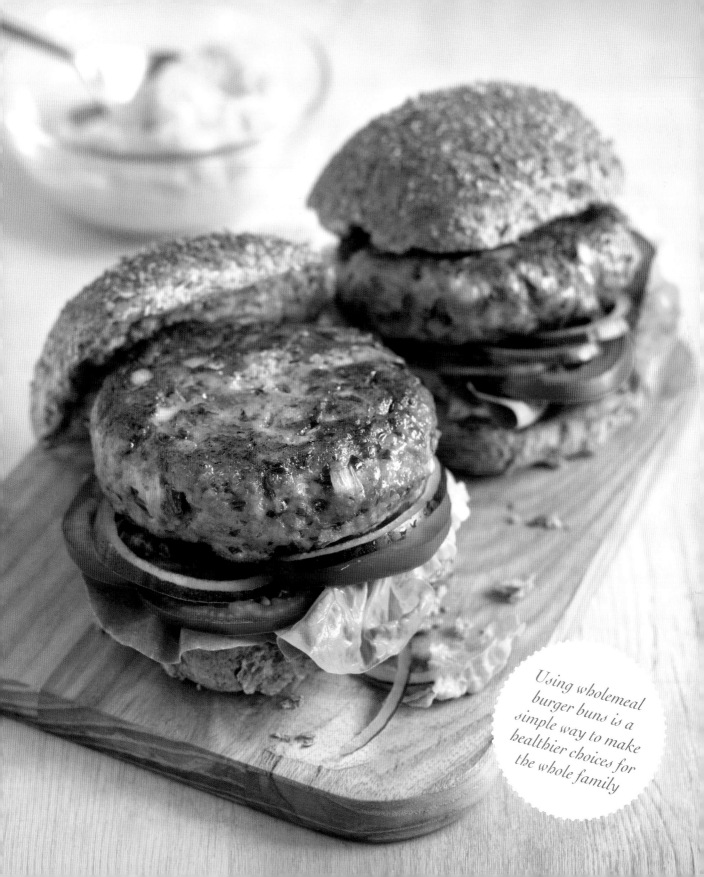

Using wholemeal burger buns is a simple way to make healthier choices for the whole family

Wholemeal Cheesy Chicken, Squash, and Chard Pasties

FULL OF PROTEIN, VITAMIN A, AND ZINC

These simple, hearty pasties turn leftover chicken into a tasty, portable meal, fantastic for picnics and packed lunches. Swap the chard for shredded kale or spinach if you prefer.

Ingredients

SERVES 6 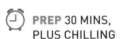 **PREP 30 MINS, PLUS CHILLING** **COOK 45–50 MINS**

For the pastry
125g (4½oz) wholemeal flour
125g (4½oz) plain flour, plus
   extra for dusting
½ tsp salt
125g (4½oz) butter, chilled
   and diced
1 egg, beaten, to glaze

For the filling
1 tbsp olive oil
½ onion, finely chopped
100g (3½oz) butternut squash,
   coarsely grated
1 garlic clove, crushed
2 tbsp plain flour
250ml (9fl oz) skimmed milk
50g (1¾oz) strong cheese, grated
100g (3½oz) Swiss chard,
   deribbed and finely shredded
250g (9oz) cooked
   chicken, shredded

1 For the pastry, sift both lots of flour and the salt into a large mixing bowl. Rub in the butter with your fingertips until the mixture resembles fine breadcrumbs. Make a well in the centre of the mixture and add 3–4 tablespoons of cold water. Bring the mixture together to form a smooth dough, using a little extra water if necessary. Wrap in cling film and chill for 30 minutes.

2 For the filling, heat the oil in a large, non-stick frying pan. Cook the onion over a medium heat for 3 minutes, until softened, but not browned. Add the squash and cook for 2 more minutes, stirring frequently, until it starts to soften and turns opaque. Add the garlic and cook for a further 1 minute.

3 Remove from the heat, sprinkle the flour over the vegetables, and mix well. Stir in the milk, a little at a time, until well combined. Cook over a low heat for 2–3 minutes, stirring frequently, until the sauce has thickened. Add the cheese and cook briefly until it melts. Fold the Swiss chard into the sauce, and continue to cook until it has wilted. Remove from the heat, stir in the chicken, season to taste, and set aside to cool. Preheat the oven to 180°C (350°F/Gas 4)

4 On a well-floured surface, cut the pastry into 6 equal pieces. Roll each piece out to a thickness of 5mm (¼in). Using a small plate or saucer (about 15cm/6in in diameter), cut out a circle from each piece of rolled pastry. Place one-sixth of the cooled chicken mixture in the centre of each circle, leaving a 1cm (½in) border around the edge. Brush the edges with a little of the beaten egg, bring them together to seal, and use your fingers to crimp the edges to make a pasty shape.

5 Place the pasties on a non-stick baking sheet, brush the outsides with a little more beaten egg, and cook in the centre of the oven for 35–40 minutes, until golden brown and cooked through. Cool for at least 15 minutes before serving warm or at room temperature.

Nutrition data per serving	
Energy	462 kcals
Protein	22.5g
Fat	28g
Saturated fat	15g
Carbohydrate	32g
Sugar	4g
Fibre	4g
Salt	1g

Roasted Chicken and Root Vegetables

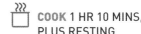

PACKED WITH PROTEIN AND BETA-CAROTENE

A good-quality chicken deserves star treatment, and here a simple tray of vegetables makes a colourful and tasty accompaniment that is also wonderfully satisfying.

Ingredients

1.5kg (3lb 3oz) whole chicken
salt and freshly ground
   black pepper
1 small lemon, halved
4 garlic cloves, skin on, crushed
   with the side of a knife
1 tbsp olive oil

For the vegetables
8 small new potatoes, halved
4 carrots, cut into 4cm (1½in)
   chunks
2 leeks, white part only, cut into
   4cm (1½in) chunks
2 parsnips, cut into 4cm (1½in)
   chunks
2 small onions, roots intact,
   trimmed and cut into quarters
2 tbsp olive oil
1 tbsp thyme leaves

SERVES 4–6   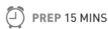 **PREP** 15 MINS   **COOK** 1 HR 10 MINS, PLUS RESTING

1 Preheat the oven to 240°C (475°F/Gas 9). Rinse the chicken, inside and out, and pat dry with kitchen paper. Season the cavity with plenty of salt and pepper, and place the lemon and the garlic inside it. Rub the chicken skin with the oil and season well. Place the chicken in an oven-proof pan and roast for 25 minutes.

2 Meanwhile, place all the vegetables, oil, and thyme in a large bowl. Season well and toss until the vegetables are well coated in the oil.

3 Remove the chicken from the oven and reduce the heat to 200°C (400°F/Gas 6). Add the vegetables to the pan and spread them evenly around the chicken. Roast for a further 45 minutes, until the vegetables are done, the chicken is golden brown, and the juices run clear when the thickest part of the thigh is pierced with a metal skewer.

4 Remove the chicken from the pan and leave to rest for 10 minutes before carving. If the vegetables need further cooking, return them to the hot oven until cooked. Turn off the heat and keep the vegetables in the warm oven while the chicken is resting.

Cook's tip: Serve as it is, or with a simple dark green, leafy salad of rocket and watercress with a citrus dressing.

Nutrition data per serving

Energy	519–346 kcals
Protein	59–40 g
Fat	15–10 g
Saturated fat	3–2 g
Carbohydrate	37–25 g
Sugar	16–11 g
Fibre	11.5–8 g
Salt	0.6–0.4 g

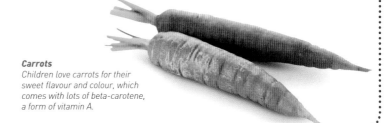

Carrots
Children love carrots for their sweet flavour and colour, which comes with lots of beta-carotene, a form of vitamin A.

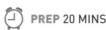

PACKED WITH PROTEIN, FIBRE, AND SELENIUM

Chicken, Vegetable, and Noodle Soup

Nothing is more comforting than a bowl of chicken soup. Perfect for when you are feeling under the weather, it is light yet tasty, warming, and nourishing.

Ingredients

For the stock

1 onion, peeled and quartered
1 celery stick, roughly chopped
1 large carrot, roughly chopped
2 leeks, green parts only, roughly chopped
$1/4$ tsp black peppercorns
pinch of sea salt
1 bay leaf
sprig of thyme
2 large or 3 medium chicken legs, about 400g (14oz), skinned

For the soup

2 tbsp olive oil
1 onion, finely chopped
1 large carrot, finely chopped
1 celery stick, finely chopped
2 leeks, white parts only, finely chopped
2 garlic cloves, finely chopped
2–3 tbsp finely chopped flat-leaf parsley
salt and freshly ground black pepper
150g (5½oz) egg noodles

Nutrition data per serving

Energy	354 kcals
Protein	25.5g
Fat	12g
Saturated fat	2.5g
Carbohydrate	37g
Sugar	10g
Fibre	7.5g
Salt	0.7g

SERVES 4　　**PREP** 20 MINS　　**COOK** 1 HR 30 MINS

1 Place all the ingredients for the stock in a large, heavy-based saucepan and cover with 2 litres (3½ pints) of cold water. Bring to the boil, then reduce to a simmer, and cook uncovered for 1 hour, until the stock is well flavoured and reduced to about 1.5 litres (2¾ pints). The top may need to be skimmed occasionally if foam forms on the surface.

2 Pour the stock through a colander, retaining the liquid, and set aside the cooked chicken to cool. Discard the vegetables. When the chicken is cool enough to handle, separate the meat from the bone, and shred it roughly.

3 For the soup, clean out the saucepan and return it to the heat. Heat the oil, then add the onion, carrot, celery, and leeks and cook over a low heat for 10 minutes, until softened. Do not brown. Add the garlic and cook for 1 minute. Then add the strained stock and the parsley and season well. Bring to the boil, reduce to a low simmer, and cook, uncovered, for 15 minutes.

4 Meanwhile, cook the noodles according to packet instructions. Drain well in a sieve and use a pair of kitchen scissors to snip them across in several places to make them easier to eat.

5 Add the chicken to the soup and cook for 5 more minutes. Then add the cooked noodles and heat thoroughly before serving.

Cook's tip: If you are cooking the egg noodles in advance, rinse them under a cold tap and drain them well. Tossing the noodles in a little oil will help them to stay separate, and not stick together, when they cool.

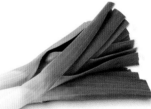

Leeks
Giving a gentler allium hit than the traditional onion, leeks are nonetheless rich in fibre and antioxidants.

Chinese Chicken and Rice

RICH IN PROTEIN, ZINC, AND FIBRE

Long, slow cooking brings out the delicious, warming flavours of this clay-pot style of Chinese dish, leaving the chicken soft and more-ish. Brown rice and seeds add a lovely nutty texture.

Ingredients

1 tsp sesame oil
2 tbsp Chinese rice wine
   or dry sherry
1 tbsp soy sauce
450g (1lb) skinless and boneless
   chicken thighs, cut into
   3cm (1¼in) chunks
2 tbsp sunflower oil
1 red onion, finely chopped
2 garlic cloves, finely chopped
5cm (2in) piece of fresh root
   ginger, finely chopped
1 green chilli, deseeded and
   finely chopped
1 tsp five-spice powder
1 litre (1¾ pints) chicken stock
300g (10oz) brown basmati rice
200g (7oz) small broccoli florets
200g (7oz) frozen edamame
   (soya beans)
2 tbsp pumpkin seeds
2 tbsp sunflower seeds

SERVES 4   **PREP** 10 MINS   **COOK** 1 HR 10 MINS

1 Place the sesame oil, rice wine, and the soy sauce in a large bowl and mix well. Marinate the chicken in the mixture for at least 1 hour.

2 Heat the sunflower oil in a lidded, heavy-based saucepan. Drain the chicken from its marinade and fry for 2–3 minutes, until coloured all over. Add the onion, garlic, ginger, and chilli and cook for 2 more minutes. Add the five-spice powder and cook for 1 more minute.

3 Pour the stock and any remaining marinade into the pan, then stir in the rice. Bring to the boil, then reduce to a low simmer, and cook, covered, for 50 minutes, stirring occasionally.

4 Meanwhile, blanch the broccoli and edamame in boiling water for 1 minute, then drain. Dry-fry the pumpkin and sunflower seeds in a non-stick frying pan for 2–3 minutes, until they start to colour and make a popping sound.

5 Stir the blanched vegetables into the rice and cook for a further 5–10 minutes, until the rice is cooked and all the liquid has evaporated. Remove from the heat and leave it to rest, covered, for 5 minutes before mixing in the toasted seeds to serve.

Nutrition data per serving

Energy	649 kcals
Protein	40.5g
Fat	22g
Saturated fat	3g
Carbohydrate	69g
Sugar	3.5g
Fibre	7g
Salt	1g

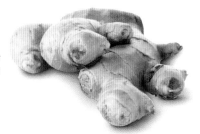

Fresh root ginger
Grated or finely chopped ginger is one of the three foundations of so many Asian dishes, along with garlic and fresh chillies. It also eases digestion.

Falafel Burgers with Rocket and Tzatziki

FULL OF FIBRE, ZINC, AND SOME USEFUL IRON

These herby vegetarian burgers make a great alternative to a traditional burger, and are quick and easy to make. Wrapped in pitta, they're also perfect for picnics and packed lunches.

Ingredients

For the falafel
400g can cooked chickpeas
75g (2½oz) fresh breadcrumbs
1 small egg, beaten
2 large spring onions, trimmed and finely chopped
1 large garlic clove, crushed
2 tbsp plain flour
2 heaped tbsp each of roughly chopped flat-leaf parsley, fresh coriander, and mint
½ tsp each of ground cumin and coriander
salt and freshly ground black pepper
2 tbsp olive oil

For the tzatziki
170g (6oz) low-fat Greek-style yogurt
1 garlic clove, crushed
handful of mint leaves, finely chopped

To serve
4 fresh pitta breads
70g (2¼oz) bag of rocket
1 lemon, quartered

SERVES 4

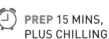 **PREP 15 MINS, PLUS CHILLING**

COOK 8 MINS

1 For the falafel, drain and rinse the chickpeas and place all the ingredients, except the oil, in a food processor and process to form a rough paste. Roll the mixture into 4 balls and flatten them to make 1.5cm (³⁄₄in) thick patties. Cover and chill in the fridge for 30 minutes, to help the patties hold together when cooking.

2 Heat the olive oil in a large, non-stick frying pan. Fry the patties, over a low heat, for 3–4 minutes on each side, until golden brown and crispy on the outside and cooked through.

3 For the tzatziki, mix together the yogurt, garlic, and mint, and season well. Heat or toast the pitta bread slightly to soften it (this can be done in a toaster), then use a small, sharp knife to split one side to make a pocket. Stuff each pitta pocket with a quarter of the rocket leaves and a falafel patty. Top with a little of the tzatziki, to taste. Serve the burgers with some lemon squeezed over, and hot sauce, if you prefer.

Cook's tip: These burgers are delicious served with Cajun ketchup (see p225).

Nutrition data per serving

Energy	454 kcals
Protein	21g
Fat	10.5g
Saturated fat	2g
Carbohydrate	71g
Sugar	5g
Fibre	6g
Salt	1.6g

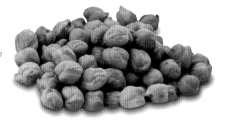

Chickpeas
Pwulses are a useful standby to keep in your kitchen. Rich in fibre and protein, chickpeas give a creamy, satisfying hit to any meal.

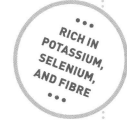

Root Vegetable Crumble

This creamy, homely dish is an easy and deliciously satisfying way to increase the amount of autumnal and winter vegetables in your family's diet.

RICH IN POTASSIUM, SELENIUM, AND FIBRE

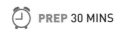

SERVES 4   **PREP** 30 MINS   **COOK** 50 MINS

Ingredients

1kg (2¼lb) mixed root vegetables, such as carrots, potatoes, turnips, parsnips, celeriac, sweet potatoes, swede, and squash, cut into 1.5cm (¾in) chunks
50g (1¾oz) butter
50g (1¾oz) plain flour
450ml (15fl oz) skimmed milk
100g (3½oz) grated strong cheese
1 tsp Dijon mustard, or more to taste
1 tsp grain mustard, or more to taste
salt and freshly ground black pepper
50g (1¾oz) fresh white or wholemeal bread, torn into rough chunks
25g (scant 1oz) rolled oats
25g (scant 1oz) grated Parmesan cheese
1 tbsp olive oil

1 Preheat the oven to 180°C (350°F/Gas 4). Cook the vegetables in a large pan of boiling, salted water for 10 minutes, until partially cooked. Drain them well and return to the pan.

2 Meanwhile, make the sauce. Melt the butter in a small, heavy-based saucepan. Reduce the heat to low and whisk in the flour. Cook the mixture over a low heat, whisking constantly, until it bubbles and separates under the whisk.

3 Remove the pan from the heat and slowly whisk in the milk, a little at a time, until it is incorporated and smooth. Return the pan to the heat and cook the sauce over a medium heat, stirring constantly, until it thickens. Reduce the heat to low and continue to cook, stirring occasionally, for 3–5 minutes. Add the cheese and both mustards, and season well. Cook for a further 1–2 minutes, until the cheese has melted.

4 Pour the sauce over the cooked vegetables, and gently turn them so they are well coated. Pile the vegetables into a 20cm x 25cm (8in x 10in) ovenproof dish (or similar) and smooth the top down.

5 For the topping, place the bread chunks, oats, and Parmesan in a food processor and season well. Process until the mixture resembles rough breadcrumbs. Tip the mixture onto the vegetables and smooth them over. Drizzle with the olive oil and bake in the oven for 35–40 minutes, until the top is golden brown and crispy and the vegetables are bubbling.

Nutrition data per serving

Energy	467 kcals
Protein	19 g
Fat	26 g
Saturated fat	14 g
Carbohydrate	39 g
Sugar	15 g
Fibre	11 g
Salt	1.4 g

Quick and Spicy Mixed Bean Soup

FULL OF FIBRE, LYCOPENE, AND PROTEIN

A meal in a bowl, this richly satisfying soup is packed with vegetables and pulses. Mildly spicy, it's even tastier the next day, and perfect in a flask to go.

Ingredients

2 tbsp olive oil
1 onion, finely chopped
1 celery stick, trimmed and finely chopped
2 garlic cloves, finely chopped
1 tsp smoked paprika
½ tsp cayenne pepper
½ tsp dried oregano
400ml (14fl oz) passata
400ml (14fl oz) vegetable stock
2 tbsp roughly chopped flat-leaf parsley
400g can mixed beans, drained and rinsed
2 tbsp finely chopped coriander

SERVES 4   **PREP** 10 MINS   **COOK** 30 MINS

1 Heat the oil in a large, heavy-based saucepan. Add the onions and celery, and cook over a medium heat for 5 minutes, until softened, but not browned. Add the garlic and cook for 1 more minute.

2 Add the paprika, cayenne pepper, and oregano to the pan and cook for 1–2 minutes to release the flavours of the spices. Then add the passata, stock, and parsley, and bring to the boil. Reduce to a low simmer and cook, uncovered, for 15 minutes.

3 Add the beans and cook for 5 more minutes. Stir in the fresh coriander just before serving with crusty bread.

Cook's Tip: For a hearty, non-vegetarian twist, try adding 50g (1¾oz) of diced pancetta to the onions in step 1, and replacing the vegetable stock with chicken stock.

Nutrition data per serving

Energy	165 kcals
Protein	5.5g
Fat	6.5g
Saturated fat	0.9g
Carbohydrate	16g
Sugar	6.5g
Fibre	6.5g
Salt	1.4g

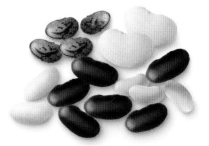

Mixed beans
Stock up on a selection of dried or canned beans for tasty soups, stews, and salads. They're good value and full of satisfying fibre and protein.

Angel Hair Pasta with Cherry Tomatoes and Rocket

A simple summery way with pasta that brings together the colours of Italy, this dish should be made with sweet, ripe tomatoes and plenty of freshly grated Parmesan cheese.

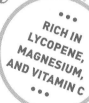

••• RICH IN LYCOPENE, MAGNESIUM, AND VITAMIN C •••

Ingredients

300g (10oz) angel hair
    pasta (spaghettini)
4 tbsp olive oil
50g (1¾oz) butter
2 large garlic cloves, crushed
400g (14oz) cherry tomatoes,
    halved, or quartered if large
salt and freshly ground
    black pepper
100g (3½oz) rocket leaves
grated Parmesan cheese,
    to serve

SERVES 4   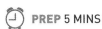 **PREP** 5 MINS   **COOK** 5–10 MINS

1 Boil a large pan of salted water and cook the pasta according to packet instructions. Meanwhile, make the sauce. Heat the oil and butter in a large frying pan over a medium heat. When it is bubbling, add the garlic and tomatoes and cook for 1–2 minutes, until the tomatoes soften slightly, but maintain their shape. Remove from the heat and season well.

2 Drain the pasta, then return to the pan, and pour over the tomatoes. Add the rocket and toss well to combine. The heat from the pasta will wilt the rocket. Stir well to combine the sauce, adjust the seasoning, and serve with plenty of grated Parmesan.

Cook's Tip: It is important to use ripe, flavourful tomatoes at the height of the season. Look for dark red, glossy skins and a slightly yielding texture when gently pressed.

Nutrition data per serving

Energy	470 kcals
Protein	10 g
Fat	23 g
Saturated fat	8 g
Carbohydrate	56 g
Sugar	6 g
Fibre	4.5 g
Salt	1.2 g

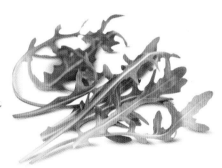

Rocket leaves
Garden rocket adds a sweet, peppery bite and a healthy dose of calcium, iron, and vitamin C to this dish.

Roasted Butternut Squash and Mushroom Lasagne

This colourful winter warmer is a healthy twist on a family favourite. For a richer, earthy flavour, try wholemeal lasagne sheets and a mild blue cheese.

PACKED WITH FIBRE, VITAMIN A, AND POTASSIUM

SERVES 4–6   **PREP** 20–25 MINS   **COOK** 1 HR 15 MINS

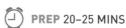

Ingredients

600g (1lb 5oz) butternut squash, peeled and cut into 1.5cm (½in) cubes
400g (14oz) chestnut mushrooms, halved or quartered
2 red onions, roughly chopped
4 tbsp olive oil
2 tbsp finely chopped sage
salt and freshly ground black pepper

For the sauce

50g (1¾oz) butter
50g (1¾oz) plain flour
450ml (14fl oz) skimmed milk
75g (2½oz) grated strong cheese, such as Cheddar
100g (3½oz) (about 6 sheets) precooked lasagne

1 Preheat the oven to 200°C (400°F/Gas 6). Mix the squash, mushrooms, and red onions in the oil, and toss together with the sage, salt, and pepper. Spread the vegetables out in a large roasting pan, and roast them at the top of the oven for 30 minutes, turning them once, until soft. Remove from the oven and set aside to cool.

2 For the sauce, melt the butter in a small, heavy-based saucepan. Remove from the heat and whisk in the flour. Whisk in the milk, a little at a time, until the sauce is smooth. Return the pan to the heat and cook, stirring constantly, until the sauce has thickened. Reduce the heat to low and continue to cook, stirring occasionally, for 5 minutes. Add two-thirds of the grated cheese, season well, and cook for a further 2–3 minutes until thick and creamy.

3 Reduce the temperature to 180°C (350°F/Gas 4). To construct the lasagne, spread one-third of the sauce at the bottom of a 20cm (8in) square ovenproof dish. Cover with half the vegetables, then a layer of lasagne. Repeat the process, finishing with a layer of sauce on top. Sprinkle the remaining cheese over the top and bake in the oven for 45 minutes – 1 hour, until it is well browned on top and soft when pierced with a knife. Remove from the oven and allow it to rest for 5 minutes before serving.

Cook's tip: Lasagne can be time-consuming to make. Get ahead by roasting the vegetables (step 1) up to a day before, and store them in the fridge in an airtight container until needed.

Nutrition data per serving

Energy	519 kcals
Protein	17 g
Fat	29 g
Saturated fat	12 g
Carbohydrate	48 g
Sugar	15 g
Fibre	7 g
Salt	0.7 g

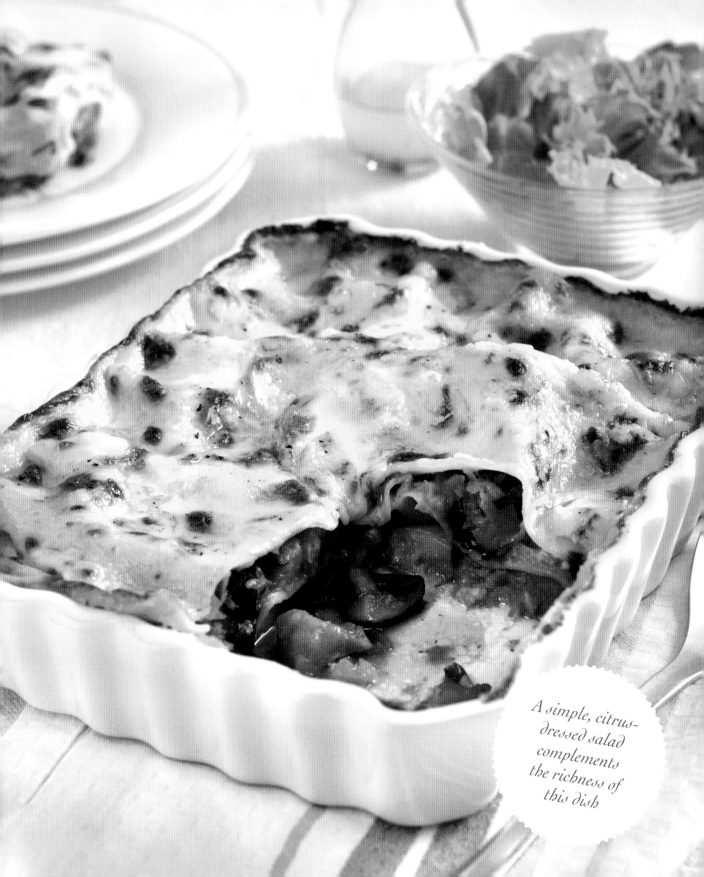

A simple, citrus-dressed salad complements the richness of this dish

A GOOD SOURCE OF VITAMINS C AND K AND FIBRE

Orzo "Risotto" with Pea Pesto

Try this shortcut risotto, made of pasta instead of rice. Children love this tasty, colourful dish, which makes a quick midweek supper and an equally delicious lunch if you have leftovers.

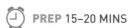

Ingredients

For the pesto
200g (7oz) frozen peas
1 handful mint leaves
100ml (3½fl oz) vegetable stock
salt and freshly ground
    black pepper

For the pasta
800ml (1¼ pints) vegetable stock
1 tbsp olive oil
1 tbsp butter
1 small onion, finely chopped
2 garlic cloves, finely chopped
300g (10oz) orzo pasta
50g (1¾oz) grated Parmesan
    cheese, plus extra to serve

SERVES 4   **PREP** 15–20 MINS   **COOK** 25 MINS

1 For the pesto, boil the peas in a large pan of salted water for 2 minutes, until just cooked. Drain them well, rinse under cold water, and allow to cool completely. Once cooled, place the peas, mint leaves, and vegetable stock in a food processor, season well, and process until smooth. Set aside.

2 Gently heat the stock in a small saucepan over a low heat. Meanwhile, heat the olive oil and butter in a large, non-stick frying pan. Cook the onion over a low heat for 5–7 minutes, until softened, but not browned. Add the garlic and cook for a further 2 minutes. Add the orzo and cook for a further 1–2 minutes, stirring until well coated in the oil.

3 Add the stock to the pasta, a ladleful at a time, stirring constantly, until well absorbed. Continue the process for at least 10 minutes, until the pasta is nearly cooked and most of the stock has been used up.

4 Add the pea purée to the pan and continue to cook, stirring constantly, for a further 2–3 minutes, until the excess moisture evaporates and the pasta is cooked through. Remove from the heat, stir in the Parmesan, and adjust the seasoning. Serve with extra Parmesan, if preferred.

Cook's tip: Any leftovers can be quickly reheated in a frying pan with a tablespoon or two of water to loosen the pasta as it cooks. Reheat thoroughly before serving.

Nutrition data per serving

Energy	463 kcals
Protein	17 g
Fat	12 g
Saturated fat	5 g
Carbohydrate	61 g
Sugar	4 g
Fibre	6.5 g
Salt	0.9 g

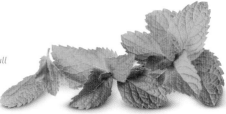

Mint
This aromatic herb adds amazing flavour. It is also full of vitamin C and used as a traditional aid to digestion.

Thai Rice Noodle Salad

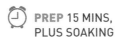

PACKED WITH FIBRE, POTASSIUM, AND VITAMIN C

Thai salads are hot, sour, sweet, and spicy all at once. Serve as a vegetarian main – or, if your family is happy to eat meat, add griddled chicken, prawns, or oily fish such as salmon.

Ingredients

200g (7oz) thin Chinese rice noodles
1 large carrot, finely shredded with a potato peeler
10cm (4in) cucumber, cut in half lengthways, deseeded and finely sliced on the diagonal
150g (5½oz) cherry tomatoes, halved, or quartered if large
1 celery stick, trimmed and finely sliced on the diagonal
½ red onion, very finely sliced
100g (3½oz) beansprouts
handful each of fresh coriander and mint, roughly chopped

For the dressing

juice of 2 limes
2 tbsp rice wine vinegar or white vinegar
1 tbsp Thai fish sauce
1 tsp caster sugar
½–1 tsp chilli flakes (optional)
pinch of salt
3 tbsp cashew nuts, roughly chopped, to serve

SERVES 4

PREP 15 MINS, PLUS SOAKING

1 Place the noodles in a large bowl and cover them with boiling water. Leave to soak for 5–15 minutes, depending on the type of noodles used, until they are soft but still have a bite to them. Drain well and refresh them under cold water.

2 While the noodles are soaking, place the rest of the salad ingredients in a bowl. Add the cold, drained noodles to the vegetables and herbs.

3 For the dressing, whisk together all ingredients, except the cashew nuts, in a bowl. Add it to the salad, toss it through, and serve, scattered with the chopped cashew nuts.

Nutrition data per serving

Energy	296 kcals
Protein	6 g
Fat	6 g
Saturated fat	1 g
Carbohydrate	50 g
Sugar	9 g
Fibre	3 g
Salt	1 g

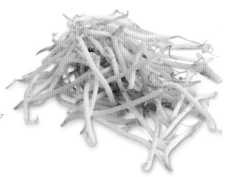

Beansprouts
Fun for children to grow their own (see p89), beansprouts are lovely and crunchy and full of vitamin C.

Sweet Potato and Coconut Curry

● ● ●
FULL OF
CALCIUM,
POTASSIUM,
AND VITAMIN A
● ● ●

This simple curry takes minutes to prepare and is ideal for a quick midweek supper. The mild spices and sweet potato complement the creamy coconut perfectly.

Ingredients

2 tbsp sunflower or coconut oil
1 onion, finely chopped
3cm (1¼in) piece of fresh root ginger, finely chopped
2 garlic cloves, finely chopped
1 large mild green chilli, deseeded and finely chopped
2 tomatoes, skinned, deseeded, and finely chopped
½ tsp ground cumin
½ tsp ground coriander
1 tsp garam masala
200ml (7fl oz) vegetable stock
400ml (14fl oz) coconut milk
1 tsp salt, plus extra to taste
400g (14oz) sweet potato, diced into 2cm (¾in) cubes
100g (3½oz) frozen peas
100g (3½oz) baby spinach
freshly ground black pepper, to taste
2 tbsp roughly chopped fresh coriander

SERVES 4–6   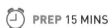 **PREP 15 MINS**   **COOK 25 MINS**

1 Heat the oil in a medium-sized, heavy-based saucepan. Cook the onion for 5 minutes over a medium heat, until softened. Do not brown. Add the ginger, garlic, and chilli and cook for 1 more minute.

2 Add the tomatoes and cook for 2–3 minutes, until they start to soften and break down. Then add the cumin, coriander, and garam masala and cook for 1–2 minutes.

3 Pour in the stock and coconut milk, season with the salt, and bring to the boil. Then add the sweet potatoes and reduce to a low simmer. Cook for 10–15 minutes, until the sweet potato is nearly cooked.

4 Increase the heat to a steady simmer, add the frozen peas, and cook for 2 more minutes. Add the baby spinach and cook for 2 more minutes, stirring frequently, until the spinach has wilted and the sauce has reduced and thickened. Remove from the heat and adjust the seasoning if necessary. Stir in the coriander and serve with steamed rice.

Nutrition data per serving

Energy	362–242 kcals
Protein	7.5–5g
Fat	24–16g
Saturated fat	16–11g
Carbohydrate	30.5–20g
Sugar	9–6g
Fibre	7–4g
Salt	1.2–0.8g

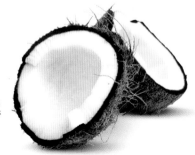

Coconut
Rich in monounsaturated good fats, coconut milk gives a lovely, "good for the heart" creaminess to anything it touches.

Macaroni Cheese with Butternut Squash

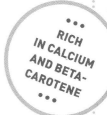

RICH IN CALCIUM AND BETA-CAROTENE

The ultimate in comfort food, here the velvety cheese sauce is made even more nourishing with the addition of puréed butternut squash.

SERVES 4–6   **PREP 20 MINS**   **COOK 1 HR**

Ingredients

400g (14oz) dried macaroni
300g (10oz) butternut squash, peeled, deseeded and cut into 2cm (³/₄in) chunks
500ml (16fl oz) skimmed milk, plus 2 tbsp extra
pinch of nutmeg
salt and freshly ground black pepper
1 heaped tbsp plain flour
125g (4¹/₂oz) grated strong cheese, such as Cheddar

1 Preheat the oven to 190°C (375°F/Gas 5). Boil a large pan of salted water and cook the macaroni according to packet instructions. Drain well and set aside.

2 Place the butternut squash in a medium-sized, heavy-based saucepan and cover with the milk. Add the nutmeg and season well. Bring to the boil, reduce to a low simmer, and cook, covered, for 10–15 minutes, until the squash is soft. Use a hand-held blender to purée the squash into the milk and make a smooth sauce.

3 Place the flour and 2 tablespoons of milk in a small bowl and mix. Whisk the flour and milk mixture into the sauce. Bring the sauce to the boil, stirring frequently, then reduce to a low simmer. Cook for 2–3 minutes, until it thickens. Add three-quarters of the cheese and whisk until it melts.

4 Pour the sauce over the cooked macaroni and mix well. Adjust the seasoning to taste. Place the macaroni in a 20cm x 25cm (8in x 10in) ovenproof dish, sprinkle over the remaining cheese, and bake in the centre of the oven for 30–35 minutes, until golden brown and bubbling. Cool for 5 minutes before serving.

Nutrition data per serving

Energy	560–373 kcals
Protein	26–17g
Fat	13–9g
Saturated fat	7–5g
Carbohydrate	86–58g
Sugar	11–7g
Fibre	6–4g
Salt	0.7–0.5g

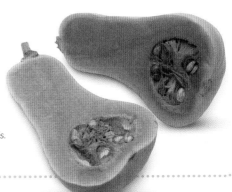

Butternut squash
Bursting with beta-carotene, this squash's warm colour, sweet flavour, and smooth texture tantalize the taste buds.

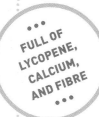

••• FULL OF LYCOPENE, CALCIUM, AND FIBRE •••

Mediterranean Vegetable and Mozzarella Bake

Meat-free meals should be a weekly event for the whole family. Underneath the crispy topping, these scrumptious vegetables are rich in vitamins, minerals, and fibre.

Ingredients

2 tbsp olive oil, plus extra
   for the vegetables
1 onion, finely chopped
2 garlic cloves, finely chopped
400g can chopped tomatoes
2 tbsp roughly chopped
   flat-leaf parsley
salt and freshly ground
   black pepper
2 tbsp roughly chopped basil leaves
2 red peppers
1 large aubergine, about
   450g (1lb), thinly sliced
2 courgettes, about 200g (7oz)
   each, thinly sliced lengthways
125g (4¹/₂oz) ball of mozzarella
   cheese, thinly sliced

For the topping

4 slices wholemeal bread,
   roughly torn
60g (2oz) pine nuts
50g (1³/₄oz) grated
   Parmesan cheese
handful of basil leaves

Nutrition data per serving

Energy	505 kcals
Protein	21g
Fat	33.5g
Saturated fat	9.5g
Carbohydrate	30g
Sugar	13.5g
Fibre	10.5g
Salt	1.1g

SERVES 4 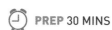 **PREP** 30 MINS **COOK** 1 HR

1 Preheat the oven to 220°C (425°F/Gas 7). Heat the oil in a small, heavy-based saucepan. Cook the onion for 5 minutes over a medium heat, until softened, but not brown. Add the garlic and cook for 1 more minute. Then add the tomatoes and parsley, season well, and bring to the boil. Reduce to a low simmer and cook, uncovered, for 30–40 minutes, until the sauce has thickened and reduced. Remove from the heat and add the chopped basil.

2 Rub the peppers with a little oil and cook in the oven for 25–30 minutes, turning them over occasionally, until they have softened and the skin has blistered in parts. Transfer them to a heatproof bowl and cover tightly with cling film. Remove the cling film after 5 minutes and drain off any water, carefully as it will be hot. When the peppers are cool enough to handle, deseed and skin them, leaving them in large pieces.

3 Reduce the oven temperature to 180°C (350°F/Gas 4). Heat a griddle pan over a high heat. Brush the aubergine slices with a little oil and chargrill for 2 minutes on each side, until they have scorch marks and are softened, but not cooked through. Do the same with the courgettes and set aside.

4 For the topping, place the bread, pine nuts, Parmesan, and basil in a food processor and season well with pepper and a little salt, as the Parmesan will be salty, Process the mixture until it resembles breadcrumbs.

5 To assemble the bake, grease a 20cm (8in) square baking dish with a little oil and place half the aubergines at the bottom. Cover them with half the peppers, and then half the courgettes. Spread over half the tomato and basil sauce and top it with the mozzarella slices. Repeat the process with the remaining vegetables, finishing with the last of the tomato sauce.

6 Spread the breadcrumb topping over and bake in the oven for 45 minutes until the top is golden brown and crispy. If the topping begins to over brown, cover the dish loosely with foil, but remove the foil for the final 5 minutes of cooking time, to crisp up the top. Remove from the oven and cool for 5 minutes before serving with a green salad and crusty bread.

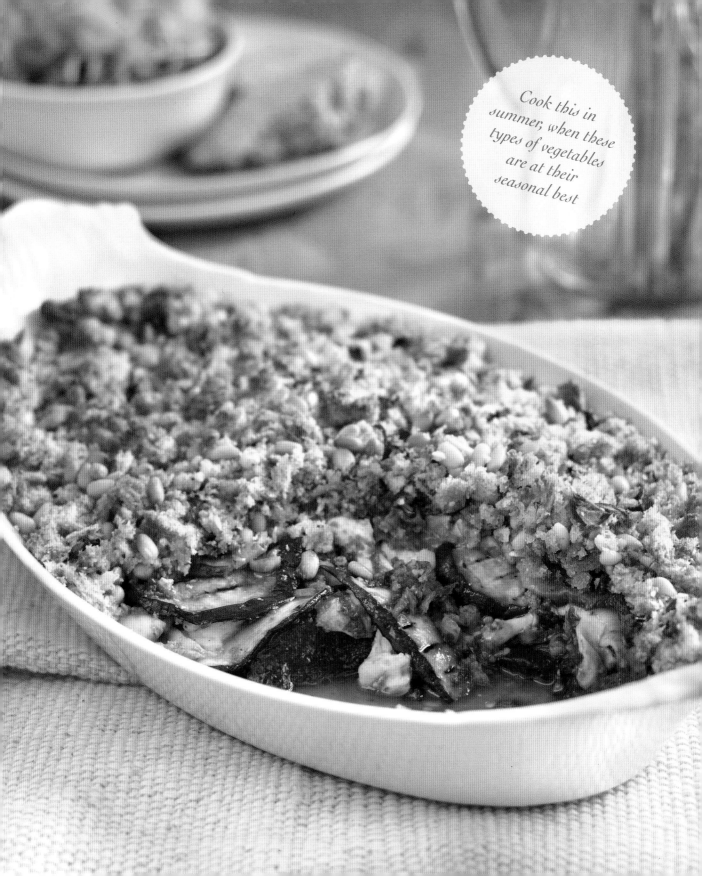

Cook this in summer, when these types of vegetables are at their seasonal best

Herby Hummus with Spiced Flatbread Crisps

Making your own hummus is easy – with handfuls of fresh herbs adding colour and flavour, it is ready in a flash, and a great staple to keep in the fridge for those peckish moments.

PACKED WITH PROTEIN, FOLATE, FIBRE, AND CALCIUM

Ingredients

For the flatbreads
½ tsp cumin seeds
½ tsp coriander seeds
½ tsp dried thyme
¼ tsp paprika
salt and freshly ground
    black pepper
4 large tortillas
2 tbsp olive oil

For the hummus
400g can chickpeas, drained
    and rinsed
1 large garlic clove, crushed
1 heaped tbsp tahini
½ tsp smoked paprika
juice of 1 lemon
100ml (3½fl oz) olive oil
large handful of fresh herbs,
    such as flat-leaf parsley, mint,
    and coriander, leaves only

SERVES 4   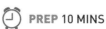 **PREP** 10 MINS   **COOK** 7 MINS

1 Preheat the oven to 200°C (400°F/Gas 6). Place the cumin, coriander, thyme, and paprika in a mortar and use the pestle to grind to a fairly coarse powder. Season with salt and a little black pepper.

2 Lay the tortillas out on a work surface and brush both sides evenly with the oil. Scatter the spice mix on both sides, patting it down to make sure it sticks to the surface. Pile the tortillas on top of one another, and cut them into 8 equal wedges. Spread them out in a single layer over two large baking sheets, making sure they do not overlap.

3 Bake the tortillas at the top of the oven for 5–7 minutes, until golden brown, puffed up, and crispy. Watch them carefully, as they burn easily. Remove from the oven and cool on a wire rack. They will crisp up further as they cool.

4 For the hummus, place all the ingredients in a food processor, season well, and process to a smooth texture. Serve alongside the tortilla crisps in a small bowl.

Cook's tip: You can of course serve your hummus with raw vegetable sticks, too, such as carrot, celery, and cucumber.

Nutrition data per serving	
Energy	492 kcals
Protein	10 g
Fat	29 g
Saturated fat	4 g
Carbohydrate	50 g
Sugar	1 g
Fibre	6 g
Salt	0.9 g

Tortillas
Yeast-free flatbreads are among the oldest breads in the world. Tortillas (Spanish for "small cakes") come from Mexico – your home-made crisps are great for guacamole, too.

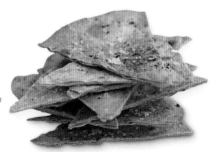

Sweet Potato Wedges with Cajun Ketchup

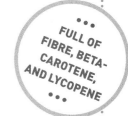

FULL OF FIBRE, BETA-CAROTENE, AND LYCOPENE

For a nourishing treat, try these smoky sweet potato wedges, with a tasty, additive-free homemade ketchup that the whole family will enjoy.

Ingredients

For the ketchup
150g (5½oz) tomato paste
100ml (3½fl oz) rice wine vinegar
4 tbsp maple syrup
¼–½ tsp cayenne pepper, to taste
½ tsp smoked paprika
¼ tsp garlic salt
¼ tsp salt

For the potato wedges
3 sweet potatoes, about 600g
   (1lb 5oz) in total
2 tbsp olive oil
1 tsp smoked paprika
½ tsp dried oregano
salt and freshly ground
   black pepper

SERVES 4   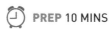 **PREP** 10 MINS   **COOK** 20 MINS

1 Preheat the oven to 220°C (425°F/Gas 7). For the ketchup, place all the ingredients in a small, heavy-based saucepan. Cover with 100ml (3½fl oz) of cold water and whisk together. Bring to the boil, reduce to a low simmer, and cook, whisking occasionally, for 15–20 minutes until the mixture has thickened and reduced. Remove from the heat and cool.

2 Cut each sweet potato into one-eighths, lengthways, to make 8 equal-sized wedges. In a large bowl, whisk together the oil, paprika, and oregano and season well. Add the potato wedges to the oil mixture and toss well until coated.

3 Spread the wedges out in a single layer on one or two non-stick, metal baking trays. Bake in the oven for 20 minutes, turning once, until golden brown and cooked through. Serve with the cooled ketchup.

Cook's tip: This recipe will make more ketchup than you need. You can store the remaining ketchup, in a jam jar or airtight container, in the fridge for up to 2 weeks.

Alternative dip: For a milder, less spicy dip, this delicious alternative takes just 5 minutes. Place 250g (9oz) of roughly chopped, cooked beetroot in a food processor. Add 1 crushed garlic clove, 2 heaped tablespoons of sour cream, and a small handful of dill. Season well and process the ingredients until smooth. Taste and adjust the seasoning if necessary. Serve alongside the potato wedges.

Nutrition data per serving

Energy	256 kcals
Protein	4 g
Fat	6 g
Saturated fat	1 g
Carbohydrate	45 g
Sugar	22 g
Fibre	6 g
Salt	0.9 g

Couscous-Stuffed Roast Peppers with Hazelnut Pesto and Feta

RICH IN VITAMIN C AND BETA-CAROTENE

These deep-red roasted peppers provide a light, comforting case for the couscous. The filling can also be served alone as a salad or side dish.

Ingredients

2 large red peppers
salt and freshly ground
   black pepper
2 tbsp olive oil
½ red onion, finely chopped
1 garlic clove, crushed
75g (2½oz) giant couscous
100ml (3½fl oz) vegetable stock
75g (2½oz) feta
   cheese, crumbled

For the pesto

15g (½oz) basil leaves
20g (¾oz) skinned
   hazelnuts, chopped
1 garlic clove, crushed
20g (¾oz) grated
   Parmesan cheese
60ml (2fl oz) extra virgin
   olive oil

SERVES 4   **PREP 30 MINS**   **COOK 45 MINS**

1 Preheat the oven to 200°C (400°F/Gas 6). Slice the red peppers into two, lengthways through the stems. Deseed them carefully to preserve the bowl-like structure. Rub the halved peppers, inside and out, with 1 tablespoon of oil and season well. Bake, cut-side up, in an ovenproof dish for 30 minutes or until softened and the edges slightly charred.

2 For the pesto, place all the ingredients, except the oil, in the small bowl of a food processor and process until they are well combined. With the motor running, pour the oil in slowly until the mixture is bright green and fairly smooth. Season to taste and set aside.

3 To prepare the couscous, heat the remaining 1 tablespoon of oil in a small, heavy-based saucepan, and cook the onion for 5 minutes over a medium heat until softened, but not brown. Add the garlic and cook for 1 minute. Then add the dry couscous and cook for 1–2 minutes, until it starts to colour slightly. Add the stock to the pan, bring to the boil, reduce to a simmer, and cook for 4–5 minutes until the couscous has absorbed all the stock. When it is cooked, transfer it to a bowl and leave to cool.

4 Mix the pesto into the couscous, along with two-thirds of the crumbled feta, reserving the rest for the tops of the peppers. When they are cool enough to handle, fill each pepper shell with the mixture, sprinkle the remaining feta on top, and bake for a further 15 minutes until heated through. These peppers are best eaten warm or at room temperature.

Cook's tip: The peppers can be roasted up to 2 days before and chilled until needed. Simply remove from the fridge, bring to room temperature, stuff, and cook as in step 4. You can also make double the delicious pesto and store it in the fridge for a quick pasta topping another day.

Nutrition data per serving	
Energy	325 kcals
Protein	8 g
Fat	25.5 g
Saturated fat	6 g
Carbohydrate	16 g
Sugar	6 g
Fibre	2.5 g
Salt	0.8 g

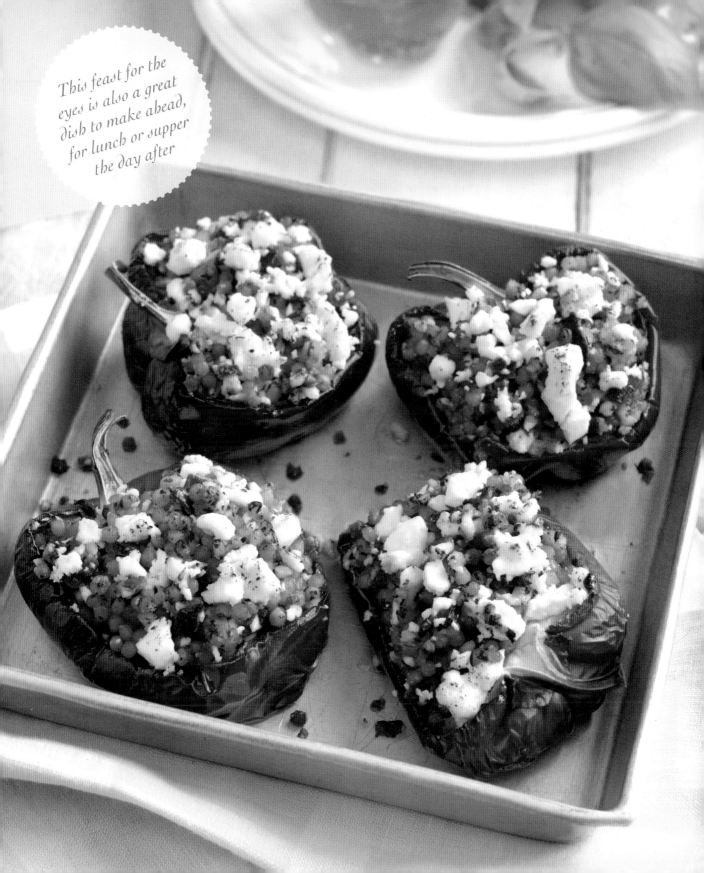

This feast for the eyes is also a great dish to make ahead, for lunch or supper the day after

Pea, Mint, and Feta Frittata

This simple, colourful frittata takes minutes to prepare and can be served hot or cold for a summer lunch or supper. A great dish to make ahead and put in the fridge for hungry teenagers to tuck into.

A GOOD SOURCE OF PROTEIN AND CALCIUM

Ingredients
2 tbsp olive oil
1 onion, finely chopped
2 garlic cloves, finely chopped
150g (5¹/₂oz) frozen peas
3 tbsp chopped mint leaves
salt and freshly ground
    black pepper
100g (3¹/₂oz) feta
    cheese, crumbled
6 eggs, beaten

SERVES 4   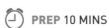 **PREP 10 MINS**   **COOK 25–30 MINS**

1 Preheat the oven to 200°C (400°F/Gas 6). Heat the oil in a 25cm (10in) ovenproof, non-stick frying pan. Cook the onion over a low heat for 10 minutes, until softened, but not browned. Add the garlic and peas and cook for 2 more minutes, until the peas have defrosted.

2 Remove the pan from the heat. Add the mint, season well, and spread the mixture evenly around the pan. Spread the feta over the peas and then gently pour the eggs over the top. Shake the pan gently to ensure that the egg settles into the mixture.

3 Return the pan to a low heat and cook for 2–3 minutes, until the sides start to set a little. Then place the pan in the oven and cook for 10–15 minutes, until the frittata is just set.

4 Turn the frittata out onto a plate and allow it to cool for at least 5 minutes before serving warm or at room temperature.

Cook's tip: Chunks of cold frittata make an easily portable lunch or picnic food. It is equally delicious sliced as a sandwich filling, with some crusty bread and a handful of salad leaves.

Nutrition data per serving

Energy	289 kcals
Protein	18 g
Fat	21 g
Saturated fat	7 g
Carbohydrate	6 g
Sugar	2.5 g
Fibre	3 g
Salt	1.2 g

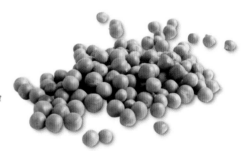

Peas
A useful standby to keep in your freezer, peas take minutes to cook, have a sweet taste that children love, and boost their vitamin C levels.

Roasted Mediterranean Vegetables with Lemon Basil Pesto

A tasty way to give the whole family their five a day, these roasted vegetables make a fabulous side dish for a barbecue. Serve as a vegetarian main with rice or couscous.

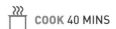

FULL OF VITAMIN C AND BETA-CAROTENE

Ingredients

1 aubergine, cut into quarters lengthways, and then into large chunks
1 red pepper, deseeded and cut into large chunks
1 yellow pepper, deseeded and cut into large chunks
2 small red onions, peeled and quartered
2 small courgettes, cut into large chunks
3 tbsp olive oil
salt and freshly ground black pepper

For the pesto

25g (scant 1oz) basil leaves
zest and juice of ½ lemon
1 garlic clove, crushed
1 heaped tsp capers
25g (scant 1oz) grated Parmesan cheese
100ml (3½fl oz) olive oil

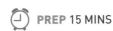

SERVES 4   **PREP** 15 MINS   **COOK** 40 MINS

1 Preheat the oven to 200°C (400°F/Gas 6). Place all the vegetables in a large, metal roasting tin. Drizzle over the oil, season well, and toss them together until well coated. Spread them out in a single layer and roast in the centre of the oven for 40 minutes, turning them occasionally, until cooked through and charred in places.

2 Meanwhile, make the pesto. Place all the ingredients, except the oil, in a food processor or blender and season well. Process the ingredients, adding the oil in a thin stream until well combined. You may need to scrape down the sides occasionally.

3 Remove the vegetables from the oven and allow to cool until they are warm, or at room temperature. Toss in the dressing to serve.

Cook's tip: This pesto is very versatile and can be used as a sauce for a summery roast chicken, grilled steaks, or fish.

Nutrition data per serving

Energy	329 kcals
Protein	5 g
Fat	29 g
Saturated fat	5 g
Carbohydrate	11 g
Sugar	10 g
Fibre	5.5 g
Salt	0.2 g

Aubergine
This versatile vegetable readily absorbs whatever flavours it is cooked with and makes a tasty substitute for meat.

PACKED WITH
FIBRE AND
VITAMIN A
AND C

The Perfect
Summer Salad

This salad benefits from using young, raw vegetables at their best – small, young fennel and crisp, bright sugar snaps dressed in a citrussy vinaigrette.

Ingredients
150g (5¹/₂oz) bag of mixed-leaf salad, such as baby leaves, baby spinach, and rocket
handful of mint leaves
1 small fennel bulb, trimmed, halved, and finely sliced
10cm (4in) piece of cucumber, halved and thinly sliced
4–8 radishes (depending on size), washed and finely sliced
50g (1³/₄oz) sugar snap peas, trimmed and finely sliced on the diagonal
handful of edible flowers, such as pansies or nasturtiums, to serve (optional)

For the dressing
2 tbsp extra virgin olive oil
1 tbsp freshly squeezed lemon juice
1 tsp Dijon mustard
salt and freshly ground black pepper

SERVES 4   **PREP 10 MINS**

1 For the dressing, place the oil, lemon juice, and mustard in a large salad bowl and season well. Whisk together, until well combined.

2 For the salad, place the remaining ingredients in the bowl and toss gently to coat. Make sure the heavier ingredients are evenly distributed amongst the leaves. To serve, scatter edible flowers on top, if available.

Cook's tip: A salad can be made of whatever ingredients you have at hand, but for a salad with layers of flavour and texture, try to choose at least one of each of the following catagories:
• **Lettuce** loose-leaf or crunchy, well washed and drained, and torn into bite-sized pieces.
• **Salad leaves** try stronger leaves, such as rocket, mizuna, or mixed leaves, for their extra flavour, colour, and texture.
• **Salad herbs** go for soft-leaved herbs such as mint, flat-leaf parsley, coriander, or more unusual ones such as loveage and chervil.
• **Salad vegetables** thinly sliced raw vegetables such as cucumber, radish, courgette, or fennel work well, as do baby peas or halved cherry tomatoes. Cutting the vegetables very finely makes sure they don't sink to the bottom of the bowl when you toss the salad.

Nutrition data per serving

Energy	71 kcals
Protein	1.6g
Fat	6g
Saturated fat	0.8g
Carbohydrate	3g
Sugar	2.5g
Fibre	2.5g
Salt	0.1g

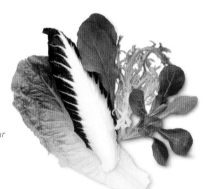

Mixed salad leaves
A bag of mixed leaves adds a bright, spicy flavour to your salads, as well as colour, texture, and gentle fibre.

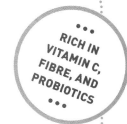

Red Cabbage, Fennel, and Apple Slaw

This simple, modern take on traditional coleslaw takes minutes to put together and is bursting with vibrant colours and fresh flavours.

RICH IN VITAMIN C, FIBRE, AND PROBIOTICS

Ingredients

2 tbsp low-fat Greek yogurt
2 tbsp good-quality mayonnaise
1 tsp lemon juice
1 tbsp finely chopped mint
1 tbsp finely chopped fennel fronds and 75g (2¹/₂oz) fennel bulbs, very finely sliced
1 spring onion, trimmed and finely chopped
salt and freshly ground black pepper
1 large apple, peeled, quartered, and cut into thin matchsticks
125g (4½oz) red cabbage, very finely sliced

SERVES 4   **PREP** 5 MINS

1 Place the yogurt, mayonnaise, and lemon juice in a large mixing bowl and whisk until thoroughly combined.

2 Add the mint, fennel fronds, and spring onions and season well. Then fold in the apple, fennel bulbs, and red cabbage and serve immediately.

Cook's tip: If preparing ahead, make the dressing and leave it, covered, in the fridge. Shred the apple and fennel, toss them in a little lemon juice, cover, and chill until needed. Cut the red cabbage and store it separately.

Nutrition data per serving

Energy	83 kcals
Protein	2 g
Fat	6 g
Saturated fat	1 g
Carbohydrate	6 g
Sugar	6 g
Fibre	3 g
Salt	0.1 g

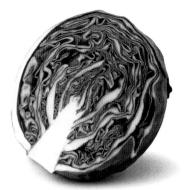

Red cabbage
These crunchy, burgundy-red leaves are loaded with protective phytonutrients called polyphenols, and 6–8 times more vitamin C than green cabbage.

• • •
FULL OF
FIBRE, BETA-
CAROTENE,
AND CALCIUM
• • •

Summer Berry Layered Compôte

A scrumptious source of vitamins and antioxidants, a few punnets of berries can be turned into a dessert in a matter of minutes with this easy, creamy layering and cheat's brûlée on top.

Ingredients

400g (14oz) mixed soft fruit, such as raspberries, blueberries, and strawberries
1 tbsp lemon juice
2 tbsp caster sugar
150ml (5fl oz) double cream
150g (5¹/₂oz) low-fat Greek yogurt
1 tsp vanilla extract
4 heaped tsp soft, light brown sugar

SERVES 4

 PREP 20 MINS, PLUS MACERATING AND CHILLING

1 If you are using strawberries, dice them so that they are roughly the same size as the other berries. Mix all the fruit with the lemon juice and 1 tablespoon of caster sugar in a non-reactive bowl, and set aside for 30 minutes to macerate.

2 Place the double cream in a bowl and whisk to form stiff peaks. Fold in the yogurt, vanilla extract, and the remaining caster sugar.

3 Using 4 wide-mouth glasses, place one-eighth of the fruit at the bottom of each glass. Top this with a tablespoon of the whipped cream mixture, and spread it out evenly. Repeat the process until you have two layers of fruit and cream.

4 Sprinkle 1 heaped teaspoon of the brown sugar over the top layer of cream in each glass, spreading it out lightly with the back of a teaspoon. Place the desserts in the fridge and chill for at least 30 minutes, or until the sugar has melted into the creamy topping, before serving.

Cook's tip: This also works well with seasonal soft stone fruit, such as plums, greengages, peaches, or nectarines. And if you want to keep the fat down, use more Greek yogurt instead of the double cream.

Nutrition data per serving

Energy	294 kcals
Protein	5.5g
Fat	21g
Saturated fat	13g
Carbohydrate	22g
Sugar	22g
Fibre	2.5g
Salt	trace

Blueberries
•Brimming with goodness, blueberries freeze well, too. A small bowlful makes a delicious snack at any time of year.

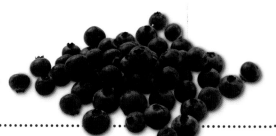

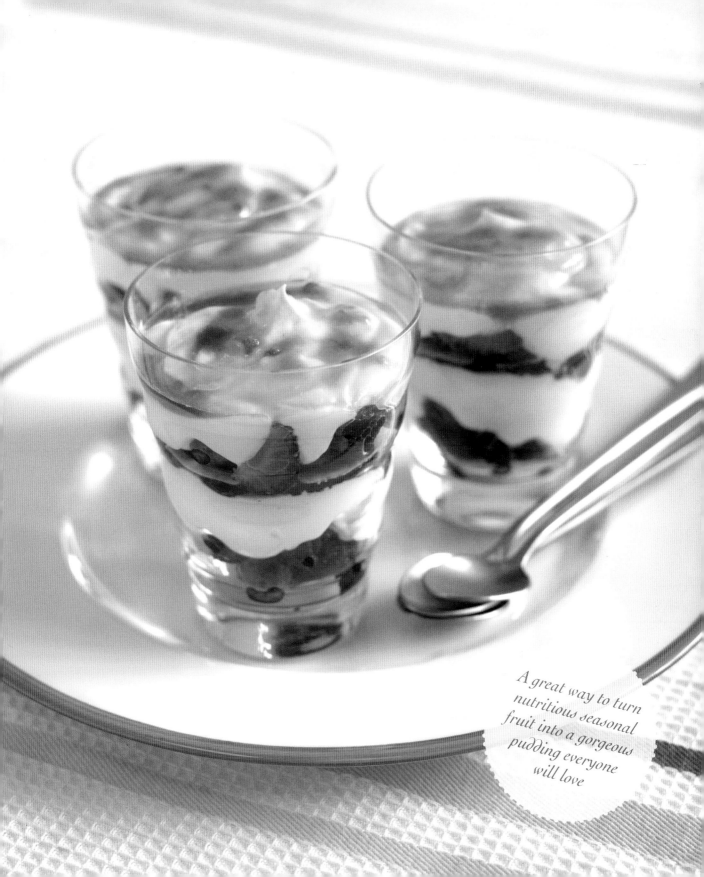

A great way to turn nutritious seasonal fruit into a gorgeous pudding everyone will love

FULL OF VITAMIN C AND BETA-CAROTENE

Vanilla, Honey, and Thyme Roasted Peaches

During the height of the summer season, try roasting perfectly ripe peaches for a quick yet elegant dessert, with just a little yogurt and crème fraîche to add at the end.

Ingredients

30g (1oz) butter
1 tbsp honey
1 tbsp lemon juice
¼ tsp vanilla extract
4 ripe peaches, halved
 and stones removed
2 tbsp soft, light brown sugar
4 sprigs of thyme

For the cream

4 tbsp crème fraîche
4 tbsp low-fat Greek yogurt
1 tbsp honey

SERVES 4   **PREP 10 MINS**   **COOK 20–30 MINS**

1 Preheat the oven to 200°C (400°F/Gas 6). Gently heat the butter in a small saucepan and whisk in the honey, lemon juice, and vanilla extract. Remove from the heat and set aside. Place the peaches, cut-side up, in a shallow ovenproof dish that fits them snugly and pour the honey mixture over. Sprinkle the brown sugar over and tuck the thyme sprigs between the peaches.

2 Bake in the oven for 20–30 minutes, depending on the ripeness of the peaches, until the fruit is soft and the edges caramelised in places. Remove from the oven, discard the thyme sprigs, and set aside.

3 For the cream, place the crème fraîche, Greek yogurt, and honey in a bowl and whisk well to combine. Serve the peaches warm, or at room temperature, with a little of the cream on the side and any baking juices drizzled over.

Nutrition data per serving	
Energy	226 kcals
Protein	3.5g
Fat	12g
Saturated fat	8g
Carbohydrate	26g
Sugar	26g
Fibre	3g
Salt	0.2g

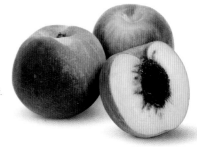

Peaches
These are at their juiciest best from June through August. To ripen to perfection at home, store them in a paper bag.

Apple and Blackberry Crisp with Oaty Almond Topping

Keep a bag of blackberries in the freezer so you can make this family favourite in any season. Sharper-tasting apples, such as granny smiths, add a more intense flavour.

••• RICH IN VITAMIN C, VITAMIN E, AND MAGNESIUM •••

SERVES 4 **PREP 15 MINS** 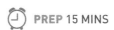 **COOK 40 MINS**

Ingredients
300g (10oz) blackberries
4 apples, about 300g (10oz) in total, peeled, cored, and roughly chopped
1 tsp sugar
1 tsp cornflour

For the topping
75g (2½oz) flaked almonds
75g (2½oz) rolled oats
25g (scant 1oz) soft, light brown sugar
25g (scant 1oz) caster sugar
1 tsp cinnamon
75g (2½oz) butter, softened

1 Preheat the oven to 180°C (350°F/Gas 4). Place the blackberries and apples in a large mixing bowl. Sprinkle over the sugar and cornflour and toss well to coat. Place the fruit in a 20cm x 2cm (8in x ¾in) shallow ovenproof dish.

2 For the topping, place all the dry ingredients in a bowl. Rub in the butter with your fingertips until well combined and there are no more large lumps of butter. Spread the topping over the fruit.

3 Bake in the centre of the oven for 40 minutes, until golden brown and bubbling. Remove from the oven and rest for at least 5 minutes before serving with cream or vanilla ice cream.

Nutrition data per serving	
Energy	435 kcals
Protein	7.5 g
Fat	28 g
Saturated fat	11 g
Carbohydrate	40 g
Sugar	26 g
Fibre	7 g
Salt	0.2 g

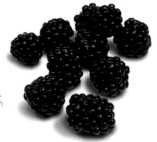

Blackberries
Whether frozen or fresh from the garden or hedgerow, these berries are bursting with sweetness and vitamin C.

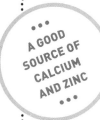

A GOOD SOURCE OF CALCIUM AND ZINC

Wheat-Free Chocolate and Pecan Brownies

These rich, dark, and delicious brownies make a fantastic gluten-free dessert. Small but intensely chocolatey, a little goes a long way.

Ingredients
200g (7oz) good-quality dark chocolate, at least 70 per cent cocoa solids, roughly chopped
100g (3½oz) unsalted butter, plus extra for greasing
200g (7oz) caster sugar
125g (4½oz) ground almonds
4 eggs, separated
100g (3½oz) chopped pecans

MAKES 12–16 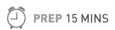 **PREP** 15 MINS **COOK** 35 MINS, PLUS COOLING

1 Preheat the oven to 170°C (325°F/Gas 3). Grease and line a 20cm (8in) square brownie tin or shallow baking tray. Place the chocolate and butter in a heatproof bowl over a small saucepan of simmering water. Stir it frequently until it is just melted, making sure the water does not touch the bottom of the bowl. Remove from the heat and allow to cool.

2 Once the chocolate and butter is cool enough, whisk in the caster sugar and ground almonds. Then add the egg yolks and beat until the mixture is smooth. In a separate bowl, whisk the egg whites to form stiff peaks. Whisk one-third of the egg whites into the chocolate mixture to loosen it, then gently fold in the remaining egg whites, taking care not to lose too much air.

3 Fold the pecans into the brownie batter, then pour it into the prepared tin. Bake the brownie in the centre of the oven for 30–35 minutes, until the edges are set, and a toothpick inserted into the centre comes out with a little batter attached.

4 Leave the brownie to cool completely in the tin. Now, turn it out and cut into 12–16 equal pieces. Dust with icing sugar or cocoa powder to serve, if you prefer.

Cook's tip: For a softer surface, cover the brownie tin tightly with foil as it cools.

Nutrition data per serving	
Energy	362–272 kcals
Protein	6–5 g
Fat	25–19 g
Saturated fat	8–6 g
Carbohydrate	28–21 g
Sugar	27–20 g
Fibre	1–0.8 g
Salt	trace

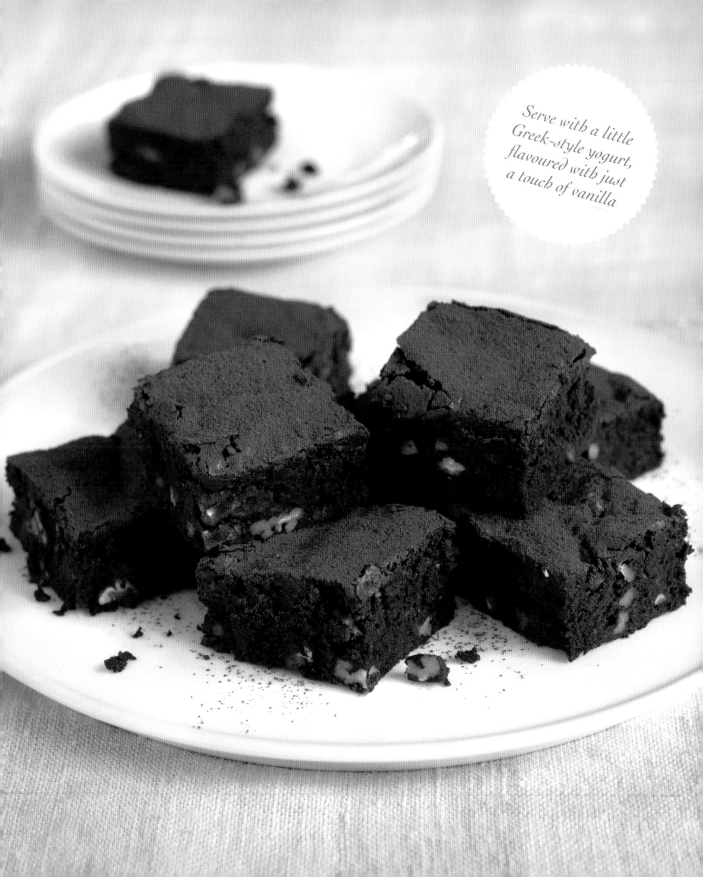

Serve with a little Greek-style yogurt, flavoured with just a touch of vanilla

Brown Bread Autumn Fruit Pudding

FULL OF POTASSIUM, B VITAMINS, AND FIBRE

For a seasonal twist on the more usual summer pudding, try this nourishing version with brown bread, gently poached autumn fruit, and a hint of cinnamon.

Ingredients
6 tbsp apple juice
2 tbsp soft, light brown sugar
¼ tsp cinnamon
2–3 apples, about 200g (7oz) in total, peeled, cored, and cut into 1cm (½in) cubes
1 large pear, about 125g (4½oz) in total, peeled, cored and cut into 1cm (½in) cubes
150g (5½oz) blackberries, cut in half if large
7–8 thick slices good-quality day old brown bread, crusts removed

SERVES 4   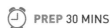 **PREP** 30 MINS   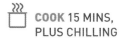 **COOK** 15 MINS, PLUS CHILLING

1 Heat the apple juice, brown sugar, and cinnamon in a medium-sized, heavy-based saucepan. Add the apples and pear and cook, covered, over a low heat for 5 minutes, until they start to soften. Add the blackberries and cook for a further 5 minutes, until the fruit is soft. Strain the fruit through a sieve, reserving the juice in a shallow dish.

2 Line a 1 litre (2 pint) pudding bowl with cling film, leaving at least a 10cm (4in) overhang on all sides. Take each slice of bread and briefly dip one side into the juice. Use the bread, dipped-side down, to line the bowl. Press it firmly to fit the shape of the bowl, making sure the slices overlap slightly and there are no gaps. Leave 2 slices for the lid.

3 Pour the fruit into the bread-lined bowl. Then pour over most of the leftover juice, reserving a little for the top. Use the final two slices of bread to make a lid for the fruit, making sure it is well sealed. Patch up any gaps with small pieces of bread, if needed. Brush the top with the reserved juice.

4 Fold the overhanging cling film over the top of the pudding. Place a small plate or saucer on top of the pudding and weigh it down with heavy cans. Place the weighted pudding in the fridge overnight to set.

5 To serve the pudding, peel back the cling film from the top and place a serving plate on top of the bowl. Invert the bowl to turn the pudding out onto the plate and gently peel the cling film away from the pudding. Serve with Greek yogurt or whipped cream.

Nutrition data per serving

Energy	213 kcals
Protein	6.5 g
Fat	2 g
Saturated fat	0.3 g
Carbohydrate	44 g
Sugar	21 g
Fibre	8 g
Salt	0.8 g

Quick Banana Ice Cream with Candied Pecans

A GOOD SOURCE OF POTASSIUM AND ZINC

This simple, creamy ice cream is studded with caramelized pecan pieces and takes just minutes to make – without the need for an ice-cream maker.

Ingredients

4 ripe bananas
1 tsp vanilla extract

For the candied pecans
25g (scant 1oz) unsalted butter
2 tbsp maple syrup
1 tsp cinnamon
pinch of sea salt
100g (3½oz) pecans
1 tbsp soft, light brown sugar

SERVES 4

 PREP 10 MINS, PLUS FREEZING

COOK 10 MINS, PLUS FREEZING

1 Peel the bananas, chop into 2cm (³/₄in) chunks, and freeze for 1 hour. Meanwhile, preheat the oven to 180°C (350°F/Gas 4). Line a large baking sheet with baking parchment and set aside.

2 For the candied pecans, melt the butter, maple syrup, cinnamon, and sea salt in a small, heavy-based saucepan, until it bubbles briefly. Remove from the heat and add the pecans. Stir them well, until completely coated in the mixture. Add the sugar and stir to coat again.

3 Spread the pecans on the prepared baking sheet. Try to make sure they are not touching each other, as far as possible, to avoid big, sticky clumps. Bake for 10 minutes in the oven, until they darken and start to smell delicious. Remove from the oven and transfer to a wire rack to cool completely. Roughly chop them when cool.

4 Place the frozen bananas and vanilla extract in a food processor and process, until you have a smooth, thick ice cream. You may need to scrape down the sides quite vigorously to ensure a smooth mixture. Fold the cooled candied pecan pieces into the ice cream mixture by hand. Return the ice cream to the freezer to firm up for at least 30 minutes or until needed.

Cook's tip: The candied pecans can be prepared in advance and stored in an airtight container for up to 1 week.

Nutrition data per serving

Energy	347 kcals
Protein	3.5g
Fat	23g
Saturated fat	5g
Carbohydrate	32g
Sugar	29g
Fibre	3g
Salt	0.35g

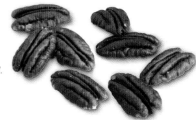

Pecans
The intense nuttiness of pecans gives this ice cream a luxurious feel. They are also rich in nutrients, with far more good fats than bad fats.

FULL OF CALCIUM, FIBRE, AND B VITAMINS

Classic Irish Soda Bread

Irish soda bread is the simplest bread to make, needing no yeast or rising and proving time, and is the perfect bread to get children interested in baking. It is best eaten the same day.

Ingredients
300g (10oz) wholemeal flour
100g (3¹/₂oz) plain flour, plus extra for dusting
1 tsp fine salt
1 tsp bicarbonate of soda
350ml (12fl oz) buttermilk

SERVES 8 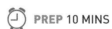 **PREP** 10 MINS 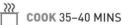 **COOK** 35–40 MINS

1 Preheat the oven to 200°C (400°F/Gas 6). Place both lots of flour, the salt, and bicarbonate of soda in a large bowl and mix thoroughly to combine.

2 Make a well in the centre of the dry ingredients, pour in the buttermilk, and stir to mix. On a well-floured surface, use your hands to bring the mixture together into a loose, sticky dough. Work gently, without kneading, only until it is smooth.

3 Shape the dough into a roughly round shape and transfer to a heavy baking sheet. Use a sharp, serrated knife to cut a cross into the surface of the loaf, dust with a little extra flour, and bake in the middle of the oven for 35–40 minutes, until well risen and golden brown. The bottom of the loaf should sound hollow when tapped.

4 Remove from the oven and allow the bread to cool on a wire rack for at least 20 minutes, before serving with some butter and home-made soup, such as spicy bean soup (see p214).

Cook's tip: Do not be tempted to cut into the bread as soon as it comes out of the oven. The hot air inside continues to cook the bread, and cutting into it too soon will result in a damp, compressed loaf.

Nutrition data per serving

Energy	175 kcals
Protein	7.5g
Fat	1g
Saturated fat	0.3g
Carbohydrate	34g
Sugar	3g
Fibre	5g
Salt	0.9g

Buttermilk
If you don't have any available, buttermilk is easy to make. Just add 1 tablespoon of lemon juice per 200ml (7fl oz) of whole milk and leave to thicken for 5–10 minutes before using.

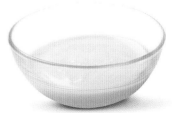

Pumpkin, Feta, and Rosemary Rolls

••• PROVIDES LOTS OF FIBRE, CALCIUM, AND VITAMIN A •••

A herby, cheesy twist on soda bread, these simple rolls are perfect with a home-made soup, freeze well, and make a satisfying snack after school.

Ingredients

200g (7oz) plain flour
200g (7oz) wholemeal flour
1¹⁄₂ tsp finely chopped rosemary
1 tsp bicarbonate of soda
¹⁄₂ tsp fine salt and freshly
   ground black pepper
100g (3¹⁄₂oz) pumpkin
   or butternut squash,
   coarsely grated
100g (3¹⁄₂oz) feta
   cheese, crumbled
300ml (10fl oz) buttermilk

MAKES 8 **PREP** 20 MINS **COOK** 20–25 MINS

1 Preheat oven to 200°C (400°F/Gas 6). Sift both lots of flour into a large bowl. Mix in the rosemary, bicarbonate of soda, salt, and a good grinding of black pepper.

2 Toss the grated pumpkin and feta through the flour mixture. Make a well in the centre and pour in the buttermilk. Use a wooden spoon and then your hands to bring the mixture together to form a rough dough.

3 On a lightly floured surface, knead the dough very briefly, until it is a smooth ball. Cut it into 8 equal-sized wedges and form each into a roll, with any joins underneath the roll.

4 Bake the rolls in the centre of the oven for 20–25 minutes, until golden brown. The bottom of the rolls should sound hollow when tapped. Remove from the oven and allow to cool for at least 10 minutes before serving.

Cook's tip: Make double the amount of dough and open freeze half the rolls, unbaked, on a tray. Then pack them in a freezer bag for storage. These can be baked straight from the freezer for 40 minutes.

Nutrition data per serving

Energy	212kcals
Protein	9g
Fat	3.5g
Saturated fat	2g
Carbohydrate	37g
Sugar	3.5g
Fibre	4g
Salt	1.1g

Pumpkin
There are so many varieties of sweet-tasting squash to use here. Pumpkin is softer and milder than butternut squash, but both bring lots of colour and beta-carotene.

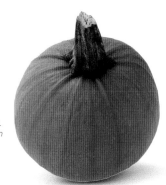

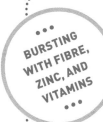

BURSTING WITH FIBRE, ZINC, AND VITAMINS

Cranberry and Hazelnut Chewy Oat Cookies

These soft, chewy cookies are full of nourishing oats, nuts, and dried fruit. Try changing the fruit and nuts to suit your favourite combinations.

Ingredients
150g (5½oz) butter
100g (3½oz) caster sugar
75g (2½oz) self-raising flour
50g (1¾oz) wholemeal flour
100g (3½oz) rolled oats
50g (1¾oz) dried cranberries, roughly chopped
50g (1¾oz) hazelnuts, roughly chopped
1 tsp bicarbonate of soda

MAKES 16–18 **PREP 15 MINS** 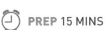 **COOK 12–15 MINS**

1 Preheat the oven to 180°C (350°F/Gas 4). Melt the butter in a large saucepan, then remove from the heat and allow it to cool. Add the sugar, flours, rolled oats, cranberries, and hazelnuts into the melted butter and stir well to combine.

2 Mix the bicarbonate of soda with 1 tablespoon of boiling water until it dissolves, then mix it into the biscuit mixture. Take tablespoons of the mixture and roll them into balls. Flatten them slightly and place them on a baking tray, spaced well apart, as they will spread when baking.

3 Bake in the centre of the oven for 12–15 minutes until they turn golden brown. Remove the cookies from the oven and leave them to cool on their baking sheets for 5 minutes, before transferring them to a wire rack to cool completely.

Cook's tip: These cookies will keep in an airtight container. Or you can make up the mixture ahead and freeze uncooked, for up to one month, then bake.

Nutrition data per serving

Energy	172–153 kcals
Protein	2–1.8 g
Fat	10–9 g
Saturated fat	5–4.5 g
Carbohydrate	18–16 g
Sugar	9–8 g
Fibre	1.5–1 g
Salt	0.36–0.3 g

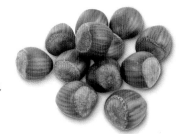

Hazelnuts
Crunchy hazelnuts, rich in B vitamins, give added texture to these indulgent, chewy cookies.

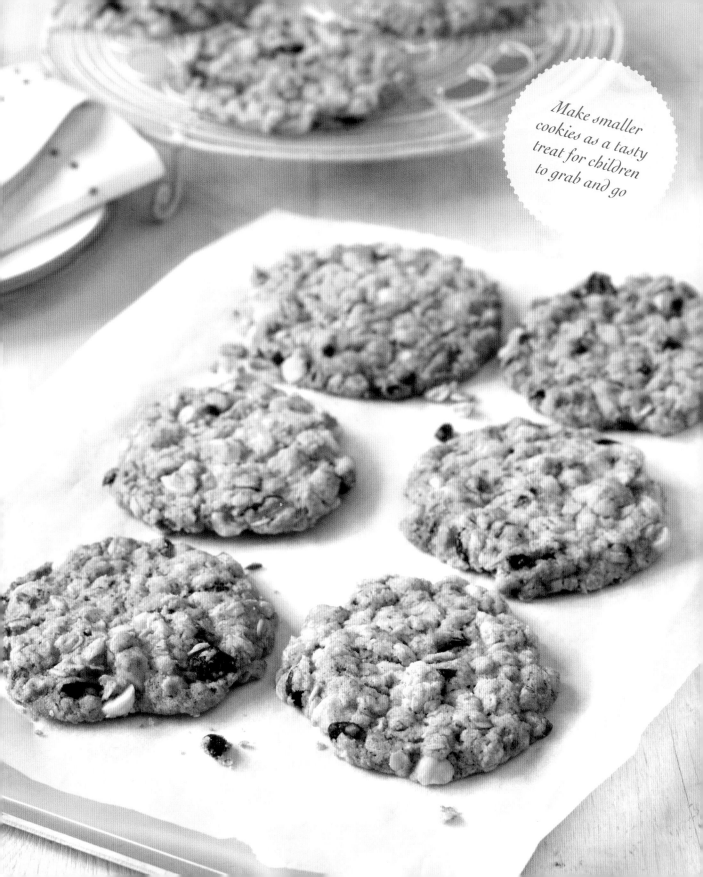

Make smaller cookies as a tasty treat for children to grab and go

Blueberry Muffins with Oat and Almond Streusel Topping

A GOOD SOURCE OF FIBRE AND POTASSIUM

These eye-catching muffins are soft and fruity underneath, delicately crunchy on top, and make a deliciously wholesome treat.

Ingredients

For the topping
25g (scant 1oz) rolled oats
25g (scant 1oz) flaked almonds
25g (scant 1oz) butter
50g (1³/₄oz) soft, light brown sugar
1 tsp cinnamon

For the muffins
150g (5¹/₂oz) self-raising flour
100g (3¹/₂oz) wholemeal flour
1 heaped tsp baking powder
¹/₄ tsp salt
125g (4¹/₂oz) caster sugar
200ml (7fl oz) buttermilk
50ml (1¹/₂fl oz) sunflower oil
1 egg, beaten
1 tsp vanilla extract
100g (3¹/₂oz) blueberries

MAKES 12 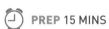 **PREP** 15 MINS **COOK** 15–20 MINS

1 Preheat the oven to 200°C (400°F/Gas 6). Line a 12-hole muffin tin with paper cases and set aside. For the streusel topping, place the oats, almonds, butter, brown sugar, and cinnamon in a food processor and process, until the mixture resembles rough breadcrumbs. Set aside.

2 Place both lots of flour, baking powder, salt, and sugar in a large bowl and mix well. Pour the buttermilk and sunflower oil into a jug, then add the egg and vanilla extract, and beat together thoroughly.

3 Make a well in the centre of the dry ingredients, pour the liquid mixture in, and mix with a wooden spoon until just combined. Gently fold in the blueberries, being careful not to over-mix. Divide the mixture equally between the paper cases and top each muffin with a sprinkling of the streusel mixture.

4 Bake the muffins in the middle of the oven for 15–20 minutes, until lightly brown and well risen. Remove from the oven and allow them to cool in the tin for 5 minutes before transferring to a wire rack to cool completely.

Nutrition data per serving	
Energy	206 kcals
Protein	4g
Fat	7g
Saturated fat	2g
Carbohydrate	32g
Sugar	16g
Fibre	2g
Salt	0.4g

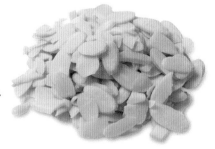

Almonds
These nuts bring a sweet, marzipan flavour and a host of nutrients – calcium, protein, vitamin E, and magnesium, to name but a few.

Peanut Butter and Maple Muesli Bars

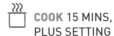

For a more-ish home-made treat, try these muesli bars – they're ideal for children's packed lunches, and make a handy after-school or pre-activity snack.

Ingredients

200g (7oz) rolled oats
100g (3¹/₂oz) smooth peanut butter
100ml (3¹/₂fl oz) maple syrup
200g (7oz) mixed dried fruit, nuts, and seeds, such as dried cranberries, raisins, flaked almonds, chopped hazelnuts, pumpkin seeds, sunflower seeds, and unsweetened shredded coconut

MAKES 8   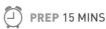 **PREP** 15 MINS   **COOK** 15 MINS, PLUS SETTING

1 Preheat the oven to 200°C (400°F/Gas 6). Spread the oats out over a large baking sheet and toast in the oven for 10–15 minutes, turning them over after 5 minutes, until lightly golden and crisp.

2 Place the peanut butter and maple syrup in a medium-sized saucepan and heat it briefly, whisking constantly, until it softens and combines to form a smooth consistency.

3 Remove the peanut butter mixture from the heat and mix in the toasted oats and the dried fruit, nut, and seed mixture. Mix well and turn it out into a greased 20cm (8in) square baking tin. Press the mixture down firmly, making sure that the edges are well pressed in.

4 Refrigerate the mixture for at least 4 hours, until set. Turn it out onto a chopping board and use a sharp knife to cut the slab into 8 bars. Wrap each bar in cling film and store in the fridge until needed. These will keep for up to 1 week in the fridge.

Cook's tip: Replace peanut butter with almond butter, if you prefer – see the nut butter recipe on p185.

Nutrition data per serving	
Energy	317 kcals
Protein	9g
Fat	15g
Saturated fat	2g
Carbohydrate	37g
Sugar	16g
Fibre	3g
Salt	0.15g

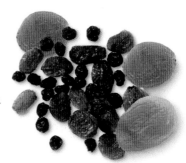

Mixed dried fruit
Intensely sweet, dried fruit can be so much more than sultanas or raisins. Try adding apricots, too, or dried cherries, blueberries, and cranberries, for a more complex and tasty mix.

Pecan Carrot Cake with Orange and Mascarpone Frosting

FULL OF BETA-CAROTENE AND CALCIUM

Eating healthily shouldn't mean cutting out all treats.
This cake is loaded with carrots and nuts, and made with
sunflower oil as a lighter alternative to butter.

Ingredients

150g (5½oz) self-raising flour
150g (5½oz) wholemeal flour
1 tsp baking powder
1 tsp cinnamon
¼ tsp ground cloves
¼ tsp grated nutmeg
200g (7oz) caster sugar
100g (3½oz) soft, light
   brown sugar
200ml (7fl oz) sunflower oil,
   plus extra for greasing
4 eggs
250g (9oz) finely grated carrot
50g (1¾oz) pecans,
   roughly chopped
50g (1¾oz) raisins
zest of 1 orange

For the frosting

225g (8oz) mascarpone
100g (3½oz) cream cheese
300g (10oz) icing sugar
zest of 1 orange

SERVES 12   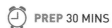 **PREP** 30 MINS   **COOK** 35–40 MINS

1 Preheat oven to 180°C (350°F/Gas 4). Grease and line two 20cm (8in) round cake tins. Sift the flours, baking powder, and spices into a large bowl. Add both lots of sugar and whisk the mixture with a large balloon whisk until it is well combined. In a separate bowl, whisk together the oil and the eggs. Make a well in the centre of the dry mixture and pour the egg mixture in. Beat until thoroughly smooth.

2 Fold the grated carrot into the batter. Then add the pecans, raisins, and orange zest, and fold gently to combine. Pour the batter into the two prepared cake tins. Bake in the centre of the oven for 35–40 minutes, until well risen and golden brown – a wooden toothpick inserted into the centre of the cake should come out clean. Remove the cakes from the oven and leave them to cool in their tins for 5 minutes, before transferring them to a wire rack to cool completely.

3 For the frosting, process all the ingredients together in a food processor or whisk together with a hand-held whisk until well combined. Use about one-third of the frosting to sandwich the two cake halves together. Cover the top and sides of the cake with the rest of the frosting. Chill in the fridge for 1 hour to help set the frosting.

Cook's tip: Any cake with a dairy-based frosting such as this should be stored in an airtight container, in the fridge.

Nutrition data per serving

Energy	575 kcals
Protein	7g
Fat	30g
Saturated fat	10g
Carbohydrate	71g
Sugar	55g
Fibre	3g
Salt	0.4g

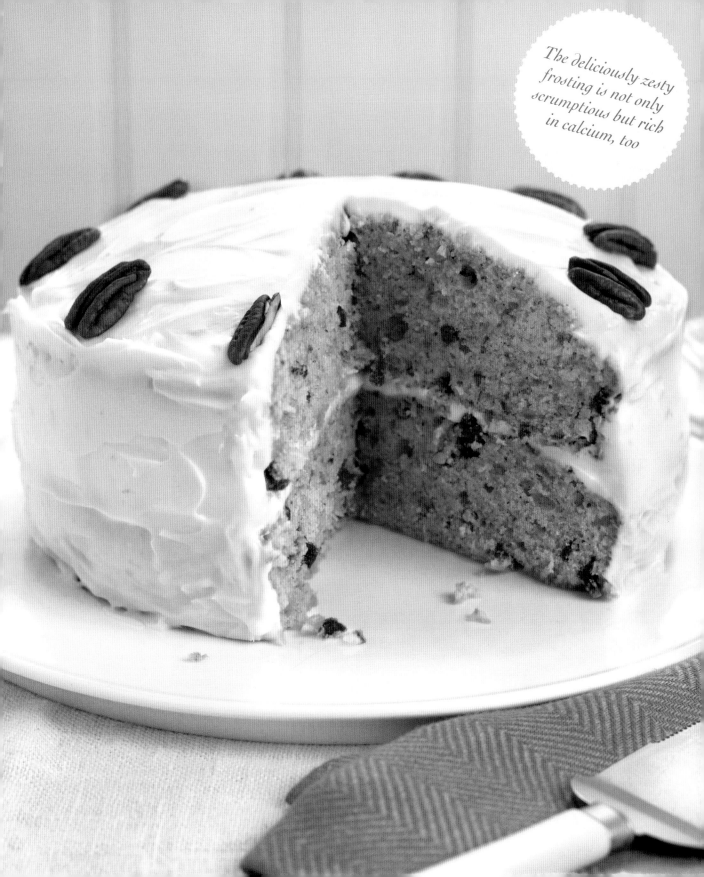

The deliciously zesty frosting is not only scrumptious but rich in calcium, too

Index

Page numbers in **bold** indicate a fuller discussion of a topic. Recipe titles are in *italic*.

Acknowledgments

About the author

Jane Clarke BSc (Honours) SRD is one of the UK's most trusted nutritionists and a trained Cordon Bleu chef. As a practising nutritionist, dietitian, and Harley Street consultant, Jane advises top sports professionals, treats young children, teenagers, and adults with a wide range of medical conditions, and runs a cancer and nutrition practice. She has written several books and cutting-edge articles on nutrition and health, is a regular contributor to the media, and is continually inspired by her young daughter's zest for food and for life.

The author would like to thank

My cherished family and friends, Sarah Brady, Ronan Faherty, David and Sam Galer-Rose, Dr Andy Gayer, Ruth and Theodore Gillick (along with their adorable family, Gus, Louis, Inigo, Florence, and Raphael), Lesja Liber, Dej Mahoney, Carole Neuhaus, Pauline and Clive Pitts, Caroline Radford, Dr Martin Scurr, Sara Silm, Drs Richard and Clare Staughton, Professor Justin Stebbing, Cat Vinton, Gill and Mike Walsh, and Paul and Caroline Weilland, and my professional rocks, Paul Chiappe and Susan Hutter.

DK would like to thank

Katy Greenwood for testing the recipes; Fiona Hunter for nutrition data; Isabel de Cordova, prop stylist; Jane Lawrie, food stylist; Kate Fenton for design assistance and illustration; Elizabeth Clinton for editorial assistance; Fiona Wild for proofreading; and Marie Lorimer for the index.

All images © DK Images. For more information, see **www.dkimages.com**

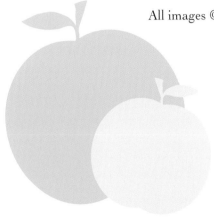